THE REVISED NEO PERSONALITY INVENTORY

CLINICAL AND RESEARCH APPLICATIONS

THE PLENUM SERIES IN SOCIAL/CLINICAL PSYCHOLOGY

Series Editor: C. R. Snyder

University of Kansas
Lawrence, Kansas

Current Volumes in the Series:

ADVANCED PERSONALITY
Edited by David F. Barone, Michel Hersen, and
Vincent B. Van Hasselt

AGGRESSION
Biological, Developmental, and Social Perspectives
Edited by Seymour Feshbach and Jolanta Zagrodzka

AVERSIVE INTERPERSONAL BEHAVIORS
Edited by Robin M. Kowalski

COERCION AND AGGRESSIVE COMMUNITY TREATMENT
A New Frontier in Mental Health Law
Edited by Deborah L. Dennis and John Monahan

THE IMPORTANCE OF PSYCHOLOGICAL TRAITS
A Cross-Cultural Study
John E. Williams, Robert C. Satterwhite, and José L. Saiz

PERSONAL CONTROL IN ACTION
Cognitive and Motivational Mechanisms
Edited by Miroslaw Kofta, Gifford Weary, and Grzegorz Sedek

THE PSYCHOLOGY OF VANDALISM
Arnold P. Goldstein

THE REVISED NEO PERSONALITY INVENTORY
Clinical and Research Applications
Ralph L. Piedmont

SOCIAL COGNITIVE PSYCHOLOGY
History and Current Domains
David F. Barone, James E. Maddux, and C. R. Snyder

SOURCEBOOK OF SOCIAL SUPPORT AND PERSONALITY
Edited by Gregory R. Pierce, Brian Lakey, Irwin G. Sarason, and
Barbara R. Sarason

A Continuation Order Plan is available for this series. A continuation order will bring delivery of each new volume immediately upon publication. Volumes are billed only upon actual shipment. For further information please contact the publisher.

THE REVISED NEO PERSONALITY INVENTORY

CLINICAL AND RESEARCH APPLICATIONS

RALPH L. PIEDMONT

Loyola College in Maryland
Baltimore, Maryland

PLENUM PRESS • NEW YORK AND LONDON

Library of Congress Cataloging-in-Publication Data

Library of Congress Cataloging in Publication Data

Piedmont, Ralph, L., [DATE]
    The revised NEO Personality Inventory: clinical and research applications / Ralph L.
Piedmont.
      p.   cm.—(The Plenum series in social/clinical psychology)
    Includes bibliographical references and index.
    ISBN 0-306-45943-4
    1. NEO Personality Inventory. 2. NEO Five-Factor Inventory. I. Title. II. Series.
BF698.8.N46P54   1998   98-42281
155.2'83—dc21   CIP

Figures 3.1–3.4, 4.1–4.7, 5.1–5.7, and the appendices on pages 111 and 157 are
reproduced by special permission of the Publisher, Psychological Assessment
Resources, Inc., 16204 North Florida Avenue, Lutz, Florida 33549, from the
NEO Personality Inventory-Revised, by Paul Costa, and Robert McCrae,
Copyright 1978, 1985, 1989, 1992 by PAR, Inc. Further reproduction is
prohibited without permission of PAR, Inc.

ISBN 0-306-45943-4

© 1998 Plenum Press, New York
A Division of Plenum Publishing Corporation
233 Spring Street, New York, N.Y. 10013

http://www.plenum.com

Printed in the United States of America

To Rose P., Joanna P., and Dominic P.,
Three of the most endearing NEO PI-R profiles
I have ever come across

FOREWORD

The assessment of individual differences has a long history. As early as 2200 B.C. the Chinese were employing methods to select candidates for civil service positions. Over the ensuing centuries philosophers, theologians, and the nobility all noticed and debated the role of "character" in shaping the destiny and quality of individual lives. This interest spawned widely different methods of evaluating the timbre of temperament—bumps on the head, lines on the hand, shape of the body—all of which were employed in attempts to gain insight into basic human motives. The emergence of the scientific method and its application to this endeavor reinvigorated society's efforts in this direction, and an abundant variety of assessment instruments consequently became available.

The outbreak of World War I created a need for the efficient assessment of individual differences in large groups. Such instruments as the Woodworth Personal Data Sheet and the Army Alpha Test resulted in genuine breakthroughs in assessment technology. These tests provided standardized sets of items that permitted quantitative comparisons among people. Over the years, numerous scales have been developed which have been based on widely differing levels of psychometric sophistication. Today, personality scales, clinical assessment devices, and batteries of cognitive tests are established and accepted in society. It is surprising how many people know their "type" or have taken an MMPI or CPI at some point in their lives. Just about everyone in America today has taken at least some form of aptitude test (e.g., SAT, GRE). Assessment appears to be here to stay, at least for the foreseeable future.

Unfortunately, the sheer number of such instruments has created new problems for the field of assessment, not the least of which is the problem of establishing a meaningful taxonomy for classifying the different measures. The diverse collection of currently available instruments and scales reflects the variety of theoretical perspectives on personality and temperament held by professionals. New scales and instruments are being developed to fill identifiable gaps between assessment theory and assessment practice. Other scales are being developed in an attempt to keep pace with the new adaptive styles that have emerged in response to the rapid changes created by postindustrial society. In addition, the very number of these scales, together with their potpourri of underlying constructs, is likely to baffle and bewilder even the most sophisticated assessment professional.

Fortunately, an important paradigm shift in the field has occurred during the past ten years with the emergence of the five-factor model of personality (FFM). The FFM is a robust taxonomic model that has organized the myriad of existing scales just described with respect to five superordinate dimensions: Neuroticism, Extraversion, Openness, Agreeableness, and Conscientiousness. These broadband dimensions of personality provide a useful and succinct summary of the various qualities that personologists have found to be important, relevant, and predictive of life events. The FFM also provides an organizing framework for understanding and interpreting ongoing discussions about personality. This volume focuses on a single instrument, the Revised NEO Personality Inventory (NEO PI–R), which is currently the only commercially available instrument explicitly designed to measure the dimensions of the FFM. However, the model underlying the NEO PI–R is part of the much broader history of personality assessment.

The first chapter details a review of the FFM and outlines what this model can and *cannot* do. This treatment provides an empirical and theoretical context for understanding the constructs embodied in this instrument. It is important to realize that this book is not merely a "cookbook" of NEO PI–R interpretations. Instead, the author makes every effort to provide the reader with a context and a foundation for understanding how and why the instrument was developed, and how and when it should be applied. The wide-ranging coverage of the research literature in ensuing chapters illuminates the versatility of the NEO PI–R in differing contexts that emphasize clinical, applied, cross-cultural, and psychometric considerations. I believe that this book really hits its mark and that it will prove to be an effective resource for anyone who wishes to develop a deeper understanding of the area of personality assessment. The book is delightfully reader-oriented and user-friendly. Dr. Piedmont has a flair for presenting technical issues in clear, readable prose that should be both accessible and engaging to a wide audience of both students and professionals.

The chapter on profile analysis provides insight into addressing the multidimensionality of personality represented in the NEO PI–R. The challenge in this case is to learn how to integrate the wide personological spectrum covered by 35 scales into cohesive, interpretively useful, and predictively salient "chunks." Again, Dr. Piedmont provides a practical and understandable framework for making these kinds of interpretations that are so imperative for sound assessment practice.

The chapter on using observer ratings opens still another door to assessment. Although the availability of a validated rater form is a rarity among current instruments, there are many advantages to this form of assessment. This is most clearly evident in the discussion of Cross-Observer Agreement analysis with married couples. The logic and empirical utility of this approach is nicely outlined and the case histories demonstrate the value of the interpretive process.

Finally, the chapter on research applications provides an excellent articulation of sound empirical strategies for using the NEO PI–R, or any other assessment protocol. Useful materials are provided to help both clinicians and researchers formulate relevant theoretical and applied questions. Regardless of one's view on the utility of the FFM, this book will be useful for learning about both profile interpretive approaches to personality assessment and about the manner in which test validation should proceed. There is no question that this book will assist the reader in developing proficiency in the use of the NEO PI–R. More important, it will provide instruction in conducting the general enterprise of personality assessment and research.

Paul T. Costa, Jr.
Baltimore, Maryland

PREFACE

The mental health field is going through a number of important transformations. One such development is the field's increasing theoretical diversity. There are many different types of practitioners who are applying a broad range of therapeutic paradigms, from the more traditional behavioral and cognitive frameworks to the emerging areas of spirituality and holistic medicine. The philosophies and treatment approaches are as numerous as the professionals themselves. Another reality is the growing concern over health care and how it will be managed. The rise of managed care companies is an outgrowth (or impetus) for this new trend. These organizations have emphasized the need for clinicians to provide effective treatments in a timely and cost-efficient manner. Finally, with the increasing awareness of the ethical dimensions of practice, there is the recognition that practitioners need to be made accountable for their services, both to the consumers of their services and to themselves. Therapists must be able to provide evidence of the efficacy of their services to consumers. Certainly, many factors influence how much success a client will experience; some of these are beyond the reach of the therapist, but consumers have the right to know just how much improvement they are likely to experience in therapy. Clients, like consumers in other areas, are entitled to valid assurances that their therapy will have a potential benefit. The responsibility of therapists to themselves is to maintain a high level of clinical expertise. This requires that the therapist receive useful feedback on the effects of his or her interventions. Therapists must be aware of such factors as the overall extent of improvement experienced by clients as a result of interventions, whether interventions are more effective with certain types of problems than with others, and whether certain intervention strategies are working better than others.

All of the forces just mentioned are moving the mental health field toward a recognition of the need for better documentation of clinical efficacy. The mental health field needs to provide support for what it does [quantitatively] in an objective, substantive manner. The technology best suited for providing this kind of information is psychological assessment. Traditionally, measures of clinical practice have been the purview of psychology. Psychologists usually receive extensive training in the application and interpretation of psychological measures. In fact, many clinical assessment instruments are usually restricted to psychologists who have had detailed graduate training in testing. Therefore, many nonpsychologists believe that they do not have access to *any* types of psychological measures and thus do not employ testing as part of their practice, nor do they see it as part of their clinical identity. This is unfortunate, because there is a wide range of nonclinical psychological measures that are appropriate for nonpsychologists and that would also be relevant to, and helpful for, their practice. Being unaware of these measures deprives such therapists of important sources of information that could be useful for client assessment, for documenting clinical efficacy, and for obtaining valuable clinical feedback.

The measures to which I refer are instruments designed to assess normal personality qualities. Such scales are less restricted by test publishers. Usually, a graduate course in psychological assessment and/or some supervision in their use is all that is required to gain access to these materials. Personality questionnaires can be very useful in telling a therapist about a wide range of client dispositions, needs, and motivations. Although they may not be diagnostically revealing in their own right, these individual-difference variables set important parameters for any therapeutic interaction. For example, a person who is closed and rigid, who does not experience a wide range of emotions, and who requires much structure may not benefit from insight therapy. Conversely, an individual who is open and has very permeable inner boundaries may keenly experience whatever negative affect is dominant. By assessing a client's personality, a therapist can gain insight on how the client sees the world and copes with it. Depending on the constructs being measured, a therapist may also be able to anticipate therapeutically relevant outcomes. For example, a client high on Machiavellianism may have trouble in establishing trust, while a client high on Anxiety may need a great deal of reassurance and support.

There is a wide range of personality questionnaires that span numerous constructs. These measures vary from assessing specific constructs (e.g., Fear of Fat Scale) to more global, multidimensional inventories (e.g., the California Personality Inventory). Personality measures are usually easy-to-use scales that, with some reading and practice, can be used by most mental health professionals. The purpose of this book is to introduce clinicians to a general personality measure that is most relevant for the clinical context—the Revised NEO Personality Inventory (NEO PI–R). This well-developed instrument is designed to measure the five major dimensions of personality: Neuroticism, Extraversion, Openness to Experience, Agreeableness, and Conscientiousness. These constructs define what is known as the five-factor model of personality (FFM)—a trait-based taxonomy of personality dispositions. These five factors represent independent constructs that have been shown to provide a comprehensive description of normal personality. There is an extensive and constantly expanding research literature that continues to document the utility of this model for predicting real-life outcomes in a number of applied contexts. This book shows how the FFM can provide a very useful framework for conceptualizing people and for anticipating the directions in which they will move.

This book therefore introduces clinicians to the FFM and the instrument designed explicitly to measure it—the NEO PI–R. My goal is to challenge the ways readers think about personality and to familiarize them with an empirically sound method for concretizing those conceptualizations. Strategies are presented for using the instrument in clinical contexts. The research applications of the NEO PI–R are also discussed. Paradigms for approaching many of the most salient issues in research are provided. Every attempt has been made to provide information that is as current as possible. I hope that this book will prove the clinical value of personality assessment and interest readers in employing this technology in their own clinical work. The eventual benefit to our field will be the accumulation of a body of knowledge that demonstrates the efficacy of our interventions and the value of our services.

Ralph L. Piedmont, Ph.D.
Baltimore, Maryland

ACKNOWLEDGMENTS

In the writing of any book, there are numerous people who contribute to the project even though there may be only one author. In this case, I am indebted to a number of colleagues and friends who contributed information and material, as well as moral support. First and foremost, I would like to thank my wife, Rose, who read and reread the manuscript several times to check structure and grammar. I would also like to thank Gail Worrall, who edited the entire manuscript. The manuscript was certainly made more "user friendly" because of the efforts of Rose and Gail. I would also like to express my gratitude to Drs. Joseph Ciarrocchi and Thomas Rodgerson, who shared with me some of their clinical experiences using the NEO PI–R. Special thanks go to Reg Watson, who created the NEO PI–R profile forms used in this book. I would also like to thank those individuals who consented to have their NEO PI–R profiles included as examples throughout the book. I would like to thank Dr. Robert Wicks, my colleague and friend, who provided the initial inspiration for doing this book. Finally, I would like to thank Paul T. Costa, Jr. and Robert R. McCrae for all they taught me about the NEO PI–R in particular, and about good science in general.

CONTENTS

Chapter 3

PERSONALITY AND ITS ASSESSMENT

Every time I teach a course in personality theory, I begin the class by asking the students, "What is personality?" Given the newness of the class situation and the perennial need of college students to remain anonymous to teachers, this question is always followed by a long silence. In order to jump-start this social interaction, I follow up with a request. I ask students to raise their hands if they believe they have a personality. Invariably, there are muffled coughs, eyes begin to dart around the room, and perhaps two or three people will, grudgingly, raise their hands. "Good," I say. "It seems that some people are certain that they have a personality but others are not as sure as to whether they have one or not. Perhaps some people may have had a personality at some time in the past, but do not have one currently, while still others may be engaged in an ongoing search to find one."

On a good day, these comments will elicit not only several good chuckles, but some hands will be raised in an attempt to define the term "personality." The variety of definitions I get for the term clearly tells me that we all know personality when we see it, but we cannot put our fingers on what exactly we mean by "it." Personality is something that defines who we are as people, yet some believe that it is always changing. Some people are said to have "personality"; others seem to lack it. Some believe that personality is the aggregate of our behaviors and attitudes, yet others see personality as something more fundamental: It is the "why" to our behavior. No doubt a course on personality theory is exactly what these students need! Personality is a central concept in the social sciences because it speaks about people: Who they are, how they come to be, and where they are heading in their lives. It is the foundation for building theories of psychopathology and treatment.

1

The purpose of this chapter is to outline some of the important issues surrounding current notions of personality and to describe a model of personality that is becoming quite prominent in the field: the Five-Factor Taxonomy. The development and application of this model in the social sciences is discussed. The remaining parts of this book are concerned with the psychometric and clinical utility of the NEO Personality Inventory–Revised (NEO PI–R), a measure designed explicitly to capture the dimensions underlying this personality model. It is hoped that this volume will assist users of the NEO PI–R in developing their interpretive skills as well as providing strategies for using the instrument in a research context.

WHAT IS PERSONALITY?

Before beginning, it seems appropriate to offer a working definition of personality that can be amended as we go along. For our purposes, personality can be defined as the intrinsic organization of an individual's mental world that is stable over time and consistent over situations. There are three important points to this definition. First, personality represents some structured system by which individuals organize themselves and orient to the world around them. This system is clearly located *within* the person and is not imposed by the environment. Second, personality is stable over time. This means that there is something about who we are and what we are like that remains consistent through our lives. There is more to say about personality change, but for now we can modestly say that despite all the "change" we may have experienced over our lifetimes, there is some thread that seems to be consistent over all the years. There is something about who I was as a child or adolescent that lingers with me today. Finally, personality is consistent from one situation to another. As the old saying goes, "Wherever you go, there you are." Although specific behaviors may change from one context to the next, who we are inside and how we perceive the world remains the same. Although our behaviors may change, the personal goals we may be pursuing remain essentially the same.

This person-centered definition should not be construed as denying the role of the environment in shaping our personalities. Culture, context, and situation all have an influence on our development. But there lies within us some kind of psychological "stuff" which provides the basis for the needs we have, the ways in which we perceive and interpret the outer world, and the goals we ultimately pursue in our lives. Nor should this definition be thought of as reflecting personality as a static quality. Quite the contrary; personality is a dynamic structure. It is always responding to needs that arise from within and without the individual. Further, there is a developmental aspect to personality. Just as we are not born physically mature, so, too, personality is something that begins in a simple form and becomes progressively more sophisticated over time. These changes also follow a lawful, orderly path.

This definition is saying there is something inside us that emerges over our lifetimes that comes to define us as unique individuals. This inner system helps to orient us toward the world and enables us to adapt to the demands of our environment. This inner structure has an inherent lawfulness to it, in that different personalities will lead individuals to follow different life paths. Further, the process by which personality unfolds will also follow certain regularities that can be known and understood. Thus the process of change is complex and there is a need to differentiate between changes that reflect superficial, adaptive modifications and changes that reflect more fundamental, structural shifts.

Genotype and Phenotype

To understand personality, one needs to have an appreciation of the various levels on which personality comes to exist and be expressed. This is particularly true when one wishes to evaluate personality change. We need to know what it is that is changing and what that represents about one's personality. To begin this analysis we need to understand the concepts of genotype and phenotype and their relevance for personality.

A genotype refers to the fundamental organization of the individual; the basic "stuff" that a person has been endowed with through their genetics. Genotypes are latent dimensions that establish for an individual a trajectory through time. Phenotype, on the other hand, refers to the expression of the genotype at any given moment in time. Put all the phenotypes together, and you have the genotype. These two concepts tell us that there is a lawfulness to change. Certain quantities or qualities may vary over time, but such variability may not necessarily reflect any fundamental change. Rather, change may be indicative of a gradual unfolding process for a given characteristic.

A good example of this is physical characteristics. Some readers may remember a fellow named Jack La Lane. Back in the 1950s he was one of the first to bring exercise and fitness to television. I remember watching his show when I was very little. Jack is an enthusiastic person (one could say he had a great personality) who was very muscular. He would always wear a tight jumpsuit that would clearly show off his well-developed biceps, muscular chest, and angular waist. No doubt he was a physically well-developed individual. Recently I saw a photo of him (at the time of this writing he is still alive and in his 80s), and he was still wearing that tight jumpsuit! He is still energetic, still works out and stays fit. If you were to see him today, you would most certainly say that he is a muscular man. But there is no doubt that Jack's body today is quite different from what it was 40 years ago. His body has experienced the inevitable changes of aging: There is more body fat, muscles are not as "tight" as they once were, and the skin appears looser around the body. But despite these very obvious changes, Jack is still described as a muscular man. The reason for this consistency in labeling is that we recognize that what is meant by "muscularity" is different at different stages of development. Phenotypically he is different, but genotypically he has not changed at all.

The same can be said for personality. We can think of many different qualities, but these qualities may mean different types of behaviors at different ages. For example, being an extravert in college may mean going to many different parties and staying out late. It may mean being "rowdy" and loud. However, at age 40 this quality may take on a quite different form. Rather than the raucous college parties, it may be hosting formal sit-down dinner parties for friends and coworkers. It may mean getting involved in community activities. Clearly extraversion may take a more conventional form later in life. But there is no doubt that the person remains an outgoing, socially active person.

It is important when we apply measurement instruments to assess individuals that we have some understanding of the level of analysis being assessed. Measures of phenotypic behavior may be very prone to changes, either over short periods of time or even across different situations. For example, measures of state anxiety (e.g., State-Trait Anxiety Inventory, Speilberger, Gorsuch, & Lushene, 1970) or of depressive symptomatology (e.g., Hamilton Depression Inventory, Reynolds & Kobak,1995) are designed to detect fluctuations in very specific aspects of functioning over relatively short time intervals. They are useful for understanding treatment impact or individual responses to specific situations. Changes on this level, although adaptively important for specific situations, may be less diagnostic of more fundamental, broad-based change. Genotypic measures, on the other hand, aim at uncovering the basic psychological strata of the person. A measure such as the NEO PI–R is designed to access a person's more fundamental temperaments, those qualities that drive, direct, and select behaviors. Scores on this type of scale are more likely to remain constant over time and across situations. However, changes on this level may indicate more profound shifts in personality. Thus, change needs to be evaluated carefully.

Another important realization related to this is the diversity of human behavior through which genotypes can be expressed. People have developed extensive behavior repertoires for fulfilling their needs. They adapt by means of behaviors that are successful in specific environments. Therefore, changes in behavior may not necessarily signal a corresponding change in the need being expressed. For example, consider the trait of dominance. What types of behaviors characterize a dominant person? Is a dominant person one who acts in a controlling, directive, forceful manner? Or is a dominant person one who receives acts of submission from others? The answer is, of course, "it depends." It depends on the situation. In either situation the apparently different phenotypic behaviors reflect the same personality quality. Perhaps Freud had it right when he said that any need can be expressed through any number of behaviors, and any specific behavior can gratify any number of needs.

The concepts of genotype and phenotype have important implications for how we need to conceptualize change in the individual. Certainly we should not be fooled into thinking that behavior changes reflect deeper shifts within the person. But we also need to rethink how our clinical interventions are aimed at influencing our clients. This raises important issues that we discuss later in this book about the goals of therapy. Does therapy aim to make genotypic or phenotypic changes in the person? Are genotypic changes possible? Before we proceed to those questions, we first look at how change and stability are assessed.

CHANGE AND STABILITY IN PERSONALITY

Change, like most things, seems to be a very straightforward matter. But experience teaches us otherwise. Things that look simple on the surface usually contain many nuances and subtleties. Such is the case for understanding change. There are two issues that need to be considered: rank order stability and mean level change (see Caspi & Bem, 1990, for a more extensive evaluation of personality change).

Rank Order Stability

Perhaps one of the most frequently used procedures for determining whether someone has changed on some dimensions is to obtain scores from two time periods and correlate them. A high positive correlation would show that those who scored high at Time 1 continued to score high at Time 2. This would be evidence of temporal stability or test–retest reliability for the scores. Could it be concluded from such a finding that scores did not change? Have scores remained stable? The answer to the first question is "no" and to the second, "yes."

Let's take a look at this from another perspective. Imagine that you are a therapist interested in documenting the impact of your therapy on improving the mental health of your clients. To this end, each client is assessed on a mental health inventory when entering therapy. A high score indicates mental distress. After completing therapy each client completes the mental health inventory again. After treating about 100 clients, you "crunch" the numbers; you correlate Time 1 scores on the inventory with Time 2 scores. If you were successful in treating your clients, what would you expect to find? Should there be (a) a high positive correlation (i.e., high scores at Time 1 continued to be high at Time 2), (b) a high *negative* correlation (i.e., high scores at Time 1 became low scores at Time 2), or (c) should there be *no* correlation (i.e., no relationship between scores at the two time periods)?

Finding a zero correlation would not be helpful for drawing any types of inferences. Such a result could be the product of many influences, including the lack of reliability of your assessment instrument. A negative correlation seems to be a desirable outcome, with those scoring high at first becoming much lower at the end of treatment. However, the reverse equally applies: Those who were low at Time 1 (indicating a degree of mental health) scored higher at Time 2 (indicating that the treatment made them less healthy). The most desirable result would be to find a positive correlation. This would indicate some reliability in your assessment instrument.

But if you found a high *positive* correlation between the two sets of scores would that mean you were not as successful as you thought in helping your clients? That scores are basically the same at the end of treatment as they were at the start? Not necessarily. In evaluating a correlation, it is important to appreciate what that correlation tells you about your data. Correlation is a measure of *rank order stability*. That means that if you obtain a high positive correlation, the ranking of scores at Time 1 are similar to the ranking of scores at Time 2. In terms of our example, those who were more mentally distressed upon entering therapy were also among the more mentally distressed when leaving therapy. The term "more" is a relative term. More distressed in comparison to whom? Well, the others in the study. How distressed were they? That question is *not* answered by correlation.

Remember that rank order is an ordinal level of measurement. It tells you position but not magnitude. Thus, the person who ranked number one in mental distress at Time 1 could have improved greatly over treatment, resulting in a much lower score at Time 2. However, if everyone else in the sample improved at a similar rate over treatment, then this person may again be ranked number one at Time 2. If everyone else also keeps the same rank order, then the correlation between these two sets of scores will be perfect (i.e., +1.0), even though there were significant decreases in the *amount* of psychological distress. Therefore, it is possible to obtain a high positive correlation between Time 1 and Time 2 mental health scores even when there are large changes in scores.

Correlation tells us about the relative standing of cases in a distribution. Maintaining relative standing will create higher correlations. Correlations around zero indicate that the relative standing of cases is changing in a nonpredictable way. So, if you are interested in determining whether scores have changed, then correlation would *not* be the best way to analyze your data. But if you were interested in knowing whether change over time proceeded in an orderly manner, such that all individuals are changing at a constant rate, then correlating scores would be helpful.

In terms of understanding personality stability, one needs to have a critical eye on test–retest coefficients that are presented by test manuals. High test reliability does not mean, on the face of it, that individuals' personalities are not changing. Personality may indeed be changing, but at an equal rate throughout the group. To evaluate whether there have been shifts in the magnitude of various qualities, you need to consider the notion of *mean level change*.

Mean Level Change

Mean level change refers to actual changes in the magnitude of a quantity over time. As noted in our example, it is possible to have a high level of stability while also evidencing a large amount of change. Therapy may indeed reduce the actual amount of "distress" experienced by clients. This would be reflected in a comparison of *means* for the two time periods. Any type of repeated measures analysis would certainly accomplish this task.

In terms of personality assessment the question of mean level change seeks to understand whether various aspects of the individual increase or decrease. Do individuals become more conventional as they age? Do levels of negative affect decrease as one gets older? The question of change in magnitude has important implications for both genotype and phenotype. Our need is to identify not only increasing adaptive fit with the environment, but also to determine whether the underlying qualities of our personality also vary in degree over time. If genotype changes, then the issues are how much and over what time frame?

What the data seem to indicate at this time is that there is a large amount of genotypic plasticity in personality from birth to about age 30 (e.g., J. Block, 1971; Haan, Millsap, & Hartka, 1986; Helson & Moane, 1987; Jessor, 1983; Siegler et al., 1990). That means that the underlying qualities of our personality continues to evolve over the first third of the life span. Between the periods of 17 to 30 years of age there is a tremendous amount of "personality" change in terms of both rank order stability and mean level. Levels of negative affect and extraversion decrease while levels of conventionality increase. After age 30, though, there is little or no genotypic change, although phenotypic variability will continue to be noticed over the entire life span. However, even this phenotypic variability can be meaningfully related to genotypic standing (e.g., Kaiser & Ozer, 1997; Ormel & Wohlfarth, 1991). This means that much phenotypic variation can be linked to the operation of underlying, stable qualities of the individual.

To summarize the discussion, personality is an important concept for guiding our understanding of individuals. We recognize that there is some internal structure that organizes who we are and the goals we pursue. This internal structure develops and matures over time, creating a real sense of change within us. The things we value and the situations we seek evolve over time. However, we reach a point at which this internal growth stops. We reach a point where any change reflects not so much an internal reorganization as a modification of more superficial aspects of our character that maximize our adaptiveness to the particular environment we occupy.

Perhaps an equally important understanding is the realization that this entire process follows a lawful plan. Our temperament, or personality, creates for us a trajectory through time. Our needs, desires, wants, and goals evolve in a specific direction. We can see this when we look back on our own lives, and recognize the pattern in our behaviors, decisions, and preferences. Even though we have changed genotypically from childhood to adulthood, there is still a sense of connectedness. Life appears to progress as a series of building blocks, one laid on top of the other, creating a structure that we call our identity.

Knowing that there is this orderly process can provide us with important information about ourselves and others. Understanding how personality is organized and the major qualities that constitute that organization can provide insights into human functioning and, ultimately, enable us to make predictions about meaningful life outcomes. It is here that we find the great value of personality assessment for clinical work: enhancing client understanding and clinical prediction.

THE VALUE OF PERSONALITY ASSESSMENT IN A CLINICAL CONTEXT

OVERVIEW

Today's mental health care environment is undergoing rapid change. Therapy used to be an unhurried and time-consuming endeavor. It was not uncommon 15 years ago for a client to be in therapy for years. With the rise of managed health care systems, this way of operating is quickly coming to an end. Although this new system is making counseling and psychotherapy available to more individuals than ever before, the price for this new availability is a level of cost consciousness heretofore unexperienced in the social sciences. Third-party payers are expecting therapists to do more, in less time, with greater impact. In common parlance, these service providers are looking for greater "bang for the buck."

The result of this process has been a greater emphasis on short-term therapies. Under the traditional system it would not be uncommon for the first 6 months of therapy to focus on getting to know client and problem. Today, in 6 months the therapy should be coming to an end. Therefore, clinicians do not have the time for understanding the client that they once enjoyed. New technologies are needed to expedite the evaluation and diagnostic process, and measures of personality can help fill this need.

There are numerous assessment devices that have recently appeared aimed at uncovering important aspects of clients. These new-generation instruments represent a high level of psychometric sophistication and can be very useful for providing clinically relevant insights. But this you already recognize; after all, that is why you are reading this book. The NEO PI–R can be very useful in a clinical context because it can make you aware of the types of needs clients seek to satisfy, their interpersonal styles, value systems, and levels of ongoing emotional distress. The NEO PI–R can also be helpful in identifying therapeutic interventions that may be particularly effective. For example, you would not want to put a social introvert in group therapy, or try insight therapy with an individual who has little or no personal insight or empathy. This book will provide you with a first step in learning to use the NEO PI–R in this way. But there is another value to personality assessment that is frequently overlooked.

As professionals we have an ethical responsibility to both ourselves and our clients to provide them with high-quality, effective interventions. As therapists, we need to have feedback on our interventions, information about what therapies work and with what type of client. To determine the amount of improvement we are able to bring about. This information is also useful to our clients, who need to be informed about the efficacy of our services in clear, concrete ways. Psychological assessment provides a straightforward method for documenting treatment efficacy. Such measures provide a standardized, quantifiable means for determining the nature and degree of change. It is important that people have access to therapists, but it is even more important that people have access to therapists who will actually improve their mental status.

You can ask any therapist whether the clients who come to see them benefit from their services, and in almost every instance the reply will be "Of course!" What other answer is there? After all, even therapists have to maintain some sense of personal efficacy and professional value. If a therapist thought that he or she was not helping clients, the therapist would certainly not stay in that line of work. But the real question is, "Do your clients get better?" Just taking a therapist's word on the matter is insufficient. Some kind of empirical documentation of benefit is needed. By how much do clients improve? In what ways do clients improve? These are important questions that health care providers, clients, and therapists themselves are increasingly asking. The answers will need to be in a language that is objective and universally understood: a quantitative one.

In this cost conscious, highly competitive environment it becomes cost effective not only to identify effective therapists (individuals who can deliver some therapeutic clout in a short period), but also to be able to match clients with therapists who are particularly adept with the kind of problem the client is facing. Therefore, health care networks are now beginning to conduct their own clinical outcome studies. Eventually, they will begin to demand from their therapists some evidence of their own effectiveness.

Obtaining such evidence will require the use of standardized tests. The paradigm for this type of study is quite straightforward. Simply give a test(s) to clients when they enter therapy and again when they exit. In this way it can be shown how much change there is over the identified dimensions. Combining these data with clinician ratings of effectiveness (simple Likert scale ratings have been developed and are frequently used), one can identify those personality characteristics of the individual noted at the beginning of therapy that are linked with ratings of treatment efficacy (these issues and methods to address them are discussed in more detail in Chapter 6).

The implications of this type of research are legion. The value they serve for improving therapy efficacy and developing new models of intervention cannot be overstated. Although many bemoan the new health care behemoth, there may be a silver lining to this dark cloud. In developing a facility with assessment technologies now, you will give yourself an edge in this developing health care landscape. When you begin to use the NEO PI–R along with other clinically relevant indices, you will not only be gathering important information about your client that can be directly applied to your therapeutic work, but you will also be creating a clinical database. This information can provide you with important feedback on the quality of your work and important documentation of your psychotherapeutic effect.

THE CLINICAL YIELD FROM PERSONALITY ASSESSMENT

The value of using structured personality instruments in a clinical context is that they provide very clear, tangible evidence of where a client is psychologically. This information is in a form that is readily understandable by a wide range of professionals and represents an objective, broad perspective on the client's functioning. Costa and McCrae (1992a) have identified six ways that this type of information can be fruitfully employed in your clinical work. These uses are outlined in Table 1-1.

The first value is for *understanding the client*. Rather than focusing exclusively on symptomatology, the NEO PI R provides a broad based assessment of the individual's personality. This includes a thorough understanding of the patient's strengths and weaknesses. The NEO PI–R provides information relevant to interpersonal style, character, levels of emotional well-being, aspiration levels, and a wide range of other psychologically relevant information. The NEO PI–R can also provide a larger context for understanding the presenting problems. Are the current distressing symptoms a reaction to recent events or are they symptoms of an enduring and pervasive maladjustment? The answer to this question can have important implications for determining the extent of improvement likely to occur over treatment.

For example, consider a client who presents with the complaint of frequent arguing with his wife. The level of marital distress is becoming so high that the marriage may be in danger of failing. What kind of man is the client? Is he someone who is habitually very argumentative and naturally encounters many interpersonal conflicts in his life? Does this person have stormy relationships with other family members, neighbors, and coworkers? Is he just naturally antagonistic? Or is he usually an easy-going guy who is mostly very pleasant and engaging? Could he just be going through a very stressful period at work? The answers to these questions have very direct implications for the type of treatment to be employed and the kind of outcome expected.

In the first scenario, the client is temperamentally antagonistic and much work will have to be done to develop a level of insight necessary to effect real change in his behavior. Even then, his wife may not be able to tolerate his curmudgeonlike persona. Much work will most likely need to

TABLE 1-1   Clinical Uses for Personality Measures

Understanding the Client
Differential Diagnosis
Empathy and Rapport
Feedback and Insight
Anticipating the Course of Therapy
Matching Treatments to Clients

Note. From "Normal Personality Assessment in Clinical Practice: The NEO Personality Inventory," by P. T. Costa, Jr. and R. R. McCrae. 1992, *Psychological Assessment, 4*, p. 5–13.

be done with both husband and wife. However, in the second scenario it is clear that the problems are situationally induced. There is a transient stressor that is turning a usually goodnatured person into an ogre. Certainly when the stressor subsides many of these problems may disappear as well. Treatment may wish to focus on developing short-term coping skills and a complete remission of symptoms is likely.

Personality instruments like the NEO PI–R can be helpful in outlining the underlying dispositions of clients and alerting you to the presence of internal motivations that may be fueling current problems.

The second clinical value concerns *differential diagnosis*. Although the NEO PI–R is not designed to assess pathology, it can be useful for providing information relevant to making a diagnosis or for ruling one out. For example, a high score on extraversion, one of the major domains assessed by the NEO, would rule out schizoid personality disorder. A high level of emotional dysphoria is a feature of all clinical patients, but the presence of only high Self-Consciousness (a facet of the NEO) would suggest a social phobia rather than depression.

Personality inventories can serve as a basis for thinking meaningfully about the kinds of diagnoses that may be relevant in a particular case. Assessing the underlying dispositions of the client leads one to see the motivational sources of behavior, which in turn can help clarify the etiology of the presenting problem. Later chapters evaluate the relations between the dimensions measured by the NEO PI–R and both *DSM-IV* (American Psychiatric Association, 1994) Axis I and Axis II clinical phenomena. These empirical relations can be very useful diagnostically.

The third value of personality assessment is *empathy and rapport*. The insights into clients that are provided can help promote understanding of and empathy with the client. A better understanding of the person's conflict, struggles, and aspirations helps to present a more nuanced portrait of the issues that surround his or her seeking of treatment. Unlike a more clinically focused scale and its emphasis on pathology, the NEO PI–R provides a more holistic, person-centered orientation that captures clients' growth potential as well as their growing edges.

Feedback and insight represents another important value of personality assessment. Providing clients with feedback on their NEOs can help provide a voice for the client to articulate his or her issues: the patient can feel understood. Many times clients feel distress or conflict but do not have the language to fully articulate their difficulties. Oftentimes, clients may feel that their problem is something unique, not understood, and therefore not treatable. Once clients receive feedback on the NEO PI–R and begin to see how their own personalities are accurately captured, they have a sense of hope. New words are learned that carry some of the nuances of their own special psychological experiences.

This new language can then be shared with the therapist and a common language for working in therapy is then established. Presenting problems, clinical issues surrounding treatment goals, problems and issues, and resistance (to name only a few) can all be framed in the dimensions of the NEO PI–R. This language can also be used by clients to monitor their own sense of change and growth throughout the therapeutic process. These insights can readily be shared with the therapist, because both partners have a common framework.

The NEO PI–R is one of a few instruments that provide a computer-generated feedback report that can be given to clients. This report is presented in easily interpreted, jargon-free terms that give the client a broad understanding of their personality. These reports are readily accepted by clients and contain little objectionable material. One of the advantages of giving feedback is that it can provide a springboard to meaningful dialogue between therapist and client.

Anticipating the course of therapy is the next value. Successful psychotherapy depends not only on a therapist's skill, but also on the client's cooperation, motivation to work, and capacity for therapeutic change. No matter what clinical school one works from, each client brings unique characteristics to the session that need to be accommodated in treatment. The NEO PI–R can provide important insights into these aspects of the individual.

For example, very low Agreeableness scores indicate a client who may be skeptical about the entire therapeutic process and expect the clinician to prove him- or herself at every turn. Such individuals may appear resistant and mistrustful. Conversely, very high Agreeableness scores can indicate an overly compliant client who may easily become dependent on the therapist. The client may smile and nod in agreement but inside be completely rejecting everything the therapist is saying. Or such a client may uncritically accept whatever the therapist says without critically judging its merits for his or her particular situation. In such situations, the treatment fails because the client does not struggle enough to tailor the intervention to his or her own needs.

Because personalty scales provide information about adaptive styles, the therapist can anticipate potential issues that may emerge in treatment and take preemptive action. Scores on the various personality scales can also be useful for identifying issues that were not part of the presenting problem but may need to be explored.

Finally, *matching treatments to clients* is perhaps the most important contribution personalty assessment can provide to practitioners. It has long been known that certain clients benefit more from certain types of therapies than others. Personality measures can facilitate this matching process. For example, individuals high on Extraversion, who are sociable and talkative, will find therapies that require interpersonal interactions more helpful than do introverts, who may prefer and benefit from behavior therapy or Gestalt approaches. Individuals high on introspectiveness, who are more willing to consider novel ideas and try out unusual problem-solving approaches, may prefer Gestalt, psychoanalysis, or Jungian analysis. Individuals who are closed to internal experiences will prefer directive psychotherapies that offer sensible advice, behavioral techniques that teach concrete skills, or client-centered therapies that provide emotional support.

By obtaining high-quality information about the basic dispositions of the client, therapists can think more precisely about the kinds of treatments that would complement the client's style. Personality assessment can help therapists better appreciate the uniqueness of clients and to think flexibly about how to intervene. As clinical outcome research progresses, we hope gains will be made in our ability to link specific treatments to particular types of individuals.

There is no doubt that measures of normal personality characteristics provide a lot of "bang for the buck." Obtaining a comprehensive sampling of personality traits can provide a pool of information that is as flexible in its application as it is informative in its descriptions. The next section outlines some of the major models of personality constructs that dominate the way personality psychologists conceptualize temperament. It also outlines the problems these approaches create. The NEO PI–R is an outgrowth of one of the solutions to these problems.

QUALITIES OF PERSONALITY

The value of personality assessment cannot be overstated. Capturing the fundamental aspects of the client provides the therapist with a broad understanding of the client and his or her psychosocial context. Symptoms can then be seen as part of a larger ongoing life process. For example, an understanding of personality can inform clinicians about the etiology of the presenting problem and about other potential weaknesses. The course of therapy can be anticipated and client resources identified. The question that arises is, "What are the personality variables that need to be assessed?"

Over the past century, numerous theorists have appeared and each has presented his or her own model of personality. Each model not only includes insights into how personality is organized, but also identifies characteristics that are the most salient for understanding underlying motivations. There is a rich literature in personality theory.

Modern scientific thought about personality finds a strong beginning with the work of Sigmund Freud, who saw two major personality dimensions: Eros (the life instinct) and Thanatos (the death instinct). For Freud these two qualities were the basic sources of all personal motivations. Every behavior or characteristic of an individual could be psychologically parsed into some combination of these two forces.

Later theorists noted many limitations to Freud's analyses of temperament and began to elaborate on other qualities of the person. A review of these theorists and their philosophical foundations is beyond the scope of this book, but Table 1-2 outlines a few of the more modern major personality theorists whose ideas continue to influence current personality theory and measurement. These theorists are merely a small sampling of personality psychologists. They were selected because they represent a spectrum of approaches to conceptualizing personality and also because the instruments that are based on their approaches are multidimensional inventories claiming to represent a comprehensive sampling of personality constructs. These theorists were selected largely because they see many more qualities of the individual as important than Freud did.

The individuals listed in Table 1-2 represent various perspectives on normal personality. Henry Murray provided a motivational approach, while Cattell, a trait theorist, based his work heavily on quantitative methods. However, the reader should be aware that there are other personality models that exist for explaining abnormal personality functioning. There are the biosocial model of Millon (e.g., Millon, 1990), the psychobiological model of Cloninger (e.g., Cloninger, 1987; Cloninger, Svrakic, & Przybeck, 1993), and a model semantically derived from the *Diagnostic and Statistical Manual of Mental Disorders* itself (e.g., Harkness & McNulty, 1994). There are numerous variables here that also need to be understood not only in relation to each other but also with respect to those constructs that define normal functioning.

Two issues emerge from Table 1-2. First, it is quite obvious that these few theorists have identified a number of personality characteristics; there are 80 constructs identified in the table alone. Yet, there are many other psychologists who have identified more circumscribed, putatively important constructs that define important aspects of personality and predict salient life outcomes. Such constructs as *cynicism, hostility, hopelessness, shyness, fear of success, fear of failure, origence, intellectence, critical parent, adult, free child, nurturing parent, altruism, well-being, coping ability, burnout, empathy, self-esteem, stress experience,* and *authoritarianism* are but a few of literally thousands of such scales that occupy the psychological literature. The

TABLE 1-2. Measurement Models of Personality and Their Constructs

Theorist	Measurement device	Constructs
Henry Murray	T.A.T./Adjective Check List/Edwards Personal Preference Schedule/Personality Research Form	Achievement, dominance, abasement, succorance, heterosexuality, play, exhibition, nurturance, order, infavoidance, autonomy, aggression, change, defendence, affiliation, harmavoidance, counteraction, sentience, understanding, rejection
Harrison Gough	California Personality Inventory/Adjective Check List	Self-confidence, self-control, personal adjustment, ideal self, creative personality, military leadership, masculinity, femininity, dominance, capacity for status, sociability, social presence, self-acceptance, independence, empathy, responsibility, socialization, self-control, good impression, communality, sense of well-being, tolerance, achievement via conformance, achievement via independence, intellectual efficiency, psychological mindedness, flexibility
J. P. Guilford	Guilford–Zimmerman Temperament Survey	General activity, restraint, ascendance, sociability, objectivity, friendliness, thoughtfulness, personal relations, masculinity
Raymond Cattell	16PF	Warmth, reasoning, emotional stability, dominance, liveliness, rule-consciousness, social boldness, sensitivity, vigilance, abstractedness, privateness, apprehension, openness to change, self-reliance, perfectionism, tension
Carl Jung	Myers–Briggs Type Indicator	Introversion–extraversion, thinking–feeling, sensing–intuiting, judging–perceiving
Hans Eysenck	Eysenck Personality Questionnaire	Neuroticism, extraversion, psychoticism

plethora of measures testifies to the richness of personality research and underscores the interpretive and predictive value that personality holds for the social sciences. However, the nearly limitless number of these scales very easily boggles the mind.

This is the second issue that emerges from Table 1-2. Given all these scales, how does one select instruments for use? Are all these constructs needed to provide a comprehensive sampling of personality? If not, then which ones should be used? As we scan the list of scales, it becomes clear that there is much redundancy among the measures. Clearly Socialization, Affiliation, Extraversion–Introversion, Personal Relations, and Privateness all seem to have something in common. But one should never rely on scale names to identify the personological content of the scale. It is entirely possible that two scales having the same name measure very different constructs. Conversely, two scales having different names may in fact be measuring the same quality. I give an example of this issue in the next chapter.

But here lies the real crux of the issue. There really is no established framework for evaluating all these diverse scales or for linking them together conceptually. As things stand now, assessors need to select scales that appear to them to be appropriate for their particular needs. However, many of these scales and inventories proceed from very different theoretical traditions. For example, if one is interested in motivational needs, then measures of Murray's constructs are appropriate. If one does not prefer such a motivational perspective, then the more empirically based constructs offered by Cattell may be preferred. Then again, one may wish to take the "folk" approach offered by Gough and use constructs he deems as being important concepts for describing important interpersonal behaviors.

In each instance, though, the selection is one of theoretical preference. Even though one's identification of a theoretical preference is based on a serious consideration of both the heuristic value of the theory and the relevant research data, unfortunately there is no larger, objective paradigm for critically comparing and evaluating the merits of these many approaches. Therefore, the field is left in a chaotic state, in that there are many different measurement models each with its own jargon and terminology but with no conceptual or empirical linkage among them. When one surveys the field of assessment instruments, it appears almost as a Tower of Babel: so many constructs, so little understanding.

What is needed is a taxonomy of personality characteristics. Such a framework would allow one to compare and contrast personality measures in terms of important, defining qualities. Ideally, this framework would not work out of any particular theoretical tradition. Rather, it would represent a more objective, preferably empirically based, system of classification. A taxonomic model would be useful in organizing the many personality constructs that exist and help in identifying areas of redundancy and uniqueness. This would make the task of developing a comprehensive assessment battery much easier.

WHAT IS A TAXONOMY?

A taxonomy is simply a framework for classifying things. As Bailey (1994) noted, "classification is merely defined as the ordering of entities into groups or classes on the basis of their similarity. Statistically speaking, we generally seek to minimize within-group variance, while maximizing between-group variance" (p. 1). In order to accomplish this, one needs to identify all the necessary qualities that distinguish the entities that are to be classified and these distinguishing characteristics must be mutually exclusive.

Taxonomies provide a better understanding of the things they classify by revealing similarities and differences among them. Taxonomies are able to do this because, as already stated, they enumerate the most important defining qualities of the things to be classified. Further, these qualities are not overlapping. Each dimension of the taxonomy provides nonredundant information. As a result, things that are located closer together in the taxonomy have more things in common than elements located farther apart.

Perhaps the best-known taxonomy is the one developed by Carl von Linne (also known as Linnaeus) in the mid-eighteenth century. This model is used to classify all living things. We are all aware, to some degree, of the major categories of kingdom, phylum, class, order, family, genus, and species. Every animal and plant receives a taxonomic classification based on these eight dimensions. Creatures located close to one another in this framework (e.g., in the same family), have more in common than creatures that are not in the same family. The introduction of this framework was a major step forward in our understanding of animal life, much of which we take for granted today.

For example, think of whales. For centuries people thought that whales were fish. After all, they swam in the ocean like fish, they looked like fish, acted like fish, smelled like fish—fish! However, when Linnaeus's system of organizing physical characteristics of animals was introduced we received quite an awakening. From his perspective whales were much more related to human beings than to fish. Why? Because both have similar characteristics, such as possessing mammary glands, lungs, and bearing live young, whales and human beings were located very close together in the taxonomic scheme (they share the class, mammalia). Fish, on the other hand, do not have any of these physical characteristics and therefore were placed very far away from both whales and human beings (fish occupy several different classes: osteichthyes, chondrichthyes, and agnatha).

From this discussion we can see that there are two important values of a taxonomy. First, as already noted, a classification framework provides an organization for understanding the elements that we wish to classify. Such systematic description can provide new insights into already "familiar" objects, as we saw with the case of whales. The second value of a taxonomic structure is that it gives us a frame of reference for evaluating new objects that may be discovered. Measuring new items in terms of the existing dimensions of the taxon allows one to determine whether the new element represents something distinct from existing elements, or overlaps them in specific ways. It is this "parsing" feature of taxonomies that can be the most value for psychological assessment.

TAXONOMY VERSUS TYPOLOGY

Perhaps a more familiar term to social scientists is *typology*. A typology is the flip side of a taxonomy. In a taxonomy one is interested in understanding some entity in terms of basic qualities or dimensions. With a typology, on the other hand, interest is in identifying the constellations of basic qualities that co-occur. Thus a typology is usually multidimensional in nature and represents a conceptual grouping of taxonomic elements.

For example, Jungian theory provides a good example of both concepts. As noted in Table 1-2, Jung sees four major qualities that describe people, Extraversion–Introversion, Thinking–Feeling, Sensing–Intuiting, and Judging–Perceiving. These qualities would constitute a taxonomy. For Jung, any behavior or motivation can be seen as some combination of these qualities. However, the way one stands on all of these domains simultaneously constitutes one's *type*. The label INTJ, a type, represents a combination of qualities into a larger whole that has its own personological implications. Using chemistry as an example, one can think of a taxonomy as representing the elements, while a typology represents compounds.

Thus taxons and types represent important ways of organizing and describing individuals. Their value is founded on the identification of important, discriminating constructs. The usefulness of taxons for personality theory and assessment has not been overlooked.

THE VALUE OF A TAXONOMY FOR PERSONALITY ASSESSMENT

Social scientists have also been very interested in developing taxonomies of personality functioning. Having such a model would help organize our understandings of how individuals come to be and the qualities they display. It would enable us to distinguish a characteristic representing a superficial quality, one that may be situationally determined, from a feature that may represent a more fundamental attribute, stable over time and situations. To borrow a metaphor from Ozer and Riese (1994), a personality taxonomy would be like the latitude and longitude markings on a map. Just as explorers would locate their new landfalls by reference to these calibrations on a globe, so, too, would personality psychologists need to identify their new individual-difference variables

using the calibrations of the taxonomy. In this way, psychological phenomena could be reliably located and competing claims identified.

Numerous social scientists have tried to establish taxonomies in order
to accomplish this important goal. As we noted earlier, Freud was perhaps
the first to specify some type of model, postulating the existence of Eros
and Thanatos. For him, these dimensions constituted the entire taxonomy.
But not all agreed with Freud. Jung proposed a separate set of dimensions
which, as already discussed, formed his typological model of personality.

As Table 1-2 reviewed, there are numerous personality models, each
with their own language and constructs of interest. However, there is no
objective manner here for selecting and interpreting psychological constructs. The theoretical basis of all these models makes any option one of
personal bias. The natural sciences always seemed to have a way to rise
above this subjectivity and to find a common reference point that all could
find acceptable and reasonable. For example, when early researchers were
in need of a temperature scale, the interval-level indices were in need of a
"zero" point. Where to put zero? It could be put anywhere, because of the
inherent subjectivity of an interval-level scale. Why not fix zero to where
water freezes? Why there? Why not? Water is a common element that all
are familiar with and, of course, like. In astronomy there is a need to talk
about distances among objects in the solar system. What metric would be
useful? What standard should be applied? The result, *the astronomical unit,*
which is the distance between the sun and earth. Why this unit? Again,
why not? The earth is a familiar place, one that all know about and feel
comfortable with. It is, after all, a reference to ourselves and what could be
more user friendly than that?

For our purposes, then, is there such a familiar standard that can be
applied in personality assessment? Is there a reference point or points that
would be meaningful to everyone? Given the plethora of personality variables and models that exist one may be tempted to think not. But where
would one begin in such a quest? Where is the common element? For Gordon Allport, that common basis was found in the English language.

THE LEXIGRAPHIC HYPOTHESIS

For the most part in personality psychology, the major resources for
identifying important dimensions of personality were the experiences and
insights of individual personality theorists. Although these theories have
important theoretical and clinical value, the fact remains that they are inherently subjective. Ellenberger (1970) has advanced the idea that many of
these influential theories find their basis in the "creative illnesses" of their

creators. In an attempt to make sense of their own social reality, theorists become absorbed in finding answers to these very personal questions. The theories that emerge, then, reflect the answers that seem to make the most sense for the theorists.

If one does not find value or meaning in these "answers," then the theory has little relevance. There is nothing compelling one to accept a theory other than available data (which may be lacking) or a personal orientation shared with the theorist. In either case, these theories are locked into a particular set of life circumstances. Ultimately, something larger and more compelling is needed for developing a catalogue of individual difference constructs.

In order to bypass this problem Gordon Allport took a different path. Instead of necessarily evaluating his own personal experiences, he decided to access the accumulated knowledge of our larger culture. The repository of this wisdom, experience, and insight was the English language itself. To understand the value of using language in this way, we need to evaluate its function.

Language is an important tool that human beings have. From an evolutionary point of view, there is no doubt that language serves an adaptive function: Having language helps us to survive and reproduce. If we could go back to primeval times and look at our evolutionary forebears, it would be clear that those who could talk and communicate survived while those who could not, died. Therefore speaking was selected "in" to our genetic stock. But what do we talk about? For language to be effective, we would need to talk about important aspects of our adaptive landscape. We would need to create words that would help us to survive. Words that would direct us away from danger and closer to food. Any object, event, or place that would relate to our survival would certainly, over time, acquire a word to represent it.

Take, for example, Eskimos. They have many different words for snow. Why? Because snow is an important part of their adaptive world. There is the type of snow to build one's igloo out of; a type of snow that is good for traveling over, and so on. How many words do we have for snow? One—snow. Why so few? Look around; how much snow do you see? Other than a possible inconvenience at times, snow is a transitory phenomenon for most of us in the United States. If you were to ask people from, say, equatorial Africa, you would find that they may not have a word for snow at all! Why? No snow.

As human beings we are also very much social animals. We live in groups and depend on others for our survival. Because of our strong interpersonal needs, it is clear that other people make up an important dimension of our own adaptive landscape. We need to distinguish the ones who will help us from the ones who will hurt us. We need to discover whom can we depend on and whom we should select as a mate. In short, to survive in the human community, one needs to be able to effectively anticipate the motivations and behaviors of others. Because the personal characteristics of others play a significant role in our own survival, it stands to reason that over time our language has accrued terms that reflect or describe these important aspects of people. Thus, the lexigraphic hypothesis asserts: "Those individual differences that are most salient and socially relevant in people's lives will eventually become encoded into their language; the more important such a difference, the more likely is it to become expressed as a single word. The analysis of the personality vocabulary represented in a natural language should thus yield a finite set of attributes that the people in the language community have generally found to be the most important" (John, Angleitner, & Ostendorf, 1988, p. 174). The view of language as a means for our species to codify important dimensions of our environments is the central element of the lexigraphic hypothesis.

The rationale for the lexical hypothesis is relatively straightforward, although there are three important limitations that need to be appreciated.

First, how words come to be developed and included in a lexicon is not well understood. Further, words that do appear may not necessarily be of importance scientifically. It is possible that some qualities of personality may not be apparent to lay observers and therefore overlooked in the language. Also, some words that are developed may be more evaluative and expressive than descriptive. Thus, language serves more than just a descriptive function.

Second, the personality attributes that are defined in a lexicon are specific to the culture that generated them. Different cultures may emphasize certain qualities over others, or may not exhibit various characteristics that are apparent in other cultural contexts. Thus, word-based models may lack generalizability.

Finally, although words do have a shared meaning within a culture, there is a broad range of descriptive and explanatory convenience for any given term. According to Allport (1961), words represent "ratbag categories," or broad ranges of qualities. For example, we can refer to two people as being dominant, but that does not mean that their levels of dominance are the same. Rather, the same term implies some level of *general* agreement in temperament; how much is not known. Thus, the same label may be applied to describe a wide array of behaviors. This lack of precision makes it difficult to isolate the phenomena described.

These three issues raise important questions that need to be addressed empirically if any lexically based taxonomy is to be found useful. For now, these issues generate questions surrounding the robustness, inclusiveness, and generalizability of any model based on language. These issues are considered again in Chapter 2. Despite these limitations, language does offer the opportunity for identifying potentially important individual-difference variables. Although these "ratbag categories" do not possess the level of precision demanded by science, they do provide a useful starting point. Science can provide more rigorous definitions as the classification progresses.

Proceeding from this perspective, Allport and Odbert (1936) went to Webster's *New International Dictionary* (1925) and extracted all terms that were able to "distinguish the behavior of one human being from that of another" (Allport & Odbert, 1936, p. 24). The resulting list included mostly adjectives and participles, although some nouns and slang words were included. This investigation netted some 17,953 different terms! This represented about 4.5% of the total number of words in the dictionary. The sheer number of terms indicates just how important others are in our adaptive environments. Our need to anticipate real interpersonal events resulted in the development of a wide assortment of descriptive labels that certainly capture the many nuances and subtleties of human functioning.

This list of words provides the basic fodder for evaluating personality dispositions. Allport and Odbert (1936) organized these terms into four general categories in order to facilitate classification. The first category included "names that seemed to symbolize most clearly 'real' traits of personality. They designate generalized and personalized determining tendencies—consistent and stable modes of an individual's adjustment to his environment" (Allport & Odbert, 1936, pp. 25–26). This category included terms such as aggressive, introverted, and sociable. The second category contained terms "descriptive of present activity, temporary states of mind, and mood" (p. 26) and included terms such as abashed, gibbering, rejoicing, and frantic. The third category was the longest of the four and contained characterological evaluations, such as insignificant, acceptable, pretentious, and worthy. The final category was a miscellaneous grouping of adjectives that had "possible value in characterizing personality, even though they have no certain place in the first three [categories]" (p. 27). This category included words such as experienced, infantile, and undisciplined.

This fourfold breakdown of terms was a useful first step in classification. However, the sheer volume of words is quite intimidating, especially from sorting and interpretive perspectives. Nonetheless, Allport and Odbert (1936) have given us an important first step in defining a universe of qualities that are relevant for describing individuals. These terms do not reflect any theoretical point of view, nor are they the working out of some context-dependent appraisal. Rather, these words represent hundreds of

years of interpersonal activity, the culmination of centuries of human observation and wisdom. These words represent our lexical heritage. Overall, not a bad place to start for learning about ourselves.

But are all these adjectives necessary? Certainly within these lists
there are many synonyms and antonyms. Not all these words need to be
considered. There are also many infrequently used terms, such as chrema-
tistic, hagiolatrous, stultiloquent, and thersitical. They may represent qualities that are not as relevant today as they once were, or they may have
more common variants (such as greedy, saintly, foolish, and abusive). In
any case, the need is to somehow reduce this list into a more manageable
number of items. Ultimately, we need to distill these items down to their
fundamental dimensions, those basic, larger qualities that seem to capture
the essence of all these words. Identifying and naming such factors would
provide the basis for a taxonomic model of personality.

Searching for a Linguistic Structure

The process of finding an underlying structure for the adjective pool
identified by Allport and Odbert (1936) is the history of the development
of the five-factor model. Numerous individuals have been involved in this
process, and good historical accounts can be found in Digman (1996) and
John and colleagues (1988). What follows here is a basic, and necessarily
limited, overview of this ongoing story.

The first person really to take advantage of the Allport and Odbert
(1936) word list was Raymond Cattell. Although he had already been active
in analyzing personality ratings (e.g., Cattell, 1933), he was not the first do
so (see Guilford & Guilford, 1936; Webb, 1915), Cattell saw this word list as
an interesting place to identify salient personality descriptions systematically. Using a subset of 35 bipolar scales, he obtained ratings on 373 male
university students. Subjecting these ratings to the then emerging statistical
tool, factor analysis, he obtained 12 interpretable factors (Cattell, 1944). In
two additional studies using new samples of both men and women, Cattell
was able to replicate these factors and he incorporated them into his 16 PF
(Sixteen Personality Factors) Questionnaire (Cattell, 1947, 1948).

The dimensions of the 16PF (see Table 1-2) represented empirically derived, cohesive patterns of intertrait relationships derived from peer ratings. The value of this work is manifold. First, it was the first effort to
identify empirically how various personality traits are related in common
usage. Rather than relying on rational interpretation, which may miss
some important dimensions or nuances in usage, the factor analytic approach provided a relatively unbiased effort at identifying an underlying
structure already in place. A second benefit is that it allowed for a more

precise evaluation of the replicability of these factor structures in new samples. Finally, it pioneered a new technology, factor analysis, that would eventually prove exceedingly useful for condensing large amounts of information into more manageable clusters or factors.

Briefly stated, factor analysis is a data reduction tool (see Gorsuch, 1997, for a brief review). It examines the patterns of correlations among items to determine whether there are "clumps" of variables that seem to correlate more highly with each other than with other variables. These "clumps" then come to be identified as factors. Factors are latent dimensions (quantities that are not directly assessed) that are hypothesized to explain the interrelatedness of the variables. For example, descriptors such as *outgoing, talkative, gregarious, friendly,* and *happy* may correlate more strongly with each other than with other items, such as *conservative, rigid, anxious,* and *disciplined.* These five adjectives would then form a factor that we may wish to label "Extraversion." Extraverted people will be hypothesized to be outgoing, talkative, and friendly. Thus, we may choose to talk about a person's level of Extraversion rather than the five different descriptors that define the factor. We have reduced five separate things into a single dimension.

In Cattell's later work, much of his effort was focused on these 16 factors. It is interesting to note that although later research would show that these 16 factors clearly fit into the more parsimonious five-factor model (e.g., Boyle, 1989; Goldberg & Digman, 1994; Hofer, Horn, & Eber, 1997), Cattell would continue to oppose this type of integration, referring to the five-factor model as the "five big factors heresy" (Cattell, 1994, p. 8). Although Cattell did not pursue any further reduction in the number of factors, others did.

Building on the work of Cattell was Donald Fiske, who used several of the rating scales developed by Cattell. Factor analyzing results from self-reports, peer ratings, and supervisor ratings, Fiske obtained five large factors, labeled Social Adaptability, Conformity, Emotional Control, Inquiring Intellect, and Confident Self-Expression. These five factors emerged independently over the three sources of information (Fiske, 1949). Despite the fact that this study was executed well and the results were quite robust, these findings were largely ignored.

During the 1950s and early 1960s, several researchers continued to use the adjective lists developed by Cattell in their studies on personality structure (e.g., Thurstone, 1951; Tupes & Christal, 1961). In all of these studies, a consistent five-factor solution emerged. In other words, when the individual ratings were examined, the pattern of intercorrelations suggested that the items created five different "clumps" or factors. Regardless of where the information was coming from (e.g., peer rating versus self-report), five different factors would emerge, and the content of these factors remained very similar. Norman (1963) concluded from both his own work and a review of the literature that these five factors seemed to constitute an "adequate taxonomy of personality" (p. 582).

This was a pretty powerful conclusion from these data. Norman was arguing that underlying the ratings on these personality variables were only five dimensions, and no more. Many were skeptical that such a small number of dimensions could adequately describe the entire realm of personality (e.g., Digman, 1996, p. 10). But, aside from a philosophical distrust of only five factors, there was a very real limitation to the studies done by Norman and others. Simply put, they relied almost exclusively on the scales identified and employed by Cattell in his early research: 35 bipolar rating scales. Given that Allport and Odbert (1936) identified close to 18,000 adjectives, 35 bipolar ratings (70 adjectives) seemed hardly representative of the original pool of items. Certainly there could be other factors residing among those remaining 17,883 adjectives.

The reason why such a small number of adjectives were selected in the first place was that factor analysis is a very complicated and intricate statistical tool. In the years before computers, individuals had to rely on hand calculations. It was not uncommon for someone to apply for a research grant to fund such an analysis and it was equally not uncommon for such a process to take the efforts of dozens of individuals several months to complete. Therefore, having only 35 to 50 items to factor analyze was a major project. Today, with the easy availability of powerful, high-speed computers and user-friendly statistical software, it may take a single person about several moments to "do" a factor analysis. It is ironic that it takes longer to print out the results of a factor analysis than it does for the computer to actually do all the calculations. Nonetheless, the issue of the representativeness of the original selection of adjectives was a valid criticism and conceptual limitation.

In response to this, Norman (1963) went back to the original pool and identified an additional 2,800 adjectives which he was able to rationally sort into the five obtained factor dimensions. Picking up where Norman left off was Lewis Goldberg who, starting in the early 1980s, began an impressive program of research aimed at empirically evaluating the linguistic structure of these adjectives. Over the next decade using large sets of ratings based on an extensive pool of adjectives, Goldberg discovered that the five-factor structure obtained in the early research continued to be observed in these larger samplings of adjective ratings (Goldberg, 1981, 1982, 1990). By the beginning of the 1990s, after nearly four decades and uncounted computer time, it was becoming clear to most researchers that underlying the adjectives identified originally by Allport and Odbert really were five large factors (Digman, 1990; Goldberg, 1993; McCrae & John, 1992).

These five factors have come to be labeled *Neuroticism* (or Emotional Stability), representing the tendency to experience negative affect, such as anxiety, depression, and hostility; *Extraversion* (or Surgency), which reflects the quantity and intensity of interpersonal interactions; *Openness to Experience* (or Intellect, Culture), indicating the proactive seeking and appreciation of new experiences; *Agreeableness*, reflecting the quality of one's interpersonal interactions along a continuum from compassion to antagonism; and, finally, *Conscientiousness* (or Will to Achieve, Control, Constraint), which reflects the amount of persistence, organization, and motivation to succeed in goal-directed endeavors. These five factors have become known as the *Five-Factor Model of Personality* and have been shown to represent the underlying structure of the 17,953 adjectives originally defined by Allport and Odbert. Whether one is working with self-report data or observer ratings, whether one is assessing adolescents or adults, these five factors seem to explain the patterns of correlations found among adjectives in personality ratings.

From Adjectives to Sentences: The NEO Model

The emergence of the five-factor model of personality represents a true effort in the field of psychology to engage in programmatic, cumulative research. In other words, data are being obtained that build on previous findings and contribute to an ongoing informational structure. The result of these efforts is a paradigm for understanding and evaluating personality constructs. However, the obtained five-factor structure derived from the original Allport and Odbert (1936) adjective pool is but a first step in understanding how individuals describe themselves and others. There are some limitations to using single adjectives.

First, the number of adjectives found in the language for describing each personality domain is not equal. Goldberg (1992) has shown that there are more adjectives associated with Agreeableness than with any of the other five domains. Extraversion is the next most frequently represented domain. As will be discussed later in this book, these two domains together represent interpersonal styles: those characteristic ways that individuals approach others and the qualities of the relationships they form. Given the highly social nature of humans, that these two domains would garner such a large number of adjectives makes sense. Conscientiousness, Neuroticism, and Openness, in that order, are represented by fewer and fewer adjectives. Goldberg did note that there are roughly equivalent numbers of adjectives that describe each of the two poles for four of the factors; there are extremely few adjectives marking low Neuroticism.

What are we to make of this uneven distribution of adjective descriptors? Does this mean that some factors are psychologically more important than others? Or that some factors have been around human psychological functioning longer than others, therefore having more of an opportunity to emerge into more diverse synonym clusters? The answer to the second question is certainly "No." All five factors have been shown to be psychologically meaningful for understanding personality. Each domain is relatively equal in size in terms of its capacity to explain a diverse range of psychological phenomena. The answer to the third question is less clear and more open to debate and discussion. As noted earlier when discussing the lexigraphic approach, one drawback is that we do not understand how words come to enter and leave the lexicon, or the factors that influence the development of new terms.

It would be interesting to perform lexigraphic analyses of the English language as it developed over time. There are distinct periods of language development (e.g., Old English, Middle English, Modern English); one could determine the relative prevalence of adjectives representing the five dimension at each stage. It may be that interpersonal behavior, a foundation of human psychological and physical development and survival, is most preeminent. As cultures develop, both socially and technologically, new pressures are placed on humans to adapt and with this evolutionary impetus come new terms to describe the emerging personality qualities being expressed. One could formulate a number of hypotheses along this line and the results of such investigations would be interesting testimonials to human psychological development. But this takes us away from our current theme. Suffice it to say that in working with adjectives, one needs to recognize that the sheer volume of adjectives does not connote the significance of a factor.

But the fourth question that emerges from the reality of an uneven distribution of adjectives over the five factors highlights one limitation to the use of adjectives: "How many adjectives are necessary before one considers a factor to exist?" Certainly, if there is a personality quality that has adaptive significance to humans, then many adjectives would be developed to capture this quality and as a result, a factor would emerge representing these numerous related terms. But there are replicable, smaller factors that have been found beyond the "Big Five" that have not received much attention. Are these qualities as personologically trivial as their low numbers suggest? The lexical approach does not establish any quantitative index for determining whether a factor is large enough to warrant attention.

A second limitation to the use of simple adjectives is that there may be qualities of people that are too complex to be reduced to a single word; they may require several words, or a phrase or sentence in order to nuance the quality. For example, Goldberg (1990) obtained smaller personality dimensions in his data when more than five factors were rotated, but they represented very circumscribed characteristics, such as Thrift versus Intemperance, and Sensuality versus Passionlessness. An additional replicated factor obtained by Goldberg was Religiosity. It included items such as Religious versus Nonreligious and Reverent versus Irreverent. What is interesting about this small factor is that it represents a quality of people that is very difficult to define using sentences, much less single adjectives only.

Imagine a very spiritual or religious person. What adjectives come to mind? I can think of only a few, such as *spiritual, religious, holy, transcendent, mystical,* and *numinous.* I would need to consult a thesaurus to find others. Such a paucity of adjectives really underrepresents the importance of religion or spirituality in the lives of people. I have argued that spirituality may represent a separate domain of personality worthy of study in its own right (Piedmont, 1997a). However, the adjective record does not seem to support such a claim. Therefore, adjectives themselves may be inadequate to capture the full spectrum of psychologically significant personality qualities. One may need to seek recourse in phrases and sentences. Also, the use of phrases and sentences allows for greater subtlety and nuance in defining personality attributes. Such added finesse may provide greater predictive power.

A third limitation of adjectives is that they may have too much interpretive variability, making assessment difficult and imprecise, not to mention the technical psychometric problems such slippage introduces. For example, take the word *steady.* What does it represent about someone? In just evaluating this term, does it mean that someone is reliable, or emotionally stable, or closed to experience? As it stands, there really is no way to tell. If this term were to appear on a questionnaire, interpreting responses to the item would be subject to much error. Usually, to compensate for this type of interpretive latitude bipolar terms are employed. This helps to fix the interpretation of the term relative to some opposite. But again, the term selected as the reference point can greatly influence the interpretation. For example *steady versus moody* would represent qualities likely to fall on the Neuroticism domain. *Steady versus distractible* would locate itself on the Conscientiousness domain, while *steady versus changeable* may represent a quality relevant to Openness to Experience. Thus the same term can have very different personological implications depending on the interpretive context.

These three limitations to the lexical approach, (a) the lack of a clear empirical criterion for determining the number of adjectives necessary to define a significant personality factor, (b) the inadequacy of single terms to capture important qualities of individuals, and (c) the wide interpretive latitude that single terms possess, can all be circumvented by relying on sentences and phrases for describing personality qualities. Qualities of interest can be defined theoretically and operationalized through multiple sentences that provide a clear portrait of the dispositions. The personological space containing this construct can be sharply defined and nuanced by using phrases and sentences. Individuals can respond to very specific dispositional statements so that their responses can be unambiguously interpreted. Then the personality dimension can be evaluated for significance by the extent to which it predicts important outcomes.

It was this approach that Costa and McCrae (1992c) used in developing their measure of the five-factor model—the NEO Personality Inventory (NEO PI). Rather than relying on adjectives to broadly describe the five factors, they constructed sentences that captured the subtleties of each of the five domains. Further, the use of sentences enabled them to construct *facet scales* for each of the domains. These facet scales are more precise articulations of the qualities subsumed by these five broad domains. Each facet scale captures a more circumscribed psychological quality that has been shown to have theoretical significance in the field. In this way, users can enjoy more interpretive precision as well as enhanced predictive accuracy (Costa & McCrae, 1995a).

The NEO model contains six facet scales for each of the five broad personality domains. For example, Neuroticism contains the facets of Anxiety, Hostility, Depression, Self-Consciousness, Impulsiveness, and Vulnerability to Stress. These facets were selected for two reasons: first, on the basis of their historical and theoretical presence in the field; second, because they have been shown empirically to represent a broad spectrum of qualities within their given domain. These scales were created to be as nonoverlapping as possible while still remaining on the same domain (Costa & McCrae, 1992c; McCrae & Costa, 1992).

Although the presence of six facets per domain appears somewhat artificial, and it is, the NEO PI–R authors recognize that there could be other facets for a domain in addition to those already created. One example of this concerns Neuroticism where a measure of somatic complaints was explicitly *not* created, although such a scale does appropriately belong on that domain. The reason for this omission was simple: Because the NEO PI–R authors worked in a research context that would evaluate personality's role in predicting physical health, including such a measure would contaminate their research. A measure of somatization would by necessity include items relating to physical health and well-being. Such a measure would certainly correlate with any physical functioning index or health measure, not because personality was an important predictor, but because the predictor and outcome would share similar items dealing with health status. This would artificially inflate any associations between the two variables, irrespective of any substantive overlap (see D. H. Schroeder &

Costa, 1984). Therefore, this type of scale was avoided. Certainly, future research may be able to discern new specific personality constructs that are relatively independent of the existing facet scales for a particular domain, but yet belong in that personological space. This would argue for the inclusion of more facet scales.

Although the ultimate structure of the NEO model may not have been settled on, the current instrument—the NEO PI-R—contains a large amount of personological information: 30 separate facet scales combining to assess the five major dimensions of personality. The NEO PI-R is rapidly becoming one of the most popular measures of normal personality in the research literature. Psychometric reviews of the instrument are uniformly favorable (e.g., Botwin, 1995; Juni, 1995; Piedmont, 1997b), citing the robust empirical nature of the instrument as well as its impressive predictive validity in a number of applications (e.g., physical and psychological health, job success, well-being, coping ability).

But given the empirical strength of the instrument, there is still a basic question that needs to be asked: "With so many different personality inventories available, why should one use the NEO PI-R?" There are several responses to this query. First, as noted earlier, the five-factor model of personality represents a comprehensive, empirically based taxonomy of personality traits. The NEO PI-R is the only commercially available instrument designed explicitly to measure those dimensions. Although there are a number of marker scales available in the general literature for assessing these domains (e.g., Goldberg, 1992; John, 1990; Saucier, 1994), the NEO PI-R is the only instrument that also provides more specific facet scales within each domain. This allows for a more precise and differential evaluation of a person's place within each personality dimension. For example, the Extraversion domain has the facet scales of Warmth, Gregariousness, Assertiveness, Activity, Excitement Seeking, and Positive Emotions. It is possible for someone to score high on Extraversion, but possess only the interpersonal component of the domain (e.g., Warmth, Gregariousness, and Assertiveness) and none of the qualities relating to personal energy or tempo (e.g., Activity, Excitement Seeking, and Positive Emotions). Global scores miss these important distinctions.

Another reason for preferring the NEO PI-R is that the five-factor model is rapidly becoming the preeminent measurement paradigm for personality in a number of contexts, both clinical and applied (Barrick & Mount, 1991; Costa, 1996; Goldberg, 1993). The empirical basis and conceptual clarity afforded by the model makes it an ideal measure for talking about individual differences that crosses subdisciplines in the social sciences. Further, these major dimensions of personality also have been shown useful for describing both normal and clinical populations.

Finally, given the taxonomic nature of the five-factor model, it can be useful for linking information from diverse sources. Scores on the major domains can speak about an individual's interpersonal style, coping ability, needs and motives, and response to psychotherapy. The five-factor model can be useful for organizing all of this information into a cohesive psychological portrait of the individual. Especially from a clinical perspective, the NEO PI–R can help streamline the assessment process and promote a better understanding of the larger context within which the client's presenting problems develop. As Miller (1991) noted, "the five-factor model can relate patient personality, presenting complaint, treatment plan, and treatment outcome to each other in a reasonable, systematic way, without loss of empathy or compassion for the patient" (p. 432).

RECOMMENDATIONS FOR APPROACHING THIS BOOK

The purpose of this book is to provide you with a document that presents the technical and interpretive aspects of the NEO PI–R. The following chapters provide basic psychometric information about the instrument and interpretive guidelines for evaluating NEO PI–R profiles. Also covered are topics relating to the application of the instrument in a research context. After reading this book I hope that you will gain an appreciation for the potential value of the NEO PI–R for your own work. By becoming familiar with the concepts of the five-factor model you will develop a language for discussing individual differences that will enable you to dialogue with professionals from other assessment areas. The five-factor model is the direction that personality assessment is moving toward and in the future will serve as the basis for all conversations about personal dispositions.

To help you gain this expertise, many interpretive examples are presented for both individuals and couples. It is hoped that these materials will illustrate the interpretive nuances represented by each of the scales. Most important, efforts have been made to perform profile interpretations of the NEO PI–R. Profile interpretations rely on an understanding of how several different scales combine to describe one's personality. Although work examining specific NEO PI–R configural patterns is just beginning, what is available demonstrates the exciting interpretive potential the instrument possesses.

As you read through the case histories you will begin to see how interpretations are made. As you begin to develop a fluency with the terminology and its application, try to interpret the case history profiles *before* reading the evaluation. In this way you can compare your own insights with those presented. It is certainly possible for you to see things that were not included in the evaluation, so do not become concerned if some of your insights are not reflected in the interpretation. Rather, see if you can capture the most salient qualities in the profile.

Once you have completed this book, remember that there is no substitution for practice. It is recommended that you obtain the necessary NEO materials from the publisher (Psychological Assessment Resources in Lutz, FL) and take the NEO PI–R yourself. Compare your profile with your self-concept with an eye toward discerning how your character became expressed over the 35 scales. Then give the instrument to several others that you know well and see how their personalities emerge. The more you use the instrument, the better your interpretive skills will become. If you plan to use the NEO PI–R in a clinical context, at first remember not to let your interpretations of your client supersede good clinical judgment.

Complementing your use of the NEO PI–R should be a reading program of the relevant research literature. The NEO PI–R is enjoying a widespread use in research and there are literally hundreds of articles that have already been published on the instrument. An extended bibliography of these studies is available from the publisher when you purchase a manual. Review these studies, which are sorted into different areas, and select those that seem most germane to your own application. Staying familiar with the current research will add to your interpretive skills. These studies do much to extend the construct validity of the instrument, and provide interpretive nuances to the scales. An examination of the bibliography at the end of this book can point to the kinds of journals that contain these types of articles.

For applying the NEO PI–R in a research context, the final chapter highlights some of the techniques and procedures that can be used to maximize the instrument's interpretive and empirical utility. Despite a very strong quantitative record, there is still much controversy surrounding both the five-factor model in general and the NEO PI–R in particular. Much of the issue concerns the number of factors necessary to describe personality. Although this book tries to provide a conceptual framework for approaching this question, it does not provide any definitive answers. Rather, it outlines the questions that need to be asked and the kinds of results that are necessary to provide useful answers.

Another controversial area surrounds the factor structure of the NEO PI–R in different populations (e.g., its cross-cultural generalizability). A number of procedures have been used to evaluate factor comparability over samples, each with differing levels of success. Although one can debate the relative merits of each procedure (e.g., confirmatory versus exploratory factor analysis), the authors of the NEO PI–R have developed their own technique for addressing this issue. That method is presented here and is recommended for use. In this way, individuals wishing to join the ongoing dialogue on the psychometric integrity of the NEO PI–R can do so in a language that is the most relevant and persuasive for those who already use the instrument.

Overall, this book should provide a useful first step to professionals interested in developing a basic competence in the interpretation and application of the NEO PI–R. Many of the materials presented here are provided in an attempt to facilitate your efforts at finding new ways of applying both the instrument and the underlying measurement model. Many of the interpretive strategies reflect preliminary results from a few research studies. As such, you should be aware that most of the knowledge about the NEO PI–R still needs to be revealed—this book should be considered a work in progress. Ultimately, it will be up to you, the reader, operating in diverse contexts, to provide the additional information to help fill out our understanding of this instrument and to document its utility to our field.

CHAPTER 2

PSYCHOMETRIC OVERVIEW OF THE NEO PI–R

OUTLINE OF SCALES

The NEO PI–R consists of 240 items that clients answer on a (1) *strongly disagree* to (5) *strongly agree* Likert-type scale and they are balanced to control for the effects of acquiescence. The items are simple sentences describing specific behaviors or attitudes. The NEO PI–R measures the five major domains of personality and within each domain there are six facet scales that are designed to assess more specific aspects of each domain. A listing of the facets is presented in Table 2-1.

In designing these facet scales every attempt was made to create scales that were as nonredundant as possible while still assessing the same overall dimension. This was done using a technique called validimax factoring (McCrae & Costa, 1989b). This procedure establishes the structure of a scale by its pattern of correlations with external criteria. In this manner, one can have confidence that information presented in one facet is minimally redundant with information contained in other facets. The facets for each domain were selected on the basis of their being psychologically relevant and descriptively diverse (see Costa & McCrae, 1995).

Each facet scale is composed of eight items and domain scores are calculated by summing scores over the six facet scales. As will be shown later, the brevity of the scales does not compromise their reliability.

The NEO also has a rater version, Form R, which contains the same items phrased in the third person. There are different versions for rating men and women. Not many personality assessment instruments have this

35

TABLE 2-1. Domains and Facets of the NEO PI–R

Domain	NEO-PIR facet	Domain	NEO–PIR facet
NEUROTICISM	Anxiety	AGREEABLENESS	Trust
	Hostility		Straightforwardness
	Depression		Altruism
	Self-consciousness		Compliance
	Impulsiveness		Modesty
	Vulnerability		Tender-mindedness
EXTRAVERSION	Warmth	CONSCIENTIOUSNESS	Competence
	Gregariousness		Order
	Assertiveness		Dutifulness
	Activity		Achievement
	Excitement seeking		Self-discipline
	Positive emotions		Deliberation
OPENNESS TO EXPERIENCE	Fantasy		
	Aesthetics		
	Feelings		
	Actions		
	Ideas		
	Values		

capability; the NEO PI–R's provision of a rater form has several real advantages. One advantage is the ability to gather five-factor model information on an individual when a self-report cannot be trusted. Second, rater data can be used to provide another perspective to the assessment of a client. Finally, rater forms enable one to evaluate groups and their interpersonal dynamics. These issues are discussed later in this book.

RELIABILITY

Table 2-2 presents internal consistency and test–retest information for the domain and facet scales (see Costa & McCrae, 1988b, 1992c). As can be seen, the alpha reliabilities for the facets range from .56 for Tender-mindedness to .81 for Depression, and for the Domains from .86 for Agreeableness to .92 for Neuroticism. Considering that there are only eight items for each facet, these alphas are all acceptable. Further, these values tell us that the facets and the domains are quite unidimensional. From an interpretive perspective, unidimensionality is an important quality. It tells us that high or low scores represent a single, clear construct.

Column 2 in Table 2-2 provides test–retest reliabilities. It is important to note that the large majority of test–retest reliability studies use a time interval from 1 week to 6 months between tests. Such relatively small time intervals are frequent because of both the logistics involved in following people over time and the fact that the longer the interval is between test-

TABLE 2-2   Reliability Coefficients for the NEO-PI in an Adult, Mixed-sex Sample

NEO–PI Scale	Alpha reliability[a]	Retest reliability[b]
NEUROTICISM	.92	.87
Anxiety	.78	.75
Hostility	.75	.74
Depression	.81	.70
Self-consciousness	.68	.79
Impulsiveness	.70	.70
Vulnerability	.77	.73
EXTRAVERSION	.89	.82
Warmth	.73	.72
Gregariousness	.72	.73
Assertiveness	.77	.79
Activity	.63	.75
Excitement seeking	.65	.73
Positive emotions	.73	.73
OPENNESS TO EXPERIENCE	.87	.83
Fantasy	.76	.73
Aesthetics	.76	.79
Feelings	.66	.68
Actions	.58	.70
Ideas	.80	.79
Values	.67	.71
AGREEABLENESS	.86	.63[c]
Trust	.79	
Straightforwardness	.71	
Altruism	.75	
Compliance	.59	
Modesty	.67	
Tender-mindedness	.56	
CONSCIENTIOUSNESS	.90	79[c]
Competence	.67	
Order	.66	
Dutifulness	.62	
Achievement	.67	
Self-discipline	.75	
Deliberation	.71	

[a]$N = 1,539$.
[b]Six-year stability coefficients for N, E, and O domains and facets, 3-year coefficients for A and C domains, all data from NEO-PI. When adjusted for attenuation, all coefficients are greater than .90. Ns range from 63 to 127 for various subsamples of N, E, O, A, and C.
[c]Retest coefficients for A and C are from NEO-PI original domain scales.

ings, the lower the retest correlations. The passage of time attenuates the ability of a scale to correlate over two administrations. All things being equal, the minimum acceptable retest reliability values are between .5 and .6. Values between .6 and .7 are considered to be very good, between .7 to .8 are excellent, and above .9 are impressive.

The values presented in Table 2-2 are not 6-week coefficients nor are they 6-month coefficients rather, they are 6-*year* values. As can be seen, most are in the .7 to .8 range, suggesting very good stability over time. It should also be pointed out that these values were obtained from data pertaining to the NEO PI, the previous version of the NEO PI–R. The facet scales for Neuroticism, Extraversion, and Openness are essentially the same as in the current NEO PI–R. The NEO PI did not have facet scales for the Agreeableness and Conscientiousness domains; scores for these two domains are based on global 18-item scales. Data for these facets are still forthcoming. In any event, adjusting these correlations for attenuation results in reliability estimates over .90!

What these data say is that there is impressive stability in these personality domains over time for adults (i.e., individuals over age 30). Costa and McCrae (1994) provide longitudinal data on these dimensions that indicate impressive stability, both in terms of rank order and mean level: 25-year retest coefficients for these five major personality dimensions show about 80% of the variance as stable, while 50-year estimates indicate about 60% of the variance remaining stable. Based on this great stability, Costa and McCrae believe that after 30 years of age personality is "set like plaster." From this point forward, an individual's personality has crystallized and, all things being equal, will not change. A person begins now to select his or her own environments and creates a direction for his or her life to follow. Looking into this finding certainly raises a number of important issues.

First, it seems almost counterintuitive to believe that personality is unchanging in adulthood, suggesting that people are "locked" into their lives. Any adult can review the past decade of life and see many areas of personal development that have reconfigured his or her "personality." How, then, can personality be destiny?

To answer this question, we need to revisit the concepts of genotype and phenotype. Genotype refers to the basic underlying composition of our nature. It is a trajectory through time, a pathway that our development will follow. Phenotype, on the other hand, refers to the expression of the genotype at any given moment in time. Phenotype refers to a dynamic and lawful progression of change over time. One's underlying genotype remains constant, but its expression over time will change. For example, Extraversion represents a genotypic quality, but what Extraversion means, or how it is expressed, will change over the course of one's lifetime. Being an extravert in college may mean going to parties and staying out late, dating many people, and being loud and boisterous. However, extraversion in middle adulthood is something very different. Instead of going to many parties and being loud, it could be hosting formal sit-down events, vacationing with friends, spending time with family, selecting an occupation that brings one into contact with others, such as sales. Certainly the outward features of our lives change from college to middle age, but the fundamental needs that we seek to have gratified remain constant.

The dimensions of the NEO PI–R capture genotypic qualities (McCrae & Costa, 1996). Because of this, they should not vary over time and the data in Table 2-2 support this contention. However, there is a large body of evidence that documents the robustness of personality in adulthood. Using subjects who were part of an ongoing longitudinal study, Costa and McCrae (1989a) asked participants to rate the degree to which their whole personality had changed over the previous 6 years. Three groups emerged, one of those who believed that their personality had stayed pretty much the same, another of those who believed that they had changed "a little," and a final group who believed that they had changed a great deal. Costa and McCrae then compared the retest correlations between the NEO scores of these individuals taken 6 years prior and currently for the three groups. There were no significant differences among the groups in terms of stability scores. The median uncorrected retest correlation was .80 for the group that believed they had changed a great deal. Even for those who claimed to have changed, and there is no reason to believe that these peoples' outward lives did not change, their underlying dispositions remained constant.

McCrae (1993) more formally evaluated the role of several factors (personal agency, self-monitoring, private self-consciousness, and Openness to Experience) as moderators for personality change. No consistent effects were found; any noted changes were due to measurement error. Costa, McCrae, and Zonderman (1987) also failed to find any moderating effects on personality by environmental variables, such as marital status, employment status, or state of residence. Perhaps the most compelling evidence for treating the dimensions of the NEO PI–R as genotypes comes from the behavioral genetics literature which has documented the heritability of these dimensions (Bergeman et al., 1993; Heath, Neale, Kessler, Eaves, & Kendler, 1992; Viken, Rose, Kaprio, & Koskenvuo, 1994). Thus, the dimensions of the five-factor model should not be considered mere summary descriptions of behavior, but temperamental dispositions of individuals to think, act, and feel in consistent ways over time.

It should be pointed out that until adulthood, much of personality remains fluid. Evidence suggests that perhaps up to 50% of the variance in personality may be shifting throughout adolescence and early adulthood (Block, 1971; Carmichael & McGue, 1994; Costa & McCrae, 1992d; Haan, Millsap, & Hartka, 1986; Siegler et al., 1990). However, even during adulthood there may be possibilities for change in personality. The onset of a

psychiatric disorder can have an impact on personality scores, and research has shown that scores do change between periods of depression
and remission (Hirschfeld et al., 1983). However, whether this represents a
true change in personality or a distortion of the assessment process needs
to be determined. Another possibility for change concerns the experience
of catastrophic stressors, which may alter the way that one experiences the
world. Similarly, religious conversion may be another event that has the
potential for reshaping temperament. However, these are open questions
that are in need of empirical research.

A final possibility for finding personality change concerns psychotherapy. The stability coefficients noted previously really raise questions over the intent of therapy and its effect on the individual. Should
clinicians intend to affect clients by helping them make shifts in their fundamental psychological structures or through improving their psychosocial instrumentality (i.e., coping ability)? There are data that address this
issue. Several studies have been done evaluating the retest stability of
NEO PI and NEO PI–R among clinical samples. All the studies found high
retest correlations pre- and posttreatment; however, there were significant
changes in mean level noted for the dimensions (Bagby, Joffe, Parker,
Kalemba, & Harkness, 1995; Piedmont & Ciarrocchi, in press; Trull, Useda,
Costa, & McCrae, 1995). Although the extent and magnitude of the observed changes varied over the studies, the presence of shifts in scores
opens the possibility that those seeking change may be able to find it.

With these caveats noted, the reliability coefficients presented in Table
2-2 offer some important advantages to test users. First, because the NEO
PI–R scales are relatively unidimensional, obtained scores represent clear,
unambiguous qualities of the individual. The 35 scales of the NEO provide
a rich interpretive portrait of a person. The temporal stability of these
scales shows that this picture, in adulthood, will not change much over
time. Thus, the test interpreter can anticipate the kinds of life directions a
respondent will move toward and the types of outcomes likely to be experienced.

Factor Structure

The 30 facet scales of the NEO PI–R constitute five independent personality dimensions. The six facets for each domain were selected so that
there would be a sufficient number of defining variables to reliably evidence each of the domains in later factor analyses of the instrument (Costa
& McCrae, 1995a). Although having six factors for each domain appears
very "neat" and artificial, there really is nothing magical about the number. There are certainly other aspects of personality that arguably could be

considered adequate markers or facets. Nonetheless, the chosen facets were selected by the NEO PI–R's authors because of their psychological significance in the literature.

Perhaps one of the most recurring issues about the NEO PI–R is its factor structure and the orthogonality of the domains (e.g., J. Block, 1995; Borkenau & Ostendorf, 1990). The value of independent dimensions is that this structure ensures that information collected from one domain is not redundant with information obtained from another. It would serve no purpose to create 30 scales that assess the same quality. Many scales measuring the same thing, even if from different vantage points, do not provide an adequate sampling of personological content. However, a set of non-overlapping dimensions helps to guarantee that a more varied and comprehensive evaluation is made.

The dimensions of the NEO PI–R are hypothesized to represent latent, uncorrelated factors. However, factor analyses of the scale have consistently demonstrated that some of the facet scales have significant (i.e., > .30) secondary loadings (Costa & McCrae, 1992c; Piedmont, 1994), which results in some correlational overlap. This came about as a result of how the NEO PI–R was developed.

Rather than relying on a conventional varimax rotation to identify factors (this identifies factors by obtaining simple structure among the items), Costa and McCrae developed what they referred to as *validimax rotation* (McCrae & Costa, 1989b). This technique instead identifies factors by their pattern of correlations with external criteria of convergent and discriminant validity (see Costa & McCrae, in press; McCrae & Costa, 1987, for an overview of this process). It was in this way that facets for each dimension were created that were as different from one another as possible while still remaining on the same factor. While external validity was maximized, some of the internal simple structure was compromised.

This was not a problem for Costa and McCrae, who believed that the developed facets represented important psychological qualities that should be included in any assessment protocol, simple structure or not (Costa & McCrae, in press). To delete some facet scales in order to preserve simple structure would have compromised the substantive utility of the instrument.

Several of the scales on the NEO PI–R have significant secondary loadings. For example, the facet scales of Impulsiveness and Vulnerability to Stress load negatively on Conscientiousness; Openness to Feelings loads positively on Extraversion; Warmth, low Assertiveness, and low Excitement Seeking load on Agreeableness. All of these facets represent important personological characteristics of individuals, and to delete them because of their secondary loading would be counterproductive. Yet, in other ways, these secondary patterns do make some intuitive sense. Individuals who are in control of their impulses and cope well with stress are also able to compete and succeed. Individuals who experience a high degree of positive affect are open to their inner, emotional worlds. People who are warm and nonthreatening also appear very agreeable and compassionate.

Despite this conceptual overlap, it should be noted that the magnitude of these secondary loadings creates correlations that are relatively small (averaging about .20). Thus, measures obtained from each domain can be considered, for the most part, quite independent. However, truly orthogonal domain scores can be calculated from factor score weights presented in the manual. These weights are applied to each of the 30 facets and result in domain scores that are mutually independent.

For all practical purposes, the NEO PI–R provides a factor structure that it is quite robust. Minor overlaps notwithstanding, these five dimensions have consistently emerged over instruments, raters, and even cultures (McCrae & Costa, 1987; Piedmont, 1994; Piedmont & Chae, 1997). Users of the NEO PI–R can be confident that the information obtained from the five dimensions represents a relatively comprehensive selection of personological material.

THE QUESTION OF COMPREHENSIVENESS

As noted in Chapter 1, the five factors emerged from an analysis of the English language. It could be argued that the five-factor model represents only the ways in which everyday people think about and discuss others. Thus, there is no reason to believe that this lay conceptualization would have anything in common with the ways that psychologists construe human characteristics. For example, psychodynamic models of personality find the source of human behavior in unconscious drives centered around sexual and aggressive content. Eros and Thanatos represent such constructs, as do various ego needs that reflect generalized affective forces that drive, direct, and select behavior. Individuals are hypothesized to be unaware of personal qualities such as penis envy, oedipal drives, or the need for infavoidance; it seems unlikely that such constructs would become encoded in the common language. Thus, it is possible that the types of constructs that social scientists have developed to describe and explain behavior have nothing in common with those dimensions found in the common lexicon. If this is indeed the case, then any comprehensive model of personality would require *more than* five factors; the five found in the language plus any additional factors that have been discovered by the social sciences.

Correspondence Between the NEO PI–R and Other Measurement Models

In order to evaluate the true comprehensiveness of the five-factor model, a number of studies were conducted that evaluated the five-factor model in relation to measures of psychological constructs representing diverse theoretical orientations. Using most often a joint factor analytic paradigm, these studies sought to determine the number of factors necessary to explain the majority of common variance among these measures. Table 2-3 presents an overview of such studies that have used major personality instruments. What has emerged from this very large and extensive literature is that only *five* factors are necessary for explaining the lion's share of common variance in standard personality assessment inventories; those factors are Neuroticism, Extraversion, Openness, Agreeableness, and Conscientiousness.

As can be seen in Table 2-3, the list of instruments that have been evaluated includes Murray's needs, Gough's Folk Concepts, Jungian Typologics, Interpersonal Behavior, vocational interests, and even psychopathological dynamics. These five dimensions are present, to varying degrees, among these theoretically diverse instruments. This large and growing literature documents the comprehensiveness of the five-factor model. Despite its seemingly humble origins in natural language, these five personality dimensions also permeate scientific conceptualizations of personality. As can also be noted in Table 2-3, some of these findings have been cross-culturally replicated using the NEO PI–R (e.g., Chae, Piedmont, Estedt, & Wicks, 1995; Heaven, Connors, & Stones, 1994; Levin & Montag, 1991), and other measures of the model (e.g., Paunonen, Jackson, Trzebinski, & Forsterling, 1992). There are also numerous articles that have evaluated the relations between the five-factor model and scales designed to capture more circumscribed personality constructs, such as positive and negative affect, performance motivation, and health-related variables such as anger control and locus of control. Research here also demonstrates the comprehensiveness of the five-factor model: All these smaller constructs fit very nicely into the model (e.g., Costa & McCrae, 1980a, 1984; Marshall, Wortman, Vickers, Kusulas, & Hervig, 1994; Piedmont, 1995).

Table 2-3 also shows that some of these major personality instruments do *not* capture all aspects of the five-factor model. Their theoretical and sci-

TABLE 2-3.   Bibliography of Joint Analyses Using the NEO PI–R

Instrument	Study	Findings
MMPI Factor Scales	Costa, Busch, Zonderman, & McCrae (1986)	Conscientiousness not present
MMPI Items	Costa, Zonderman, McCrae, Williams (1985)	Conscientiousness not present
MMPI-PD scales	Trull (1992)	Openness not well represented
Personality Disorder Scale–R	Trull (1992)	All five factors recovered
Personality Research Form	Costa & McCrae (1988b)	All five factors recovered
Adjective Check List	Piedmont, McCrae, & Costa (1991)	All five factors recovered
Edwards Personal Preference Schedule	Piedmont, McCrae, & Costa (1992)	All five factors recovered
California Psychological Inventory	McCrae, Costa, & Piedmont (1993); Deniston & Ramanaiah (1993)	Agreeableness underrepresented
Wiggins's Interpersonal Adjective Scales	McCrae & Costa (1989c)	Extraversion and agreeableness
Holtzman Inkblot	Costa & McCrae (1986)	No personality dimensions found
Eysenck Personality Inventory	McCrae & Costa (1985a)	No Openness found
Eysenck Personality Profiler and EPQ-R	Costa & McCrae (1995b)	No Openness found
Cloniger's Tridimensional Personality Questionnaire	Costa & McCrae (in press)	Agreeableness weakly represented, scales combine elements of the other four domain
Multidimensional Personality Questionnaire	Piedmont (1994)	All five factors recovered
Self-Directed Search	Costa, McCrae, & Holland (1984)	Neuroticism not well represented
Myers–Briggs Type Indicator	McCrae & Costa (1989a); Furnham (1994)	Neuroticism not found
Myers–Briggs Type Indicator (Korean)	Chae, Piedmont, Estadt, & Wicks (1995)	Neuroticism not found
California Q-Set	McCrae, Costa, & Busch (1986); Lanning (1994)	All five factors recovered

TABLE 2-3. (*Continued*)

Instrument	Study	Findings
Comrey Personality Scales /16PF/Eysenck Personality Inventory	Boyle (1989)	CPS & 16PF evidence the five major domains EPI corresponds to N & E
Personality Psycho-pathology 5	Trull, Useda, Costa, & McCrae (1995)	All five factors recovered
Basic Personality Inventory	Levin & Montag (1991)	All five factors recovered (Israeli sample)
MMPI PD scales/Person-ality Adjective Check List/Interpersonal Adjective Scales	Wiggins & Pincus (1989)	All five factors needed to capture range of per-sonality disorders
Guilford–Zimmerman Temperament Survey	Costa & McCrae (1985); McCrae (1989)	N & E well represented, O, A, & C weakly present
MCMI I & II	Costa & McCrae (1990)	All five factors recovered
Personality Assessment Inventory	Levin & Montag (1994)	All five factors recovered
Holden Psychological Screening Inventory	Holden (1992)	All five factors repre-sented
Interpersonal Style Inventory	Lorr, Youniss, & Kluth (1992); McCrae & Costa (1994)	All five factors recovered, but Openness only weakly
16 PF	Gerbing & Tuley (1991); Hofer, Horn, & Eber (1997)	All five factors found
Comrey Personality Scales	Hahn & Comrey (1994)	Openness not represented

entific pedigree is no guarantee of comprehensiveness. For example, research with the Myers–Briggs Type Indicator (MBTI) shows that it lacks any indicator of Neuroticism (Chae *et al.*, 1995; McCrae & Costa, 1989a). This may partially explain the popularity of this instrument: It does not provide any potentially disturbing feedback to individuals about their levels of negative affect and emotional dysphoria. The California Psychological Inventory does not have any strong measure of Agreeableness. This is curious because the instrument is based on a folk conception of personality (H. G. Gough, 1987). Folk concepts are "the kind of everyday variables that ordinary people use in their daily lives to understand, classify, and predict their behavior and that of others" (p. 1). This approach is similar to the lexical approach that spawned the five-factor model. It is surprising and important to note that this omnibus test does not provide adequate coverage of this personality dimension.

It is also interesting to note that attitudinal qualities, such as vocational interests, are also related to the five-factor model. That the types of jobs that interest us are related to personality underscores the contention that the dimensions of the five-factor model represent genotypic qualities that establish trajectories that guide the general directions and patterns of our lives. This complements a growing body of research that illustrates the usefulness of these large personality dimensions for predicting job success and job satisfaction (Barrick & Mount, 1991; Mount, Barrick, & Strauss, 1994; Piedmont, 1993; Piedmont & Weinstein, 1994).

Recognizing the empirical overlap between scientific conceptions of personality and the dimensions of the five-factor model provides two important pieces of information. First, we can have increased confidence that the five-factor model is indeed a comprehensive description of individual-difference variables. Second, given its comprehensiveness, this model provides an opportunity for better understanding the personological content of any psychological measure. By examining a construct's relations with these dimensions (which, as shown previously, are clear, univocal quantities), we can derive a better understanding of the kinds of dispositions and motivations reflected in scores from the scale. Further, we can also determine similarities and differences among scales, regardless of their theoretical origin or label, by comparing their patterns of correlations with these same five dimensions. We now turn to this major value of the five-factor model.

WHAT THE NEO PI–R CAN TELL US ABOUT OTHER SCALES

It can certainly be said without hyperbole that thousands of personality variables are being assessed by hundreds of assessment tools. The field of personality is a veritable cornucopia of constructs, measuring diverse individual differences. To a novice, this diversity can be confusing, and even to professionals, this landscape appears cluttered and disjointed. With so many constructs proposed by the varied theoretical orientations in the field, it is a challenge to discern any coherence among these variables. Despite a plethora of scales, one cannot be certain that a comprehensive description of personality can be made, or that all relevant aspects of personality have been adequately sampled.

The ability to assemble a collage of variables that one can be sure are minimally redundant and comprehensively descriptive underscores the value of the five-factor taxonomy. In his critique of the five-factor model, J. Block (1995) made reference to the "jingle fallacy" and the "jangle fallacy."

These terms refer to, respectively, the tendency to see scales as being similar, or different, on the basis of their label rather than on any empirical evidence. The former sees convergence where none may exist, and the latter allows useless redundancy to develop. Perhaps the least useful place to look for a scale's meaning is its name. But these "fallacies" too often characterize the field of assessment. Without any useful, larger framework within which to evaluate scales, there is no way to disentangle the personological content of scales.

An example of this arose in my own work during graduate school. During my first years of school, I was interested in evaluating those personality variables that predicted performance on cognitive tasks. My first set of variables included measures of anxiety and achievement motivation (see Piedmont, 1988b). In selecting measures of achievement, I was very much interested in using Murray's need for achievement. Being the industrious graduate student I was, I wanted to make sure that I was doing good science by ensuring that I had multiple measures of my constructs. Thus, I used two need achievement scales: one from the Edwards Personal Preference Schedule (EPPS; Edwards, 1959) and another from the Adjective Check List (ACL; H. B. Gough & Heilbrun, 1980).

These scales were engaging because they were both established measures of Murray's need-press theory. Working from Murray's earlier work, Edwards constructed carefully worded definitions for each need scale and then selected items that clearly reflected those dimensions. H. B. Gough and Heilbrun (1980) were also interested in developing measures of Murray's needs and they used Edwards's original definitions and items as guidelines for selecting their adjectives. In short, these two scales share not only a common theoretical pedigree, but are methodological cousins as well. If there were any two scales that I would expect to be related measures of the same construct, these were the two. Thus, once my data were collected, my first "validity check" was to correlate these two scales to make sure that I found the high positive correlation that putatively should be there. When I performed the correlation, I was horrified to find that these two scales had a correlation of "0.00"! After several attempts at rechecking my scoring, data entry, and computer commands, I realized that this value was accurate. A review of the literature showed why.

As early as 1968, researchers had noted that these two scales were not related and that they should not be considered equivalent measures (Bouchard, 1968; Megargee & Parker, 1968). Yet despite this glaring lack of construct validity, professionals continued to use widely both of these instruments. In fact, the ACL and the EPPS were listed by Buros (1978) among the top 10 tests cited in the research literature, and the EPPS was one of the most popular tests used in both clinical (Lubin, Larsen, &

Matarazzo, 1984) and counseling settings (Watkins & Campbell, 1989). Despite the empirical evidence and calls to the contrary (e.g., Entwisle, 1972), both researchers and clinicians widely employed these measures and routinely interpreted them in ways consistent with their putative definitions.

There are many reasons for this, but perhaps the most salient for me was that researchers at the time had no way to resolve this issue. Empirically both these scales predicted achievement-related outcomes, but they failed the test of convergent validity. One or both of these scales was invalid. Yet there was no independent, empirical criterion to which an appeal could be made in order to determine which one was the culprit. Although rational explanations were possible (e.g., Piedmont, DiPlacido, & Keller, 1989), they lacked the kind of persuasiveness that only data can provide.

The five-factor model offers such an empirical framework for personologically parsing scales. The dimensions of the model are clear and structurally robust. As the data in the previous section have shown, the model is conceptually comprehensive, capable of organizing information from diverse theoretical orientations. These empirical realities provide a useful medium for evaluating scales. Correlations between a scale and these five factors can help to conceptually locate the measure within this well-defined space. Second, the pattern of correlations can serve as the scale's "fingerprint," so to speak, its unique blend of personological material. From here, the similarity of the scale to other measures can be determined by an inspection of each construct's pattern of correlates. Two scales can be said to be related to the degree to which they share common correlations to the five factors. Separate patterns of five-factor correlates would be evidence of discriminant validity.

Locating scales within the five-factor space provides an opportunity for overcoming the jingle and jangle fallacies by helping to identify areas of overlap among scales as well as areas that have been overlooked. Given the fact that some dimensions are better represented in the natural language than others (i.e., Agreeableness is most represented, Openness is the least; Goldberg, 1990, 1992; McCrae, 1990; Peabody & Goldberg, 1989), it is possible that the development of personality scales has followed a similar course. This would mean that some aspects of personality are better assessed than others, construct names notwithstanding. Correlations with the five-factor model would help to determine whether, and to what degree, such a distinct pattern exists.

Ozer and Riese (1994) argued that determining a scale's pattern of correlates with the five-factor model will become an essential part of determining its construct validity. As they stated, "[those] who continue to employ their preferred measure without locating it within the five-factor model can only be likened to geographers who issue reports of new land but refuse to locate them on a map for others to find" (p. 361).

An empirical example may help to highlight the value of the five-factor model. The data to be discussed are distilled from a study that looked at the relationships between the ACL and the NEO PI (Piedmont, McCrae, & Costa, 1991). The ACL was selected because it contains scales from several different theoretical perspectives. First, there are the need scales developed from Murray's (1938) theory. There are also scales developed by Gough that represent "folk concepts"; scales designed to assess Berne's (1961) transactional analysis constructs; and, finally, scales developed by Welsh (1975) to measure origence and intellectence (measures of creativity and intelligence). These theories have little in common with lexical usage and their underlying concepts appeared to have no parallels in the lay language. It was thought that they may represent factors distinct from the five-factor model.

A joint factor analysis was performed between the NEO PI and the ACL in a sample of 244 adults. These individuals were part of the Baltimore Longitudinal Study of Aging (BLSA; Shock et al., 1984). This is a sample of predominantly white, community-dwelling individuals who have agreed to return for periodic biomedical and psychological testing. Most have at least a college degree and work (or are retired from) scientific, professional, or managerial occupations.

A principal components analysis was performed followed by a varimax rotation. A scree test indicated that five factors, accounting for 74% of the variance, would adequately represent the data. The factor loadings are presented in Table 2-4. Three observations emerge. First, the five factors that are identified in this solution are each defined by one of the domains of the NEO PI. This underscores the contention that the five-factor model represents broad domains of personality and defines the majority of the variance contained in personality assessment inventories.

The second observation is that all of the ACL scales correlate with *at least* one of the factor dimensions. This shows that the diverse personological content of these scales can be adequately represented by the dimensions of the five-factor model and provides support for the comprehensiveness of the model. If the model were not comprehensive, then some of the ACL scales would not be correlated with these five dimensions, indicating that additional factors are necessary for representing that information. But these results show that at their base, all languages used to describe personality share a common foundation; scientific conceptions of individual differences are variants of the terms found in lay vocabulary.

The third observation of Table 2-4 is that the correlations of each of the ACL scales to the five-factor model provide a personological sketch. For example, the Achievement scale correlates with the Extraversion and Conscientiousness domains. The latter correlation makes conceptual sense: high achievers should be organized, disciplined, and goal-oriented. The correla-

TABLE 2-4. Joint Factor Analysis of the NEO PI Domains and the Adjective Check List

Scale	Factor				
	N	E	O	A	C
NEO-PI Factors					
Neuroticism (N)	.80				
Extraversion (E)		.70			
Openness (O)			.79		
Agreeableness (A)				.68	
Conscientiousness (C)					.75
ACL Scales					
Unfavorable				-.59	-.61
Favorable				.57	.57
Communality				.44	
Achievement		.51			.73
Dominance		.79			.44
Endurance					.91
Order					.87
Intraception				.54	.63
Nurturance				.83	
Affiliation	-.40			.66	
Heterosexuality		.79			
Exhibition		.82			
Autonomy		.45		-.71	
Aggression		.58		-.65	
Change		.59	.48		
Succorance	.49				-.61
Abasement		-.67		.40	
Deference		-.52		.67	
Self-control		-.71			
Self-confidence		.77			.45
Personal Adjustment				.62	.50
Ideal Self	-.48				.50
Creative Personality		.43	.71		
Military Leadership					.80
Masculinity		.58		-.41	
Femininity				-.64	
Critical Parent				-.80	
Nurturant Parent				.57	.65
Adult	-.40				.80
Free Child		.80	.42		
Adapted Child	.50				-.71
Welsh's A-1					-.50
Welsh's A-2			.47	-.40	-.48
Welsh's A-3				.70	
Welsh's A-4					.80

Note: N = 244. Only Loadings > |.40| are given.

tion with Extraversion also shows high scorers to be energetic and dominant. In a group they would like to be leaders and may exude positive "vibes" that others may find inviting and charismatic. Individuals high on these two dimensions are described by others as being ambitious, proud, persistent, active, and competitive (Hofstee, de Raad, & Goldberg, 1992).

It is also interesting to note the pattern of correlates found for the Dominance scale. It, too, loads on both Extraversion and Conscientiousness, although it emphasizes the surgency while the Achievement scale highlights the ambition aspects of personality. But, despite their very different labels, these two scales are measuring redundant aspects of personality.

Similar evaluations can be done for each of the ACL scales. Each time, an evaluation of their construct validity and personological uniqueness can be made. For example, the Adapted Child scale seems not to be what it claims. The high loading on Neuroticism and the low association with Conscientiousness portrays an individual who is emotionally distressed, selfish, and needy of others. This pattern of correlates hardly reflects "adapted" qualities. Thus, the name for this scale is misleading. Again, scale names should not be relied on for interpreting scale content.

Finally, the pattern of correlations shows that many of the ACL scales correlate with the Extraversion, Agreeableness, and Conscientiousness domains. Fewer correlations are found for Neuroticism and Openness. The ACL does provide a comprehensive description of personality, but does not evidence equal personological weight across the different domains. One may wish to complement the ACL with additional measures of these domains in order to ensure an adequate sampling of all relevant personality dimensions.

These factor analytic results are similar to the findings of other studies using different instruments. The studies in Table 2-3 show that the five-factor model is indeed comprehensive: Personological material from many different theoretical positions can be substantively organized under the umbrella of the five-factor model. As Ozer and Riese (1994) suggested, the correlations of scales with these domains goes far in outlining the scales' construct validity. However, the comprehensiveness of the five-factor model should not be construed as suggesting that these domains are all that are necessary for understanding personality: The five-factor model and the NEO PI–R are not intended to supplant other measures of personality. Their inclusion in an assessment battery can ensure that a broad, comprehensive description of personality is obtained, but other scales may be necessary to provide more precise measures of specific psychological phenomena.

By way of completeness, I should also add that I conducted a similar joint factor analysis of the NEO PI with the EPPS in order to establish those scales' relations to the five-factor model (Piedmont, McCrae, & Costa,

1992). It was interesting to note that the achievement scale correlated with low Agreeableness. This is not the kind of association one would expect to find. To some degree this result was due to the item content, where high scorers sought high-status positions so they could influence others. This is consistent with low Agreeable individuals, who are manipulative and controlling. Yet it was also believed that this unexpected finding was due to the ipsative nature of the instrument (ipsatization is a relatively complex mathematical process that puts the test results into a certain form—one that is characterized by the sum of all scores adding to constant value). But whatever the reason, it became clear why these two instruments did not correlate—they were assessing independent dimensions of personality! Only the presence of a larger, taxonomic structure could provide a way of understanding why these two achievement scales relate to each other in the ways they do. Further, the correlations of the EPPS with the NEO PI provide a framework for reinterpreting the previous literature employing this instrument.

THE QUESTION OF SELF-DISTORTION

The data presented have shown that the dimensions of the NEO PI–R are internally consistent, structurally robust, and stable over time. Further, these dimensions do in fact represent salient individual-difference qualities; they are present not only in our general language but also among the constructs developed by social scientists. However, the majority of the data presented so far rely on self-reports. It could be argued that the overlap demonstrated in the research just described is entirely the result of self-reported distortions. In other words, measures of the five factors overlapped with other personality measures not because of some substantive relationship but rather because of the presence of correlated error. The dimensions of the five-factor model may represent only individuals' implicit personality theories, internal fictions used to help explain the behaviors of others. These dimensions may not have any real correspondence to actual psychological dynamics (e.g., Mischel, 1968).

Determining whether the dimensions of the five-factor model represent a cognitive fiction or are real psychological quantities requires appeal to multiple information sources.

SELF–PEER CONGRUENCE

There is no doubt that self-report data is fallible; it has its strengths and, importantly, its weaknesses. Sole reliance on self-report data creates real limitations to the level of accuracy one experiences in drawing inferences. In order to establish a strong assessment foundation, a test user needs to draw information from other sources and look for where the threads of information begin to converge. Observer ratings are an ideal counterpoint to self-reports (see McCrae, 1994a); they do not share the same sources of bias as self-report data. Although observer ratings have their weaknesses (e.g., halo effects, stereotypes), these biases do not overlap with the errors inherent in self-reports. Thus, convergence between peer- and self-ratings cannot be attributable to correlated error but to a reliable effect (see McCrae, 1982; Wiggins, 1979).

A number of research studies have evaluated the cross-observer convergence of the five-factor model and found it to be quite robust (e.g., Costa & McCrae, 1992d; McCrae & Costa, 1987). An example of these data is presented in Table 2-5. These data are a continuation of the ACL study discussed previously. A subsample of individuals who completed the NEO PI and the ACL also had their spouses and friends rate them on the NEO PI. Factor scores derived from the information presented in Table 2-4 were then correlated to those ratings.

The values in bold are the convergent validity coefficients. For example, the .43 correlation between Spouse ratings of Neuroticism and Self rat-

TABLE 2-5   Correlations between Peer and Spouse Rated NEO-PI Factors and Self-Reported Joint Factor Scores

NEO–PI Rating	Factor[a]				
	N	E	O	A	C
Spouse (N = 94)					
Neuroticism	**.43**[c]	.00	−.16	−.19	−.20[b]
Extraversion	.17	**.47**[c]	−.11	.16	−.02
Openness	−.10	−.09	**.59**[c]	.03	.02
Agreeableness	.14	.05	.06	**.58**[c]	−.08
Conscientiousness	.08	−.08	.01	.03	**.40**[c]
Peers (N = 145)					
Neuroticism	**.41**[c]	.10	.03	.03	−.14
Extraversion	−.03	**.47**[c]	.00	.11	−.11
Openness	.07	.10	**.71**[c]	.01	−.02
Agreeableness	.01	−.24[b]	−.01	**.52**[c]	−.22[b]
Conscientiousness	.05	−.13	−.05	−.08	**.46**[c]

[a]Based on factors from Table 2-4. Based on "Adjective Check List Scales and the Five-Factor Model," by R. L. Piedmont, R. R. McCrae, and P. T. Costa, Jr., 1991, *Journal of Personality and Social Psychology, 60*, p. 630–637.
[b]$p < .05$
[c]$p < .001$

ings shows that how individuals perceive themselves on this dimension corresponds to how others perceive them. As can be seen in Table 2-5, these cross-observer, cross-method convergent validities are all statistically significant and of a moderate to high magnitude. The off-diagonal items are the discriminant validity coefficients. They represent the degree to which ratings reflect one and only one personality dimension. As can be seen, all the discriminant validity coefficients are quite small indicating that when individuals rate a target on these five dimensions, raters have a clear and specific idea of what these dimensions are. The ratings reflect specific aspects of personality that agree with the particular self-ratings.

These results show that the ways individuals think about themselves temperamentally is consistent with how others construe them. Thus, self-ratings cannot be seen as merely the result of some type of personal distortion or bias. In a review of the cross-observer literature, Borkenau (1992) concluded that the data clearly showed that traits are real entities that can be reliably assessed by raters. Because these ratings correspond very well with self-assessments, one can have confidence that self-reports are not solely the product of bias, distortion, or both. Individuals, at least normal volunteers, do seem to provide accurate assessments of themselves when asked.

THE REVERSE ACQUAINTANCESHIP EFFECT

One issue that comes up in connection with observer ratings is the length of time the rater has known the target. Research has shown that the more visible the trait, the better it can be rated (Funder & Colvin, 1988), and that the better the rater knows the target, the more accurate the rating (Borkenau & Liebler, 1993; Colvin & Funder, 1991; Watson & Clark, 1991). This latter finding is called the acquaintanceship effect, and is a rather straightforward dictum: The longer you know someone and the more you know about them, the more accurate your assessments of them. However, there are caveats to this in that given the right information, even strangers can make accurate assessments of a target (Borkenau & Liebler, 1992, 1993).

The acquaintanceship effect seems to be a natural corollary of rater phenomenon when the assessments are being made during a period of personality stability. However, in a recent paper (Piedmont, 1994), I questioned whether during a period of personality change and development (e.g., adolescence, early adulthood) such long-term knowledge of a target would prove more of a liability than an asset. It may be possible that a long-term acquaintance may provide less accurate ratings than a more recent acquaintance because the images of the target the former holds may not be keeping pace with the real personality changes that are occurring.

The older acquaintance may be more likely to attribute initial changes in the target to situational factors rather than to personality development. Long-term acquaintances may also be disposed to perceive more stability in the target's personality than what may actually exist in order to bring a better sense of continuity to their relationship. On the other hand, newer friends, whose perceptions are still evolving, may be able to utilize these perceptions of variability in the target better when forming their personality impressions.

In order to evaluate this hypothesis I had 101 college students complete the NEO PI–R for themselves and had two individuals who knew them for at least 6 months rate them on the rater version of the NEO PI–R. Raters knew the targets, on average, 8.6 years ($SD = 8.1$; range three months to 25 years). Raters were also believed to have known the subjects very well.

In evaluating the cross-observer convergence, raters were divided into two groups: One group knew the target for 2 years or less, the other for more than 2 years. The results showed a modest effect: The average convergent correlation for the 2-year-or-less group was .56, while for the more established raters it was approximately .47. During this period of personality transition, those who knew the targets longer were slightly less accurate in their perceptions than those who were more recent friends.

This effect may result from the same dynamics that underlie the *fundamental attribution error*—the tendency to attribute dispositional causes to the behavior of others and situational causes to our own behavior (Jones & Davis, 1965; Jones & Nisbett, 1972). Long-term acquaintances have formed well-developed and detailed conceptualizations of the targets. During periods of personality change, targets will begin to evidence dispositional shifts in their attitudes, feelings, and behaviors. The resulting lack of correspondence between the person raters believe the targets to be and the subjects' changing behaviors may lead raters to attribute these shifts to situational forces. Such a strategy guards against the formation of erroneous impressions when the target's personality is not in transition. However, during a period of change, it may lead long-term acquaintances to ignore real dispositional shifts.

More recent acquaintances, on the other hand, are still actively developing their understanding of the targets. Each new observation is used to elaborate their developing dispositional impressions. Thus, recent acquaintances are more likely to attribute shifts in behavior to dispositional dynamics. During periods of personality change, this lower threshold for attributing behavioral inconsistencies to personality characteristics enables newer acquaintances to keep pace with the actual changes that are occurring. However, when personality is stable, this tendency to make dispositional attributions results in the fundamental attribution error.

When using observer ratings of personality one needs to be sensitive to the age of the target. Younger subjects are more likely to be in a process of personality development and change. Ratings obtained from long-term informants, such as parents, may not be as accurate as the impressions garnered from newer acquaintances, such as teachers or friends.

THE LOGIC OF ASSESSMENT USING THE NEO PI–R

There is no doubt that the use of psychological testing for any purpose is complex and fraught with much potential for bias and error. Also, there are no simple solutions for addressing this formidable array of complex issues. In the previous section I addressed the issues of distortion as they may relate to self-reports. As can probably be discerned from the earlier discussion, the best way for determining whether a self-report provides accurate information or is merely the by-product of some type of cognitive distortion is to obtain an independent source of information: an informer report.

Because observers may not have the same motivations to present the target in a good or bad light, and certainly do not share the same cognitive framework, an observer rating provides a different perspective on a target. At a minimum, an observer rating can give an insight into the kinds of social impressions the target makes on others. Finding convergence between a self-report and an observer rating lends greater strength to the inferences one can draw from the profiles. If a person admits to being interpersonally awkward, and several others who know the target also indicate him or her to be socially awkward, then you can be confident that the target *is* socially awkward.

The value of observer ratings cannot be overstated. It is the value of such information that led Costa and McCrae to develop a rater version of the NEO PI–R (Form R). Items are phrased in the third person and there are separate forms for rating men and women. Psychometric analyses of this form show the scales to be very internally consistent (alpha for the domains ranges from .89 to .95, and for the facets from .60 to .90). The factor structure of Form R is comparable to its self-report sibling (Costa & Mc-Crae, 1992c; Piedmont, 1994). Finally, personality ratings on Form R have also been shown to evidence substantial temporal stability (Costa & Mc-Crae, 1992c).

Observer data should be obtained whenever possible. It can do much to help determine whether a self-report contains bias as well as provide a different perspective for understanding a client. Later chapters in this book outline the usefulness of rating data and how to incorporate such information into the interpretive process.

NORMAL VERSUS ABNORMAL PERSONALITY

OVERVIEW

In evaluating results from the NEO PI-R it is important to keep in mind that the qualities represented by these scales pertain to the normal spectrum of psychological functioning. Scores on the NEO scales reflect the motivations, tendencies, and capacities that characterize individuals' ongoing interactions with their environments. Specific configurations of scores on these domains reflect the creative adaptations individuals have made to the demands imposed on them by their life experiences. In short, when we speak of "personality," we refer to the consistent ways in which individuals perceive the universe, their role or place in it, and the directions in which they desire to move.

These broad strokes at defining personality attempt to highlight the fact that our intrinsic organization developed in response to the unique problems of adaptation we have faced. Our personalities represent creative solutions to these problems. When interpreting scores from the NEO PI-R it is important to keep this notion in mind and not impose any value judgments on the scores. One frequent mistake committed by those professionals I have trained in the use of the NEO PI-R has been to see some of these qualities as better than others.

For example, one may perceive that being low on Neuroticism is preferable to being high on the domain, or that having a high standing on Agreeableness is better than scoring low. For most of the domains one can think of "preferable poles." But this is not a productive way of construing scores on the NEO PI-R. Personalities should not be thought of as "good" or "bad." Personality is an adaptive structure; we develop the qualities we have because they enable us to survive and thrive. The opposing poles for each domain have their strengths and their liabilities, depending on the circumstances (T. Widiger & Corbitt, 1994).

One may argue that being high on Agreeableness is a positive virtue. Being compassionate, caring, helpful, and responsive to the needs of others are certainly socially desirable characteristics. In general, we all value these qualities, and respond warmly to those who seem to typify them, such as Mother Teresa or Gandhi. However, if you were to invest your life savings in the stock of a company, hoping for it to grow, would you be inclined to entrust your money to a company run by Mother Teresa or Gandhi? Or would you prefer to have someone running the company who is much more manipulative and cunning, able to outmaneuver the competition and undermine the efforts of future competitors—say, someone like Bill Gates?

Thus the question to be asked from a personality inventory is not whether an individual has a good or bad personality, but rather how well the individual's personality fits with the demands of a given situation or environment. There is a place for all different types of people, and we use personality assessment inventories to assess needs and identify complementing environments.

Because the NEO PI–R scales capture these normal, adaptive qualities, high or low scores should not be seen as representing anything abnormal. This is not a measure of psychopathology, nor is it designed to capture such types of processes. Therefore, it is inappropriate to draw such inferences from the scales. This is particularly true on the Neuroticism domain. This term was selected to define this dimension because of its historical place in the psychological literature. However, it does not refer to the kinds of dynamics the term originally reflected. High scores on these facets (e.g., Anxiety, Hostility, Depression, Self-Consciousness, Impulsiveness, and Vulnerability) do not indicate any type of Axis I disorder. For example, an individual can have a very high score on the Depression facet, but this does not mean that the person is suffering from clinical depression. However, as we shall see later, those suffering from clinical depression will tend to score high on this facet. Scoring low on Agreeableness and Conscientiousness does not mean that someone has an Antisocial Personality Disorder; although those with an Antisocial Personality Disorder do score low on those domains.

What this tells us is that the scores from the NEO PI–R need to be interpreted from a nonclinical vantage point. Scores from these scales speak to the regularities in an individual's ongoing behavior. However, to the extent that the five-factor model provides a complete description of fundamental personality dimensions, one might expect some relationship to those dynamics that define characterological impairment as well (Widiger & Frances, 1985; Widiger & Trull, 1992). The next section evaluates the relations between the five-factor model and dimensions of clinical dysfunction. The value of such correspondence for future clinical and research practices is highlighted.

THE FIVE-FACTOR MODEL AND ITS RELATIONS TO CLINICAL BEHAVIOR

Given that the five-factor model is a comprehensive description of normal personality dispositions capable of organizing individual-difference constructs from a wide array of theoretical models, and able to provide a high degree of empirical power in predicting numerous life outcomes, it is not surprising that researchers have examined the role these dimensions may play in abnormal behavior as well. Although the five factors are descriptive of nonclinical functioning, these dimensions may nonetheless have something to contribute to our understanding of abnormal functioning. In fact, several recent volumes have appeared that attempt to outline theoretically the expected linkages between traits and clinical nosology (Costa & Widiger, 1994; Strack & Lorr, 1994).

Widiger and Trull (1992) suggested four ways in which traits may be related to Axis I disorders: (a) they may predispose individuals to a disorder; (b) they may be a result of the disorder; (c) they may affect the expression of the disorder; or (d) they may share a common etiology with the disorder. McCrae (1994c) contended that the five-factor model can provide a framework for evaluating person by treatment interactions (see also Miller, 1991). Costa and McCrae (1992a) have also argued that the assessment of these normal personality dimensions can provide valuable, nonredundant information to clinical assessment protocols that rely solely on measures of symptomatology. Finally, the five-factor model is increasingly being perceived as a dimensional alternative to the current categorically based classification system (Costa & Widiger, 1994).

There are four major questions that need to be addressed when considering the utility of the NEO PI–R in a clinical context. First, does the psychometric integrity of the instrument continue to be evidenced when used clinically? Second, what are the relations between these five domains and Axis I symptomatology? Third, what are the relations between the five-factor model and Axis II symptomatology? Finally, what is the incremental validity of the NEO PI–R? Does it provide any additional, clinically relevant information over what is already available with current instruments? Each of these questions is discussed in turn.

The Psychometric Integrity of the NEO PI–R in a Clinical Setting

Given the relatively recent appearance of the NEO PI–R, there have not been many studies conducted to date evaluating the psychometric qualities of the instrument in a clinical context. However, those that are available have much to encourage its usage.

Piedmont and Ciarrocchi (in press) gave the NEO PI–R to a sample of 132 outpatient, substance-abuse clients. Descriptive statistics showed this sample to be high on Neuroticism and low on Agreeableness and Conscientiousness, a pattern characteristic of a substance-abuse disorder (Brooner, Herbst, Schmidt, Bigelow & Costa, 1993). Alpha reliabilities for the domains were all quite high (ranging from .83 to .89). Comparable values for the facets were lower than those found normatively (range from .44 for Excitement Seeking to .75 for Hostility; median = .61). A factor analysis of the scores clearly revealed the five-factor structure. In order to determine whether this obtained structure was identical to the normative factor structure, congruence coefficients were calculated (Gorsuch, 1983). Congruence coefficients are like correlation coefficients; they determine the degree of similarity between two sets of factor loadings. Using critical values provided by McCrae, Zonderman, Costa, Bond, and Paunonen (1996), it was determined that the obtained factor structure can be considered identical to the normative structure. This tells us that the NEO PI–R in a clinical context continues to manifest the same underlying factor structure that it does with nonclinical volunteers.

Retest reliability coefficients were also evaluated. Six weeks after admission to the outpatient program, participants completed another NEO PI–R as part of their discharge process. In evaluating these values, one needs to keep in mind that the respondents had just gone through a treatment program designed to impact their ways of perceiving, interpreting, and responding to the world. Correlations between scores taken pre- and postcounseling were quite high for both the domains (range .52 for Neuroticism to .79 for Openness) and facets (range .42 for Order to .72 for Aesthetics, median = .58), although these values were lower than normative values. This may have been a result of real individual-difference changes among the participants as a consequence of their treatment.

Two other studies have evaluated the reliability of the NEO PI in a clinical context. Trull and colleagues (1995) found 3-month retest coefficients averaging .85 for a sample of university-based clients receiving outpatient services. Similar findings were reported by Bagby and colleagues (1995) in a sample of depressed outpatients; they found retest reliabilities averaging about .73. In all studies, mean level changes on the domains were noted. The Piedmont and Ciarrocchi (in press) study evidenced large (about one-half standard deviation) changes on all five domains. The other two studies showed smaller and more circumscribed changes. These differences may have been a function of the type of sample and intensity of the treatment. Nevertheless, these three studies show that the NEO scales remain structurally valid and reliable in a clinical context.

The NEO PI–R's Relations to Axis I Disorders

The impetus for evaluating the correspondence between Axis I symptomatology and the five-factor model is not so much to identify the model as a clinical paradigm, but to emphasize that psychological distress does not develop in a vacuum. A client's presenting problems find a foundation in his or her larger motivational patterns. In this way, many psychosocial difficulties may be seen as problems in living associated with specific types of personality configurations. From this perspective, measures of the five-factor model can have two uses. First, obtaining a profile of a client on the five factors can help better outline the larger internal forces that have brought the individual to his or her current situation. Is the presenting problem a reaction to recent events or part of a larger, ongoing distressed lifestyle? Second, measures of the five-factor model may be useful for identifying potential psychological risks a person may face. For example, being high on Neuroticism may predispose one toward experiencing a clinical depression (Zonderman, Herbst, Schmidt, Costa, & McCrae, 1993).

Two studies have evaluated the relations between the MMPI and the NEO PI (Costa, Busch, Zonderman, & McCrae, 1986; Costa, Zonderman, McCrae, & Williams, 1985). Both studies showed that the content of the MMPI overlaps significantly with the dimensions of the five-factor model. Further, it was noted that the MMPI contained a heavy emphasis on Neuroticism in its content and had an underrepresentation of Conscientiousness. This is important to note because the MMPI is frequently relied on to provide a description of a client's personality. Because it lacks any measurement of Conscientiousness, it cannot be counted on to provide a complete description of personality.

Piedmont and Ciarrocchi (in press) provided correlations between the NEO PI–R and self-reported scores on the Brief Symptom Inventory (BSI; Derogatis, 1993), a measure designed to capture Axis I symptomatology, and the Personal Problems Check List (PPCL; Schinka, 1985) a measure of the extent and type of psychosocial difficulties encountered by the client. High Neuroticism and low Conscientiousness were the strongest and most consistent correlates of the BSI, indicating that the experience of such symptoms as Hostility, Phobic Anxiety, Interpersonal Sensitivity, and Paranoid Ideation had a strong motivational foundation. High Neuroticism and low Conscientiousness characterize an individual who experiences high levels of affective dysphoria and seeks succorance for this distress through any type of immediate gratification.

Interestingly, scores on the PPCL also correlated with high Neuroticism and low Conscientiousness. Clients with this personality configuration reported experiencing numerous problems related to social, religious, emotional, sexual, and health issues. These correlations highlight the maladaptive aspects to these five factors. Certain personality dispositions tend to increase the likelihood that individuals will experience certain types of problems with their environment. In particular, Neuroticism seems to be the single best predictor of the level and extent of problems experienced. On one level this is not very surprising, given that the dimension represents high levels of negative affect. But what is interesting is that these characteristic levels of distress will generalize into an individual's life path and create difficulties in many other areas. Research has shown that individuals high on Neuroticism are at risk for receiving a psychiatric diagnosis or experiencing depressive symptomatology (Saklofske, Kelly, & Janzen, 1995; Zonderman et al., 1993). Those high on Neuroticism are also likely to experience a lowered sense of job satisfaction and have an increased risk of burning out (Piedmont, 1993).

Scores on the NEO also have been shown to be useful in distinguishing motivationally between various nosological types. For example, scores on the NEO PI have been shown to discriminate between those with a sexual disorder and those with a sexual dysfunction (Fagan *et al.*, 1991) and are predictive of one's level of sexual functioning (Costa, Fagan, Piedmont, Ponticas, & Wise, 1992). Trull and Sher (1994) showed that scores from the NEO–Five Factor Inventory (NEO-FFI; this is a 60-item short form of the NEO PI–R—it assesses only the five global domains) were differentially sensitive to various Axis I diagnoses, such as drug addiction, anxiety disorders, major depression, and phobias.

Overall, the results of this growing body of research support the utility of the five-factor model in clinical assessment. Scores on the five factors are related to the type and amount of symptom expression. Appreciating the motivational basis of many psychological symptoms can assist a clinician in two ways. First, scores from the NEO PI–R can help establish a broader context for evaluating symptoms. Are the presenting problems a reaction to recent events or are they symptoms of enduring and pervasive maladjustment? Being able to disentangle the motivational basis of the presenting problem may aid in selecting appropriate treatments.

A second value of the NEO PI–R is that it can help establish realistic and appropriate therapeutic goals. For example, the Piedmont and Ciarrocchi (in press) study showed that individuals who were experiencing many social problems were also high on Neuroticism and low on Agreeableness and Conscientiousness. Such individuals feel very insecure and anxious in relationships with others. Their low Agreeableness and Conscientiousness indicates an interpersonal style that is selfish and manipulative. These individuals may see others as objects whose function is to provide physical gratification to assuage the individual's affective distress. Any treatment intervention needs to appreciate that individuals with this type of personality profile will always maintain an egocentric view of the world that will be characterized by a "me first" attitude. Attempting to rework this character style into one that is defined by trust and mutuality may not be possible.

The NEO PI–R and Its Relations to Personality Pathology

The application of the five-factor model to personality pathology seems a natural and logical step. Because a personality disorder is "an enduring pattern of inner experience and behavior that deviates markedly from the expectations of the individual's culture, is pervasive and inflexible, . . . is stable over time" (American Psychiatric Association, 1994,

p. 629), it is reasonable to believe that these ongoing, stable patterns find root in one's personal dispositions. Therefore, charting these maladaptive qualities in the five-factor taxonomy may help to shed additional etiological, motivational, and prognostic light on this aspect of functioning.

The interest in applying a dimensional model to the Axis II disorders stems from a dissatisfaction with the current categorical nosology of the *Diagnostic and Statistical Manual of Mental Disorders* (DSM-IV; American Psychiatric Association, 1994). A number of critics have appeared, finding fault with many aspects of the document, including its high prevalence of boundary cases, its descriptive nature, and the putative independence of the Axis I and Axis II disorders (Frances *et al.*, 1991; Livesley, Schroeder, Jackson, & Jang, 1994; Widiger & Shea, 1991). A growing controversy has developed over whether characterological pathology is better conceptualized by a dimensional or categorical model (Widiger & Costa, 1994; Widiger & Frances, 1994).

One basic assumption of the categorical model is that pathology represents a mode of functioning separate and distinct from normality. Those individuals who exhibit more than the threshold number of criteria are believed to be qualitatively different from those who meet fewer criteria. Thus, the distributions of the phenotypic features of personality disorder are discontinuous and show either a bimodal distribution or a point of rarity (Livesley et al., 1994). A dimensional model, on the other hand, assumes that the underlying qualities of personality pathology are the same as those found among nonclinical individuals. Thus, there is a continuous, normal distribution of scores for each of the traits.

Given that these two models generate very different expectations, they can be readily tested. A number of studies have shown that a dimensional model does better represent the qualities underlying the personality disorders than does a categorical model (Helmes & Jackson, 1994; Livesley, Jackson, & Schroeder, 1992; Livesley et al., 1994; Watson, Clark, & Harkness, 1994). As Schroeder, Wormworth, and Livesley (1992) have concluded, "personality disorders are not characterized by functioning that differs in quality from normal functioning" (p. 52). Not only do the same traits that describe normal behavior also describe pathological behavior, but research continues to show that the traits of the five-factor model of personality provide a strong paradigm for organizing characterological dysfunctioning—measures of the Big Five overlap heavily with ratings of personality dysfunctioning from a wide variety of Axis II assessment tools (e.g., Duijsens & Diekstra, 1996; Trull, 1992; Trull *et al*, 1995; Widiger & Costa, 1994; Wiggins & Pincus, 1989).

Widiger and Frances (1994) outlined three advantages to using a dimensional model for conceptualizing Axis II disorders. The first is its flexibility. Using continuous scores to describe functioning allows clinicians to establish various cutoff points for determining the presence of pathology that are sensitive to the context and type of clinical issues addressed. In the current clinical reality, decisions need to be made about clients concerning hospitalization, responsiveness to medication, insurance coverage, type of therapy, and so on. The current categorical nature of the *DSM-IV* provides only a single set of thresholds that may not be optimal for different types of decisions. The dimensional model allows one to determine different cutoffs that are relevant to those outcomes.

A second benefit of the dimensional model noted by Widiger and Frances (1994) is the retention of information. The polythetic nature of the *DSM-IV* gives rise to very heterogeneous diagnostic categories. For example, there are 256 different ways to meet the *DSM-IV* criteria for Borderline Personality Disorder and 99 ways to meet the criteria for Antisocial Personality Disorder, yet all receive the same diagnostic label. Although the categorical model can appreciate the diverse expression of a single pathologic process, it fails to appreciate the unique ways the disorder is expressed in a given client. And the degree to which a client may be atypical for a category will proportionally reduce the utility of the diagnostic label.

The dimensional model can reduce such stereotyping by providing much more precise information about a client. Subtleties and nuances can be detected by evaluating how much of each personality trait a client exhibits. The graduations provided by the ordinal-interval level personality scales can provide a rich source of information addressing issues of etiology, level and style of functioning, and prognosis.

The final, and perhaps most useful, advantage of the dimensional model is its ability to improve differential diagnosis. *DSM-IV* establishes behavioral thresholds for inclusion in a diagnostic category. However, the degree to which those criteria overlap will undermine one's ability to assign a client to one and only one category. Problems surrounding comorbidity and differentiation have long plagued the *DSM* and explain why the diagnosis Personality Disorder, Not Otherwise Specified is so frequently given for clients on Axis II.

For example, Livesley, West, and Tanney (1985) have noted the difficulty in differentiating between the avoidant and schizoid personality disorders. Both groups prefer solitary activities, have few social contacts or relationships, and remain interpersonally aloof. On a phenotypic level, both disorder categories may appear quite similar; the one distinguishing characteristic is that the avoidant feels his or her loneliness while the schizoid may be content with the isolation. Although *DSM-IV* has reduced the number of overlapping criteria between these two categories evidenced in previous editions, it still may be difficult for a clinician to discern whether the reticence concerning social interaction is a result of a personal sense of inadequacy or a constricted interpersonal style.

One way to resolve this issue is to plot the personality disorders in the space defined by the five major personality disorders. Then, each disorder can be understood by its characteristic pattern of loadings. As we did with understanding personality scales previously, triangulating the personality disorders with the five-factor model can not only highlight the kinds of personality qualities captured by these diagnostic categories, but also delineate the similarities and differences among the categories.

An example of this is given by Trull (1992), who presented correlations between the NEO-PI and the MMPI Personality Disorder (MMPI PD) scales in a sample of 54 psychiatric outpatients. The results of this analysis are presented in Table 2-6. Several observations can be noted from these data. The first concerns the utility of the five-factor model for making differential diagnoses. Consider the pattern of correlates for the Avoidant and Schizoid personality scales. Both have strong, negative loadings on Extraversion, highlighting the fact that both groups find themselves interpersonally distant and aloof; they tend to express little positive affect and seek solitary pursuits. Such similar interpersonal styles makes it difficult to differentiate between the two phenotypically. However, correlations with the NEO-PI domains show that the Avoidant tends to have higher levels of emotional distress than the schizoid, who may appear more placid and content. The Avoidant has inner feelings of inadequacy, anxiety, and fear. The Avoidant may wish to be in a group but is too socially phobic to initiate any interactions. The Schizoid, on the other hand, may feel perfectly content with interpersonal isolation. Because both types of individuals may be taciturn when it comes to clinical interviews, an effort needs to be made to measure levels of emotional distress.

Another example concerns the Histrionic and Narcissistic personality disorders. Both groups have strong positive correlations with Openness and Extraversion. This pattern reflects the attention-drawing, self-aggrandizing styles of these two groups. However, the Narcissistic claims a level of emotional stability and placidity that may not be present in the Histrionic, who may evidence some level of insecurity. It should also be noted that the amount of personological overlap among the personality diagnoses raises questions about the amount of redundancy reflected in these categories. Are all necessary to capture this type of disordered functioning? Could some diagnostic categories be meaningfully collapsed into others? Are there other disorders that have yet to be discovered? The relative absence of Openness among the personality disorder scales makes this a viable empirical question.

TABLE 2-6. Correlations between the MMPI-PD Scales and the Five Domains Scores of the NEO PI

Personality Disorder Symptoms	NEO PI Domain Score					
	N	E	O	A	C	R
Paranoid	.46^c	−.06	.04	−.48^c	−.05	.61^c
Schizoid	.00	−.72^c	−.27^a	−.19	.02	.73^c
Schizotypal	.45^b	−.49^c	−.21	−.40^b	−.12	.66^c
Obsessive-compulsive	.52^c	−.29^a	.03	−.27	−.14	.58^c
Histrionic	−.01	.61^c	.39^b	−.14	−.14	.71^c
Dependent	.64^c	−.21	−.01	−.08	−.33^a	.67^c
Antisocial	.29^a	−.22	−.02	−.42^b	−.27^a	.50^a
Narcissistic	−.30^a	.59^c	.43^b	−.06	.20	.73^c
Avoidant	.55^c	−.63^c	−.27	−.16	−.19	.78^c
Borderline	.61^c	.13	.18	−.45^b	−.24	.75^c
Passive-Aggressive	.56^c	−.19	.11	−.45^b	−.37^b	.68^c
multiple R	.82^c	.80^c	.54	.66^b	.66^b	

$^a p < .05$
$^b p < .01$
$^c p < .001$, two-tailed
Note: From "DSM-III-R Personality Disorders and the Five-Factor Model of Personality," by T. J. Trull, 1992, *Journal of Abnormal Psychology, 101*, p. 557. Copyright 1992 by the American Psychological Association. Adapted with permission.
$N = 54$. All correlations are two-tailed. Correlations are based on raw NEO PI scores and raw MMPI-PD scores. R's in the bottom row indicate the correlations between the 11 personality disorder scores and each NEO PI domain. R's in the last column indicate the correlation between the five NEO PI domain scores and each personality disorder. MMPI-PD = Minnesota Multiphasic Personality Inventory—Personality Disorder.

Another observation from Table 2-6 is that each of the personality disorder scales correlates with at least one of the five personality domains, demonstrating that personality qualities underlying the personality disorders are related to those dimensions that describe normal functioning. The degree of overlap is quantified by the multiple Rs that are presented in the last column and row of the table.

The multiple Rs in the last column were obtained by using each MMPI PD scale score as the dependent variable in a multiple regression analysis. The five personality factors of the NEO-PI were entered as predictors. The resulting multiple R indexes the degree of relationship between each personality disorder and the five-factor model. Squaring these values will provide the amount of shared variance. As can be seen, each of the MMPI PD scales is strongly associated with the personality domains, sharing between 25% and 61% of their variances.

The multiple Rs in the last row index the degree to which each of the personality domains is involved in the expression of deviant characterological functioning. These values were obtained by using each NEO-PI domain as the dependent variable in a regression analysis, with the MMPI PD scales entered as the predictors. As can be seen, the personality domains are heavily related with Axis II functioning. Between 29% and 67% of the variance in the NEO-PI domains overlaps with the MMPI PD scales. There is no doubt that the five-factor model of personality in general, and the NEO scales in particular, have much in common with Axis II functioning (see Widiger & Costa, 1994, for a review of several similar studies).

Another point of interest is that Openness to Experience is least involved with Axis II symptomatology; it correlated with only the Schizoid, Histrionic, and Narcissistic disorders. This may suggest, as noted previously, that there may be other disorders, as yet undiscovered, that involve facets of this domain. Because Openness is the most underrepresented of the five domains in the psychological literature, future research may wish to further evaluate how this domain may play into characterological dysfunctioning. A related observation is the strong presence of Neuroticism and Extraversion. These two domains seem to play an important role in describing Axis II functioning. Essentially, high levels of emotional dysphoria and a withdrawn, aloof interpersonal style characterize a wide variety of psychological syndromes. This may partially explain why making differential diagnoses is difficult—because many of the disorders share similar features. One way to disentangle this indistinctiveness would be to evaluate the relatedness of the facet scales to the personality disorders (Clark, 1990; Harkness, 1992; Widiger & Costa, 1994).

Facet scales can provide a more fine-grained analysis of the personological qualities expressed in the personality disorders. For example, low Agreeableness is a correlate of both the Antisocial and Borderline disorders. It may be possible that the elements of low Straightforwardness and low Compliance are defining of the Antisocial disorder while the elements of low Trust and low Altruism may define the Borderline disorder. The former reflects the manipulative self-centeredness of the sociopath while the latter captures the interpersonal alienation of the borderline. Thus, disorders that appear similar personologically at a global level of description may become distinct at a more specific level.

This leads to a final observation, that the five-factor model can be very useful for understanding Axis II functioning. The correlations of the personality disorder scales with these dimensions help to flesh out the personological implications of each. For example, the Paranoid disorder scale correlates with high Neuroticism and low Agreeableness. Such individuals are perceived as being suspicious, ill-tempered, demanding, angry, intolerant, faultfinding, quarrelsome, and cranky (Hofstee *et al.*, 1992). Certainly, the Paranoid personality possesses a high level of affective distress that fuels an active suspicion and distrust of others. The Histrionic personality reflects qualities of high Extraversion and high Openness. Such an individual can be described as being theatrical, intense, dramatic, expressive, and eloquent.

It is clear that both the five-factor model of personality and the NEO PI–R have something important to contribute to our understanding of Axis II functioning. Those personality qualities that define normal functioning are the same as those that describe abnormal functioning. As to where one may draw the line, that is a question for future research. At this point there is no cutoff score that clearly demarcates the boundary between the two levels. Scores on the NEO PI–R reflect only *normal* personality dynamics. An extreme score on any dimension does *not* indicate the presence of any type of maladaptiveness. It may be necessary to develop additional measures that capture individual-difference qualities that are more germane diagnostically. Nonetheless, scores on the NEO PI–R can be used to address Axis II–type issues in two ways. First, as Costa and McCrae (1992a) have argued, scores on these scales can be useful in making differential diagnoses. An individual high on Agreeableness is not likely to have an Antisocial Personality Disorder. Relatedly, high scores on Neuroticism can help rule out a Schizoid disorder. Second, an individual's pattern of scores on both the domains and facets can be compared to patterns of NEO PI–R profiles obtained from individuals known to possess various personality disorders. An empirical index of profile agreement can then be calculated. Very high congruence coefficients may suggest the presence of a personality disorder, or, at the least, indicate the presence of certain character styles similar to those whose disordered profile signature is being mimicked. The computer report generated for the NEO PI–R will conduct such analyses, systematically comparing the obtained profile to prototype profiles for each of the personality disorders. In this way, clinicians can be alerted to the presence of salient character traits that could significantly impact the therapeutic process.

In any event, the research findings make it clear that Axis II functioning may be better captured by a dimensional model of personality than by the current categorical system. As the research evidence mounts, future revisions of the *DSM* may move in that direction. In the meantime, the NEO PI–R has much to contribute to the clinical context; it is a very useful component of the assessment process. As the research presented in this section has shown, scores on the NEO PI–R overlap significantly with a number of clinical measures. The next question to be addressed is, "To what degree does the NEO PI–R provide information about clients that *cannot* be obtained from standard clinical instruments?" It is to this question of incremental validity that we now turn.

The Incremental Validity of the NEO PI-R

The preceding sections have demonstrated the value of the five-factor model for conceptualizing psychopathology. Although originally based in language, the five-factor constructs not only comprehensively outline normal personality dynamics, but also have relevance for organizing and understanding clinical characteristics. This linkage provides a sense of parsimony to the psychological literature: A wide range of dynamics can be usefully described by a limited set of constructs. However, efforts at linking the five-factor model to psychopathological dynamics has not been without its critics.

Ben-Porath and Waller (1992) have argued that the enthusiasm over the five-factor model earned in normal assessment should not persuade clinicians to uncritically accept such measures for clinical measurement. They argue that there already exist a large number of clinical measures that have been established as valid for such populations. These measures have been derived from extant theories of abnormal functioning and have been demonstrated to be useful in assessing such clients. They note many problems in using an instrument derived from "normal" constructs in a clinical context, not the least of which is the need to demonstrate that a scale such as the NEO PI-R "contributes incrementally to the procurement of diagnostic information beyond that which is obtained from current clinical measures" (Ben-Porath & Waller, 1992, p. 17). In other words, what is it that the NEO PI-R adds to a clinical assessment protocol that is not already obtained from existing measures?

A growing literature is developing that addresses this issue of incremental validity and consistently demonstrates that the NEO PI-R does provide clinically relevant information above and beyond what is already obtained by more standard measures of psychopathology. Trull and Sher (1994) have shown that the domains of the NEO were related to Axis I diagnoses of substance abuse disorder, anxiety disorder, and major depression, even after the effects of gender and current psychopathology were controlled. The dimensions of the five-factor model were also shown to exhibit unique patterns of relations with the various disorders. For example, Neuroticism and Extraversion were particularly sensitive to the social phobia diagnosis, while Agreeableness was less sensitive. The findings of unique personality by diagnosis interactions led Trull and Sher to conclude that the five-factor model may aid in the differential diagnosis of Axis I disorders.

Trull and colleagues (1995) evaluated the incremental validity of the NEO PI with regard to the personality disorders. Scores for each of the personality disorders were obtained using both the results of the Structured

Interview for *DSM-III-R* (DISP-R) and a self-report measure of personality pathology, the Personality Disorder Questionnaire–Revised (PDQ-R). These scores served as the criterion measures in two separate hierarchical stepwise regression analyses. On the first step of the regression, scores from the Beck Depression and Anxiety scales were entered to remove variance attributable to acute mood variation. On the next step, scores from the NEO PI domains were entered. Partial F-tests determined whether the increase in explained variance due to the five-factor domains was significant. For the SIDP-R, 8 of 13 incremental validity coefficients were significant; all 13 were significant for the PDQ-R scales. Again, the NEO domains scores provided additional explanatory power to the Axis II disorders over and above information provided by clinical measures of symptomatology.

Finally, Piedmont (1996a) used the Global Pathology Index score obtained from counselor ratings on the Derogatis Psychiatric Rating Scale (formerly known as the Hopkins Psychiatric Rating Scale) as the criterion measure in a hierarchical regression analysis involving outpatient substance abusers. On the first step of the analysis, self-report scores from the Brief Symptom Index (Derogatis, 1993), a measure of Axis I symptomatology, were entered. On the next step, domain scores from the NEO PI–R were put in. The partial F-test again revealed a significant increase in explained variance.

The results of these three studies show that clinical distress does not occur in a vacuum. The types of problems individuals encounter as well as the intensity of distress arise from underlying, stable characterological dispositions. The NEO PI–R provides a wealth of information about individuals, including their motivational aspirations, coping styles, interpersonal approaches, character styles, and levels of personal well-being. All of this information contributes significantly to clinical outcome indices above and beyond information obtained from symptom-based scales. The five-factor model can provide a salient framework for contextualizing clients' presenting problems; different personality types may be prone to experience certain types of predicaments. Therefore, merely noting the particular difficulties that clients experience without appreciating their motivational basis may undermine not only one's clinical understanding, but the effectiveness of any therapeutic intervention.

All the information presented in this section shows that the NEO PI–R can be a very useful clinical instrument. Psychometrically sound in a clinical milieu, the NEO scales can provide not only a tremendous amount of information about the personological context of a client, but can also help organize information in clinically relevant ways. Issues about differential diagnosis, intrapsychic dynamics, and treatment prognosis can all be linked together. As Miller (1991) has noted, "the five-factor model can relate patient personality, presenting complaint, treatment plan, and treatment outcome to each other in a reasonable, systematic way, without loss of empathy or compassion for the patient" (p. 432).

ROBUSTNESS OF THE FIVE-FACTOR MODEL

The data presented throughout this chapter clearly show that the five-factor model of personality is a sound paradigm for assessing individual differences. Although originally derived from the English language, the constructs represented by this model are reflected in numerous instruments that were derived from diverse theoretical orientations. The NEO PI–R provides a psychometric articulation of these constructs that is quite robust, useful in describing both normal and abnormal groups. However, the model is not without its critics (J. Block, 1995; McAdams, 1992).

J. Block (1995) criticized the five-factor model and NEO PI–R for their nontheoretical basis; the model and the instrument were founded in factor analysis. Block believed that the model, as a statistical tool, is unable to capture the subtleties of personality. Further, as with any statistical analysis, what you put into it very much determines what you pull out. If you put in sufficient information for five dimensions, then the factor analysis will retrieve only five dimensions. Broadening the inclusion criteria may result in the retrieval of additional factors. There are those who believe that there are more than five factors (e.g., Benet & Waller, 1995; Hahn & Comrey, 1994; Hogan & Hogan, 1992; Hough, 1992; Tellegen, 1993). Thus, J. Block (1995) believed that the five-factor model does not provide as comprehensive a sampling of personological content as it argues.

McAdams (1992) saw a number of limitations to the five-factor model. The bottom line here is that because of its trait-based nature, the five-factor model provides a shallow and superficial description of personality. McAdams believed that the five-factor model is essentially a "psychology of the stranger"; it provides a broad-band description of people that is useful when you do not know anything else about them.

Critics of the five-factor model argue that, at best, this paradigm captures superficial, relatively descriptive aspects of the individual that, taken at face value, can provide some useful information. However, the model lacks depth and interpretive insight. It overlooks many of the more important qualities of the individual that drive and direct the ongoing course of a person's life. In response to some of these issues, the next sections attempt to demonstrate the value and depth of the model. Rather than being surface descriptors, the five dimensions reflect fundamental dispositions of an individual to think, act, and feel. The importance of these qualities is found in the fact that they are genetically based and have also been found to be cross-culturally valid. The final section outlines McCrae and Costa's (1996) theoretical conceptualization of the five-factor model—its place in a larger metatheoretical framework.

HERITABILITY

The field of behavior genetics attempts to discover the degree to which the observed psychological qualities of individuals are linked to one's genetic makeup. Research in this area has shown that between 25% and 50% of the variance in observed personality variables is linked to genetic factors (Bouchard & McGue, 1990; Hershberger, Plomin, & Pedersen, 1995; Plomin, Chipuer, & Loehlin, 1990). These data suggest that personality traits are not mere fictions in the eyes of observers or the product of an individual's own implicit personality theory. Rather, traits spring from the person's biological foundation and hence represent a more "objective" reality.

Research on the dimensions of the five-factor model have shown that they possess significant levels of heritability (Bergeman et al., 1993; Heath et al., 1992). Jang, Livesley, and Vernon (1996b) evaluated the genetic basis of all of the NEO PI–R scales. Heritability coefficients from 41% (Neuroticism) to 61% (Openness) were found. Interestingly, the genetic component varied tremendously over the various facet scales, with Order, Self-Discipline, and Deliberation largely determined by environmental influences.

Research has shown that genetics contribute to the stability of personality in adulthood (Jang, Livesley, & Vernon, 1996a; Viken et al., 1994). Thus, the observed consistency in personality after age 30 cannot be reduced to mere consistency in self-presentation. Rather, stability of temperament reflects the emergence of underlying neurobiological processes that guide the ongoing course of development.

Given the biological basis of the five-factor model, it is difficult to interpret these factors as mere statistical artifacts; these are qualities that will certainly emerge from any comprehensive description of individuals. Further, given their biological nature, it seems equally unlikely that these dimensions reflect mere superficial aspects of the individual. It is unlikely that such peripheral features, with limited motivational implications, would become genetically imprinted into the species. Rather, the heritability of traits argues for their recognition as important qualities of the individual that serve to enhance one's ability to adapt and survive (Buss, 1991b). Not mere summary descriptions of behavior, traits represent underlying sources of motivation that organize and direct the ongoing course of human development and activity.

If there is a genetic basis to personality it also stands to reason that these dispositions should find universal expression in the human experience. The next section shows that the dimensions of the five-factor model in general, and NEO PI–R in particular, are also readily recoverable in diverse cultures.

CROSS-CULTURAL GENERALIZABILITY

The five-factor model finds its origins in the English language. These dimensions certainly represent important personality qualities for those individuals who speak English and share in its derivational experiences. This leaves the door open for the criticism that these dimensions are culturally specific and may not even generalize to other cultural contexts. If this is so, then the five-factor model represents circumspect, superficial qualities of the individual. However, if these dimensions do generalize cross-culturally, then this would be strong evidence that these dimensions address human functioning at a much more basic, fundamental level.

In addressing issues of cross-cultural generalizability, there are two major approaches: emic and etic. The first, *emic*, refers to identifying culture-specific constructs. The second, *etic*, is concerned with identifying similarities among cultures, to identify universal aspects of human functioning. Research has shown that the dimensions of the five-factor model represent discernible constructs in a variety of societies and can be useful for understanding culture-specific phenomena (Capara, Barbaranelli, Borgogni, & Perugini, 1993; Heaven et al., 1994; John, Goldberg, & Angleitner, 1984; Paunonen et al., 1992).

Numerous researchers have shown that the dimensions of the five-factor model generalize quite well to a number of different cultures, including European (*Italian*—Capara et al., 1993; Capara, Barbaranelli, & Comrey, 1995; *German*—Borkenau & Ostendorf, 1990; *Finnish and Polish*—Paunonen et al., 1992; *Spanish*—Avia et al., 1995), Indian (Narayanan, Shanka, & Levine, 1995), and Asian (*Japanese*—Bond, Nakazato, & Shiraishi, 1975, Isaka, 1990; *Chinese*—Bond, 1979; *Korean*—Piedmont & Chae, 1997; *Filipino*—Katigbak, Church, & Akamine, 1996). Research continues to document the presence of these five factors in both self-report and rater data. It is of particular interest to note that the five-factor model is recoverable in languages that do not share a common derivational or experiential history with English (see McCrae & Costa, 1997). The diversity of cultures that have developed and applied personality dispositions identical to Western-based ones is exciting evidence of the unity of human psychosocial functioning.

An even more exciting fact has been the finding that these domains operate maturationally in similar ways across cultures (McCrae, Costa,

Piedmont, *et al.*, 1996). It has long been known that adolescents and young adults (ages 17–21) have higher levels of Neuroticism, Extraversion, and Openness than older (age 30 and over) adults and lower levels of Agreeableness and Conscientiousness. There are real changes in personality that occur over the early adult years. These maturational changes have also been noted in several other cultures where the NEO PI–R has been translated (e.g., Korea, Italy, and Croatia). Finding similar developmental patterns across diverse cultures mutes criticisms that these factors are merely structural artifacts that emerge from the questionnaires themselves. If this were so, it would be unlikely that changes in the levels of these domains over the life span would follow similar forms in different cultures.

Rather than superficial descriptive qualities or statistical artifacts, the five-factor model represents broad, generalizable qualities of individuals. Measuring people on these constructs enables one to anticipate important behavioral outcomes in a variety of cultures. These data support the view that there is tremendous parsimony to human personality. That much of personality can be described by a finite set of constructs sets the stage for the development of a more inclusive and complete understanding of individual differences.

THEORETICAL FOUNDATION

McCrae and Costa (1996) have outlined a general theoretical framework within which they place the five-factor model of personality. The value of this model is that it attempts to put forth the underlying, motivational role these five dimensions play in shaping personality. Although they note that their model is only one of a large number of theories that are consistent with research on the five-factor model, its value is that it provides a series of testable hypotheses that can help extend research in this area.

There are five components of this model and they are outlined in Figure 2-1. The first is *Basic Tendencies*. This refers to the fundamental raw material of personality, the "stuff" with which we are born and from which the individual emerges. This material is genetically received and not shaped by environmental forces (e.g., Plomin & Daniels, 1987). Rather, it is internally driven through its development, with final form reached in adulthood. The content of these basic tendencies includes the five broad dimensions of personality: Neuroticism, Extraversion, Openness, Agreeableness, and Conscientiousness. These domains are hierarchically organized, with more specific facets defining more specific levels of organization. There are other aspects of functioning located here as well, including physical characteristics (e.g., physical appearance, gender, health), cognitive capacities (e.g., perceptual styles, general intelligence), and physiological drives (e.g., need for food and oxygen).

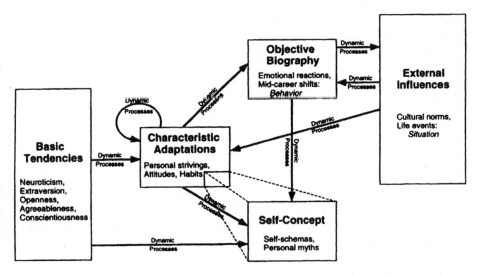

FIGURE 2-1. General Theoretical Framework for the Five-Factor Model of Personality.
Note. From "Toward a New Generation of Personality Theories: Theoretical Contexts for the Five-Factor Model," by R. R. McCrae and P. T. Costa, Jr., 1996. In J. S. Wiggins (Ed.), *The Five Factor Model of Personality: Theoretical Perspectives* (p. 73), New York: Guilford Press. Copyright 1996 by Guilford Press. Reproduced with permission.

The second component is referred to as *Characteristic Adaptations*. This component comprises the acquired skills, abilities, habits, and attitudes that emerge out of the interaction between the individual and his or her environment. It is here that the basic tendencies find their specific manifestations. Characteristic Adaptations include specific competencies, such as language, social skills, and religious beliefs and attitudes. An important element of this member is the third component—*Self-Concept*, the implicit and explicit views of the self, personal valuations of worth and value, our sense of identity. This mechanism contains an individual's self-schema, that particular affective-cognitive view of the self that is available to consciousness. This framework provides for a selective perception of one's environment and explains the unique ways that individuals orient themselves to the world.

It is important to realize this distinction between Basic Tendencies and Characteristic Adaptations. The former reflects the basic, broad qualities of human personality that are common to all people. As these qualities emerge, the individual refines their expression so that they are most adaptive to the specific demands of the immediate context. For example, different people, in different cultures may exhibit a wide variety of habits, tastes, and preferences, all reflecting the specifics of differing environments. However, it is the same set of needs that is driving these behaviors.

The third component of this model is the *Objective Biography*. This consists of every significant thing that a person has ever done. It contains the reactions one has to life events, the life paths followed, the life outcomes experienced. It is, in a sense, the testament of one's outward life. The variables in this category are usually seen as the outcomes that psychologists wish to predict. These events are the product of multiple sources of determination; factors from both within the individual and without converge to shape the direction and content of his or her life. Such variables would include whether or not one graduated college, got married, was divorced, the number of children one had, number of hospitalizations, and so on.

The fourth component of the model is *External Influences,* and refers to one's psychological environment. It includes such factors as parent–child interactions, peer socialization, and one's cultural, socioeconomic, and family groups. These outer forces exert influences on the direction and pace of development. However, individuals also select their environments and influence them in significant ways (e.g., Bandura, 1989; Hartmann, 1939/1958; M. Snyder, 1983). Thus there is an important reciprocity between the individual and the environment; people create situations that enable them to express and gratify important personal needs. The form and manner of this expression is certainly impacted by the external forces that are present.

The final component of McCrae and Costa's (1996) model is *Dynamic Processes.* This refers to the ways each of the above components interact with one another. Such processes include perceptive capacities, operant conditioning, coping and defense mechanisms, hedonic adaptation, interpersonal processes, and identity formation. This component highlights the fact that the person is an active, emergent property, always in a state of movement, development, and continual adaptation. The life process is a trajectory through time; the individual is never in the same place.

There are two types of dynamics postulated here. The first refers to universal dynamics, and reflects the fact that the "ongoing functioning of the individual in creating adaptations and expressing them in thoughts, feelings, and behaviors is regulated in part by universal cognitive, affective, and volitional mechanisms" (McCrae & Costa, 1996, p. 75). The other is differential dynamics, and refers to the reality that "[s]ome personality processes are differentially affected by basic tendencies of the individual, including personality traits" (p. 75).

This model provides for a rough sketching of how and where the five-factor model finds a home in the larger schema of personality organization. It is important to point out here that the five-factor model is *not* seen as a mere summary description of personality traits. Rather, these dimensions serve as basic temperaments that impact the entire enterprise of personality development and adaptation. The five factors take motivational precedence over all endeavors, although how these qualities become expressed in particular behaviors is certainly moderated both by external circumstances and by other intrapersonal mechanisms (e.g., self concept). Therefore, measuring these five domains and their more specific facets enables one to anticipate a wide range of important life outcomes. It is not surprising, then, that these qualities have been found cross-culturally and are relevant for understanding behavior in diverse societies.

Yet it needs to be mentioned that measuring the five factors does not provide a complete description of personality. There are many other aspects that are of value and need to be assessed. As the model just presented noted, one's characteristic adaptations and self-concept are other important aspects of functioning that have an important role to play. Understanding a person's life tasks and goals (e.g., Cantor *et al.*, 1991) can provide a real texture to the nuances of the individual's life. These constructs are predictive of important outcomes in their own right, even though they are related to one's basic tendencies (Cantor, 1990).

Nonetheless, as the information in this chapter has shown, measuring the five domains of personality provides a useful, predictively powerful way of describing personality at a broad level. The NEO PI–R can provide useful information that can help the test user anticipate a wide range of life outcomes with a relatively high degree of predictive power. The next chapter provides more interpretive information about the scales and begins to demonstrate how scores on the NEO PI–R can be used to gain useful insights into others.

Chapter 3

INTERPRETING THE NEO PI–R

Psychological test interpretation is an art. It requires of the test evaluator solid grounding in personality theory, an appreciation of the construct validity of the test being used, and a firm understanding of psychometrics. All of this information is frequently combined in ways that defy empirical quantification. No matter how advanced or skilled the interpreter, if the quality of the data for analysis is poor or invalid, then no amount of psychological acumen can create a valid interpretation. Therefore, before beginning to learn NEO PI–R interpretation, some consideration of profile invalidity and its detection is in order. The next section will first consider the role and value of validity scales for assessing profile validity.

THE USE OF VALIDITY SCALES IN ASSESSMENT

One of the most important undertakings in the enterprise of test development is the need for the test maker to demonstrate whether scores on his or her scale actually reflect important, identifiable personological constructs or are merely the by-product of response distortions, intended or otherwise. Great effort continues to be expended in order to develop scales aimed at second-guessing the response patterns of individuals on self-reports (e.g., Arbisi & Ben-Porath, 1995). The goal of these measures is to alert test interpreters to the possible presence of various response distortions that may be operating to invalidate the protocol. Such distortions can be as benign as a subject taking the test process for granted by responding randomly to items, or as serious as deliberate attempts by a respondent to manipulate his or her psychological presentation to maximum advantage. Such "validity scales" have been widely embraced by test users, and their presence in a test protocol can be quite reassuring (see Ben-Porath & Waller, 1992) if not absolutely necessary (Butcher & Rouse, 1996). The use of validity scales does raise several important questions: Do such scales provide sufficient information to justify the inclusion of additional test items, many of which can appear quite odd to test takers? Are they effective in identifying individuals who may be distorting their responses? Do the adjustments made to test scores based on these scales actually improve the validity of the measure?

Answers to these questions are important because the developers of the NEO PI–R explicitly excluded any type of validity scales. Costa and McCrae (1992c) believed that such items do not serve any empirically determined role in testing. Here we examine some issues related to the use of validity scales in personality assessment.

SOCIAL DESIRABILITY

Perhaps one of the more influential books written in the area of personality assessment was Edwards's (1957) tome on social desirability. His argument that responses on personality questionnaires were influenced to a large extent by the social desirability of the item rather than by any personological content was quickly embraced by the measurement field and has had a lasting impact. The Edwards Personal Preference Schedule (EPPS; Edwards, 1959), with its aim of eliminating biasing effects due to social desirability, represented a major shift in test construction. Even today, many test developers continue to find it noteworthy to demonstrate their scales' independence from this bias by correlating scores on their scale with measures of social desirability (Linehan & Nielsen, 1983).

One of the first efforts at uncorking the genie in the social desirability bottle surrounded the MMPI. Edwards and Heathers (1962) argued that the first factor to emerge from factor analyses of the MMPI represented a social desirability factor. The implication of this assertion was that the majority of explainable variance in MMPI responses was attributable to response distortions rather than to any kind of substantive psychological phenomenon. However, the specter of the MMPI as providing nothing more than systematic error was laid to rest with J. Block's (1965) cogent and empirically compelling analysis of the problem. He was able to demonstrate that scores on the first factor did, in fact, represent characterological aspects of the individual.

Nonetheless, the MMPI possesses a validity scale, K, that is designed to detect socially desirable responding by test takers. Several of the content scales (Hs, Pd, Pt, Sc, and Ma) are mathematically adjusted, or corrected, for K. The logic of this process is that mathematically partialing out social desirability from a test score increases its validity. However, such an assumption does not seem to be empirically justified. McCrae *et al.* (1989) have shown that *K* corrected MMPI scores are *less* valid than their uncorrected versions suggesting that rather than being only a suppressor variable, social desirability represents a substantive aspect of personality. A number of studies have shown that adjusting measures of normal personality for social desirability will compromise rather than enhance the scale's validity (Hsu, 1986; Kozma & Stones, 1987; McCrae, 1986; McCrae, & Costa, 1983b; Piedmont, McCrae, & Costa, 1992; Silver & Sines, 1962). Although the issue of social desirability as an index of response distortion has been largely refuted (see Nicholson & Hogan, 1990), interest remains keen among psychometricians to develop measures better suited for detecting response distortions. Instead of developing items whose content would reflect tendencies to manipulate one's self-presentation, efforts have focused on "content-free" validity scales. Such measures rely on response styles rather than on item content and represent the next generation of validity scales.

CONTENT-FREE VALIDITY SCALES

Early validity scales were themselves measures aimed at assessing qualities of the test taker. However, the qualities being assessed were characteristics related to a tendency to distort one's responses on other content-relevant scales. For example, Social Desirability scales contain items such as, "I always try to practice what I preach," and "I have almost never felt the urge to tell someone off" (Crowne & Marlowe, 1960) which reflect a high need for approval. Such a need to be seen in a good light was thought to dispose one to distort responses on other scales. But as shown above, measures of social desirability are confounded with personality. Need for approval is itself a substantive individual-difference variable.

In response to this, researchers began looking for other methods that were "content-free," scales that would identify aberrant responding without having to rely on items that may reflect stable qualities of the responder. One popular approach is to evaluate the consistency with which subjects respond to items (Tellegen, 1982). Tellegen (1988) outlines how such scales are developed and applied. At the heart of this approach is the belief that individuals will respond consistently to test items having similar content. Two such scales that are frequently used are the Variable Response Inconsistency (VRIN) and True Response Inconsistency (TRIN) scales. These scales have been developed for use on a number of major psychological tests (e.g., the Multidimensional Personality Questionnaire [MPQ] and the MMPI-2). VRIN scales consist of *pairs* of items with content that varies greatly from pair to pair but that is quite homogenous within each pair if both items are scored in the same direction. For example, one such pair from the MPQ is "When I work with others I like to take charge" and "I usually do not like to be a 'follower.'" Responding True to one item and False to the other item in the pair would be scored as one inconsistent response. High scores on the VRIN scale would indicate an individual who is responding to the questions in an indiscriminate manner.

The TRIN scale is made up of item pairs that are *opposite* in content. For example, one such item pair from the MPQ is "I would rather turn the other cheek than get even when someone treats me badly" and "When people insult me, I try to get even." Inconsistency is scored when an individual answers True to both items or False to both items. High scores on TRIN indicate a tendency to answer True indiscriminately (an acquiescence effect) while low scores indicate a tendency to answer False ("nonacquiescence" or "nay-saying"). In both cases, extreme scores would reflect a protocol that may be invalid, uninterpretable, or both. Tellegen and Waller (in press) have shown that the VRIN and TRIN scales are uncorrelated with each other and maintain low associations with the content scales of the MPQ. Thus, these scales are unconfounded with substantive personality and are claimed to be able to identify invalid protocols that would not be detected by the more familiar validity scales.

Interestingly, even though the NEO PI–R does not contain any validity scales, several have been developed (Schinka, Kinder & Kramer, 1997; Goldberg, personal communication, January 25, 1995). These scales assess the degree to which a subject is willing to claim positive and negative qualities as characteristic. Others evaluate the degree of consistency in responding to the items. Regardless of the content of these validity scales, their purpose is to identify protocols that are likely to be invalid. Put another way, scores on these validity scales determine the likelihood of a scale's validity. Scores on the validity scales moderate the validity of the substantive scales.

In a series of analyses conducted by Piedmont and McCrae (1998), we evaluated the validity of a number of validity scales, both those developed for the NEO PI–R and those on the MPQ. From all the analyses that were done in this study it was determined that the validity scales showed no consistent, significant pattern of effects. Scores on these response-distortion scales did not moderate the validity of either self-reports or observer ratings. Their value for use among volunteer, nonclinical samples is seriously questioned. Of course, further research is needed in this area to evaluate the utility of validity scales in clinical, forensic, and job selection samples. Until a complete answer to the value of validity scales is obtained, a reliance on self-report data will continue. In order to use such information well, some consideration of its value is necessary.

THE VALUE AND LIMITS OF SELF-REPORT DATA

The underlying assumption of a self-report is that the individual is in the best position to provide information about him- or herself (e.g., private beliefs and past behaviors) that may not be readily accessible from observers or life outcome data sources. There is also a certain parsimony to the approach: If you wish to know something about people, ask them. Yet despite such an appealing paradigm, there has always been great skepticism and mistrust of self-report information. Concerns about defensiveness, faking, and social desirability have always created a pall over such procedures and have led to the development of many different types of validity scales to correct for these sources of error.

However, data do exist that offer support for trust in self-reports. Evidence shows that more direct and "obvious" items possess better validity than subtle items (Furnham, 1986; Worthington & Schlottman, 1986; Wrobel & Lachar, 1982), suggesting that when respondents are presented with a direct query about their internal state, they will give an honest and accurate response. In perhaps the largest study to date, Hough, Eaton, Dunnette, Kamp, and McCloy (1990) concluded that applicants for a job tended not to distort their responses in the absence of any instructions to do so (see Mount & Barrick, 1995, for a review). Hogan (1991) argued that the desire by some respondents to manipulate their test image may be an individual difference variable itself worthy of study. Jackson (1989) showed convergent correlations between self-reported scores on the Basic Personality Inventory scales and professional ratings for psychiatric patients. Muten (1991) showed, with a sample of his patients, significant levels of agreement between self-reported scores and spouse ratings on the NEO PI. Taken together, these findings support the trustworthiness of self-report data. In general, people seem to respond in an honest and straightforward manner to the testing situation.

These data do not deny that there are occasions when a self-report may not provide useful data. An uncooperative client or a cognitively impaired individual may not be able to provide valid information. There may also be situations in which an individual has great incentive to distort or manipulate his or her presentation. In such scenarios, self-report data are of little use, irrespective of any validity scales or mathematical manipulations of the information. In such cases it would be more beneficial to rely on other sources of information, such as an observer rating by a friend or spouse. If you cannot trust a person to provide valid information, then do not use a self-report measure.

Observer-based data provide a useful counterpoint to self-reports. Although they have their own potential sources of error (e.g., halo effects, stereotypes), these biases do not overlap with the errors that are inherent to self-reports (McCrae, 1982). Thus, convergence between peer and self ratings cannot be attributable to correlated error but to a reliable effect (see Wiggins, 1979). Because self–peer agreement seems to be the rule in measuring the FFM, disagreements between these two sources of information may be indicative of some type of distortion. McCrae (1994c) provides a methodology for using both self and observer ratings on the NEO PI–R. But if a self-report cannot be trusted, observer data can be a very helpful stand-in. Data do support the validity of peer ratings in predicting useful outcomes such as job success and marital satisfaction (Kosek, 1996a; Mount, Barrick, & Strauss, 1994).

Believing that self-report data are relatively sound, Costa and McCrae (1992c) developed the NEO PI–R without any type of validity scales (see Costa & McCrae, 1992a). The only "validity" scale is the presence of three short items at the end of the NEO PI–R that ask the subject if he or she has completed all items in the proper way. Although such direct items may not capture subtle attempts at distortion, a "No" to any of the items would clearly indicate a questionable protocol.

NEO PI–R FACET SCALES AND THEIR INTERPRETATIONS

Recognizing that there are inherent limitations to test data, regardless of its source, we turn now to a presentation of the NEO PI–R facet scales and their definitions. Scales will be presented by domain. The facet scales can be considered partitions of the larger spectrum of qualities represented in each domain. In developing the facets every effort was made to create scales that were as nonoverlapping in content as possible while still remaining on the same domain. By minimizing redundancy among the facets, the test developers maximized the interpretability of each scale.

NEUROTICISM

Neuroticism assesses affective adjustment versus emotional instability. Individuals who score high on this domain are prone to experiencing psychological distress, unrealistic ideas, excessive cravings or urges, and maladaptive coping responses. Although high scores on this domain do not indicate the presence of any clinical disorder, individuals with a clinical syndrome do tend to have a high score here (see Costa & Widiger, 1994). In fact, high scores on Neuroticism place one at risk for receiving a psychiatric diagnosis (Zonderman, Herbst, Schmidt, Costa, & McCrae,

1993). The six facets for this domain, and their definitions are from Costa and McCrae (1992c). Adjective descriptors for each facet are taken from a variety of sources (McCrae & Costa, 1992; Piedmont & Weinstein, 1993).

N1: Anxiety. Anxious individuals are apprehensive, fearful, prone to worry, nervous, tense, and jittery. The scale does not measure specific fears or phobias, but high scorers are more likely to have such fears, as well as free-floating anxiety. Low scorers are calm and relaxed. They do not dwell on things that might go wrong. Adjectives that describe high scorers on this facet include tense, fearful, worried, apprehensive. Adjectives that describe low scorers on this facet include calm, relaxed, stable, fearless.

N2: Angry Hostility. Angry hostility represents the tendency to experience anger and related states such as frustration and bitterness. This scale measures the individual's readiness to *experience* anger; whether the anger is *expressed* depends on the individual's level of Agreeableness. Note, however, that disagreeable people often score high on this scale. Low scorers are easygoing and slow to anger. High scorers on this facet are described as being hot-tempered, angry, and frustrated. Low scorers are described as being amiable, even-tempered, and gentle.

N3: Depression. This scale measures normal individual differences in the tendency to experience depressive affect. High scorers are prone to feelings of guilt, sadness, hopelessness, and loneliness. They are easily discouraged and often dejected. Such individuals are described as being hopeless, guilty, downhearted, and blue. Low scorers rarely experience such emotions, but they are not necessarily cheerful and lighthearted—characteristics associated instead with Extraversion. High scorers on this facet are described as being seldom sad, hopeful, confident, and as feeling worthwhile.   *low ?*

N4: Self-Consciousness. The emotions of shame and embarrassment form the core of this facet of Neuroticism. Self-conscious individuals are uncomfortable around others, sensitive to ridicule, and prone to feelings of inferiority. Self-consciousness is akin to shyness and social anxiety. Such individuals are described as being ashamed, feel inferior, and are easily embarrassed. Low scorers do not necessarily have grace or good social skills; they are simply less disturbed by awkward social situations. These individuals are described as poised, secure, and feel adequate.

N5: Impulsiveness. This facet refers to the inability to control cravings and urges. Desires (e.g., for food, cigarettes, possessions) are perceived as being so strong that the individual cannot resist them, although he or she may later regret the behavior. Low scorers find it easier to resist such temptations, having a high tolerance for frustration. The term *impulsive* should not be confused with spontaneity, risk taking, or rapid decision time. High scorers on this facet are described as being unable to resist cravings, hasty, sarcastic, and self-centered. Low scorers are described as being self-controlled and able to resist temptation.

N6: Vulnerability. The final facet of N is vulnerability to stress. Individuals who score high on this scale feel unable to cope with stress, becoming dependent, hopeless, or panicked when facing emergency situations. High scorers are characterized as being easily rattled, panicked, and unable to deal with stress. Low scorers perceive themselves as capable of handling themselves in difficult situations. These individuals are described as being resilient, cool-headed, and hardy.

EXTRAVERSION

Costa and McCrae (1985) have defined this domain as representing the quantity and intensity of interpersonal interaction, the need for stimulation and the capacity for joy. This domain contrasts sociable, active, person-oriented individuals with those who are reserved, sober, retiring, and quiet. There are two qualities assessed on this domain: interpersonal involvement and energy. The former evaluates the degree to which an individual enjoys the company of others and the latter reflects the personal tempo and activity level. This dimension has been shown to capture levels of positive affect.

E1: Warmth. Warmth is the facet of Extraversion most relevant to issues of interpersonal intimacy. Warm people are affectionate and friendly. They genuinely like people and easily form close attachments to others. Such individuals are characterized as being outgoing, talkative, and affectionate. Low scorers are neither hostile nor necessarily lacking in compassion, but they are more formal, reserved, and distant in manner than high scorers. Warmth is the facet of E that is closest to Agreeableness in interpersonal space, but it is distinguished by a cordiality and heartiness that is not part of A.

E2: Gregariousness. A second aspect of E is gregariousness—the preference for other people's company. Gregarious people enjoy the company of others, the more the merrier. They are characterized as being convivial, having many friends, and seeking social contact. Low scorers on this scale tend to be loners who do not seek—or who even actively avoid—social stimulation. These individuals are described as avoiding crowds and preferring to be alone.

E3: Assertiveness. High scorers on this scale are dominant, forceful, and socially ascendant. They speak without hesitation and often become group leaders. Adjective descriptions of high scorers include dominant, forceful, confident, and decisive. Low scorers prefer to keep in the background and let others do the talking. Adjective descriptors include unassuming, retiring, and reticent.

E4: Activity. A high Activity score is seen in rapid tempo and vigorous movement, in a sense of energy, and in a need to keep busy. Active people lead fast-paced lives. They are described as being energetic, fast-paced, and vigorous. Low scorers are more leisurely and relaxed in tempo, although they are not necessarily sluggish or lazy. They are described by others as being unhurried, slow, and deliberate.

E5: Excitement-Seeking. High scorers on this scale crave excitement and stimulation. They like bright colors and noisy environments. Excitement-seeking is akin to some aspects of sensation seeking. These individuals are described as flashy, seekers of strong stimulation, and risk takers. Low scorers feel little need for thrills and prefer a life that high scorers might find boring. These individuals are described as cautious, staid, and uninterested in thrills.

E6: Positive Emotions. This facet reflects the tendency to experience positive emotions such as joy, happiness, love, and excitement. High scorers on this scale laugh easily and often. They are seen as cheerful, high-spirited, joyful, and optimistic. Low scorers are not necessarily unhappy; they are merely less exuberant and high-spirited. They are described as unenthusiastic, placid, and serious. Research has shown that happiness and life satisfaction are related to both N and E, and that Positive Emotions is the facet of E most relevant to the prediction of happiness.

OPENNESS TO EXPERIENCE

Openness to Experience is defined as the proactive seeking and appreciation of experience for its own sake, and as toleration for and exploration of the unfamiliar. This domain contrasts curious, original, untraditional, and creative individuals with those who are conventional, unartistic, and unanalytical. Of all the domains, this one is the most controversial; it is the least developed and explored. In terms of its representativeness in the language, it has the fewest number of descriptors. Nonetheless, Openness continues to show its personological value (McCrae & Costa, 1985b; McCrae, 1990, 1993–1994, 1994b). The facets for this domain are as follows:

O1: Fantasy. Individuals who are open to fantasy have a vivid imagination and an active fantasy life. They daydream not simply as an escape but as a way of creating for themselves an interesting inner world. They elaborate and develop their fantasies and believe that imagination contributes to a rich and creative life. These individuals are described as imaginative and as enjoying daydreaming. Low scorers are more prosaic and prefer to keep their minds on the task at hand. They are described as practical and as preferring realistic thinking.

O2: Aesthetics. High scorers on this scale have a deep appreciation for art and beauty. They are moved by poetry, absorbed in music, and intrigued by art. They need not have artistic talent, nor even necessarily what most people would consider good taste, but for many of them, interest in the arts will lead them to develop a wider knowledge and appreciation than the average individual. They are seen as valuing aesthetic experiences and as moved by art and beauty. Low scorers are relatively insensitive to and uninterested in art and beauty. They are described by others as being insensitive to art and unappreciative of beauty.

O3: Feelings. Openness to feelings implies receptivity to one's own inner feelings and emotions and the evaluation of emotion as an important part of life. High scorers experience deeper and more differentiated emotional states and feel both happiness and unhappiness more intensely than others. Descriptions of high scorers include emotionally responsive, sensitive, empathic, and values own feelings. Low scorers have somewhat blunted affects and do not believe that feeling states are of much importance. Descriptions of low scorers include narrow range of emotions and insensitive to surroundings.

O4: Actions. Openness is seen behaviorally in the willingness to try different activities, go new places, or eat unusual foods. High scorers on this scale prefer novelty and variety to familiarity and routine. Over time, they may engage in a series of different hobbies. They are described by others as seeking novelty and variety and trying new activities. Low scorers find change difficult and prefer to stick with the tried and true. These individuals are perceived by others as being set in their ways and preferring the familiar.

O5: Ideas. Intellectual curiosity is an aspect of Openness that has long been recognized. This trait is seen not only in an active pursuit of intellectual interests for their own sake, but also in open-mindedness and a willingness to consider new, perhaps unconventional ideas. High scorers enjoy both philosophical arguments and brain-teasers. Openness to ideas does not necessarily imply high intelligence, although it can contribute to the development of intellectual potential. These individuals are described as being intellectually curious, analytical, and theoretically oriented. Low scorers on the scale have limited curiosity and, if highly intelligent, narrowly focus their resources on limited topics. These individuals are described as being pragmatic, factually oriented, and unappreciative of intellectual challenges.

O6: Values. Openness to Values means the readiness to reexamine social, political, and religious values. High scorers on this facet are seen as tolerant, broad-minded, nonconforming, and open-minded. Closed individuals tend to accept authority and honor tradition and as a consequence are generally conservative, regardless of political party affiliation. Low scorers on this facet are seen as dogmatic, conservative, and conforming. Openness to Values may be considered the opposite of dogmatism.

AGREEABLENESS

Extraversion evaluates the degree to which a person enjoys being in the presence of others. Agreeableness examines the attitudes an individual holds toward other people. These attitudes can be very pro-person, compassionate, trusting, forgiving, and soft-hearted on one end to very antagonistic, cynical, manipulative, vengeful, and ruthless on the other. The broad interpersonal orientation captured here ranges from very Mother Teresa-ish on the one hand to Machiavellian on the other. The facets for this domain include the following:

A1: Trust. High scorers have a disposition to believe that others are honest and well intentioned. High scorers are characterized as being forgiving, trusting, and peaceable. Low scorers on this scale tend to be cynical and skeptical and to assume that others may be dishonest or dangerous. Low scorers are characterized as being wary, pessimistic, suspicious, and hard-hearted.

A2: Straightforwardness. High scorers on this scale are frank, sincere, and ingenuous. These individuals are characterized as being direct, frank, candid, and ingenuous. Low scorers on this scale are more willing to manipulate others through flattery, craftiness, or deception. They view these tactics as necessary social skills and may regard more straightforward people as naive. These individuals are described as being shrewd, clever, and charming.

A low scorer on this scale is more likely to stretch the truth or to be guarded in expressing his or her true feelings, but this should not be interpreted to mean that he or she is a dishonest or manipulative person. In particular, this scale should not be regarded as a lie scale, either for assessing the validity of the test itself, or for making predictions about honesty in employment or other settings.

A3: Altruism. High scorers on this facet have an active concern for others' welfare as shown in generosity, consideration of others, and a willingness to assist others in need of help. These individuals are seen by others as being warm, soft-hearted, gentle, generous, and kind. Low scorers on this scale are somewhat more self-centered and are reluctant to get involved in the problems of others. These individuals are seen by others as being selfish, cynical, cold, and snobbish.

A4: Compliance. This facet of A concerns characteristic reactions to interpersonal conflict. The high scorer tends to defer to others, to inhibit aggression, and to forgive and forget. Compliant people are meek and mild. High scorers are characterized as being deferential, obliging, and kind. The low scorer is aggressive, prefers to compete rather than cooperate, and has no reluctance to express anger when necessary. Low scorers are characterized as being stubborn, demanding, headstrong, and hard-hearted.

A5: Modesty. High scorers on this scale are humble and self-effacing although they are not necessarily lacking in self-confidence or self-esteem. These individuals are perceived by others as being humble and unassuming. Low scorers believe they are superior people and may be considered conceited or arrogant by others. A pathological lack of modesty is part of the clinical conception of narcissism. These individuals are seen by others as being aggressive, tending to show off, and tough.

A6: Tender-Mindedness. This facet scale measures attitudes of sympathy and concern for others. High scorers are moved by others' needs and emphasize the human side of social policies. Adjective descriptors of high scorers include friendly, warm, kind, gentle, and soft-hearted. Low scorers are more hardheaded and less moved by appeals to pity. They would consider themselves realists who make rational decisions based on cold logic. Adjective descriptors of low scorers include intolerant, cold, opinionated, and snobbish.

CONSCIENTIOUSNESS

This domain assesses the individual's degree of organization, persistence, and motivation in goal-directed behavior. This dimension contrasts dependable, fastidious people with those who are lackadaisical and sloppy. Also represented here is the amount of personal control and the ability to delay gratification of needs. The facets include the following:

C1: Competence. This facet refers to the sense that one is capable, sensible, prudent, and effective. High scorers on this scale feel well prepared to deal with life. These individuals are perceived by others as being efficient, thorough, confident, and intelligent. Low scorers have a lower opinion of their abilities and admit that they are often unprepared and inept. These individuals are perceived by others as being confused, forgetful, and frivolous. Of all the C facet scales, competence is most highly associated with self-esteem and internal locus of control.

C2: Order. High scorers on this scale are neat, tidy, and well organized. They keep things in their proper places. Adjective descriptors for high scorers include precise, efficient, and methodical. Low scorers are unable to get organized and describe themselves as unmethodical. Adjective descriptors for low scorers include disorderly, impulsive, and careless. Carried to an extreme, high Order might contribute to a Compulsive Personality Disorder.

C3: Dutifulness. In one sense, *conscientiousness* means "governed by conscience," and that aspect of C is assessed as Dutifulness. High scorers on this scale adhere strictly to their ethical principles and scrupulously fulfill their moral obligations. These individuals are described as being dependable, mannerly, organized, and thorough. Low scorers are more casual about such matters and may be somewhat undependable or unreliable. These individuals are described as being lazy, absent-minded, and distractible.

C4: Achievement Striving. Individuals who score high on this facet have high aspiration levels and work hard to achieve their goals. They are diligent and purposeful and have a sense of direction in life. These individuals are seen as being ambitious, industrious, enterprising, and persistent. Very high scorers, however, may invest too much in their careers and become workaholics. Low scorers are lackadaisical and perhaps even lazy. They are not driven to succeed. They lack ambition and may seem aimless, but they are often perfectly content with their low levels of achievement. These individuals are seen as being leisurely, dreamy, and disorganized.

C5: Self-Discipline. This term means the ability to begin tasks and carry them through to completion despite boredom and other distractions. High scorers have the ability to motivate themselves to get the job done. Adjective descriptors include organized, thorough, energetic, capable, and efficient. Low scorers procrastinate in beginning chores and are easily discouraged and eager to quit. Adjective descriptors include unambitious, forgetful, and absent-minded.

Low self-discipline is easily confused with impulsiveness. Both are evidence of poor self-control, but empirically they are distinct. People high in impulsiveness cannot resist doing what they do not want themselves to do; people low in self-discipline cannot force themselves to do what they want themselves to do. The former requires an emotional stability; the latter, a degree of motivation that they do not possess.

C6: Deliberation. The final facet of C assesses the tendency to think carefully before acting. High scorers on this facet are cautious and deliberate. High scorers are described as being cautious, logical, and mature. Low scorers are hasty and often speak or act without considering the consequences. At best, low scorers are spontaneous and able to make snap decisions when necessary. These individuals are described as being immature, hasty, impulsive, and careless.

The 35 scales of the NEO PI–R (five domain scores and the 30 facets) provide a comprehensive assessment of the individual. There is certainly a tremendous amount of information available for interpretation. As was seen in the previous chapter, this information has implications for a wide range of psychologically significant outcomes. The next section provides some examples in order to help the reader begin to work interpretively with this information.

NEO PI–R INTERPRETATIONS AND
SELECT CASE PROFILES

Now that definitions of the 30 NEO PI–R facets has been provided, this section presents three case profiles for interpretation. This provides the reader an opportunity to apply these definitions to actual scores and begin to develop a "feel" for how individuals come to be represented by these scales.

In evaluating a NEO PI–R profile, <u>I find it useful to proceed domain by domain.</u> I first evaluate a person's standing on the overall domain, say Neuroticism, to gain an overview of the kinds of global dynamics that characterize the person. Then I evaluate the facet scales for that domain in order to isolate those aspects of the larger domain that are the most defining. Keep in mind that although the facet scales for a domain are all related, they were designed to be as nonredundant as possible (see Costa & McCrae, 1995a). This can result in a high degree of interscale scatter within each personality dimension. It is not uncommon for an individual to score high (or low) on a domain, but be low (or high) on several of the facet scales. Facet analysis can be very revealing and provide a more intimate understanding of a client (Miller, 1991).

In evaluating the elevation of scores on each scale, <u>T-scores between 45 and 55 are considered average or normative. There is usually no real interpretation of such scores, because the individual can be equally likely to exhibit behaviors characteristic of the high and low poles.</u> T-scores below 45 are considered low and scores below 35 are seen as being very low. Conversely, T-scores above 55 are seen as being high and those above 65, very high. When scores move into these regions, they carry interpretive value; a respondent begins to reflect more consistently the characteristics defining that end of the pole. <u>When T-scores for a facet or domain go above 80 or below 20, this may indicate the presence of real deficits in an individual's ability to function in his or her environment.</u> Therefore, one needs to consider the real possibility of the presence of some pathological process.

The 35 scales of the NEO PI–R present a tremendous amount of information to process. This is both good and bad. It is good because of the vastness of insights revealed by the scales. There are many personological implications for scores from each scale, presenting a rather fine-grained analysis of the respondent. The down side is really not that bad. So much information means that it will take time to develop a working knowledge of all the facet and domain scales and what they represent about a client. Learning the 30 facet names can be its own challenge. With practice, however, one can quickly master this task and become quite fluent in the language of the NEO PI–R. Aside from facilitating interpretation, the personality qualities represented by the NEO PI–R will also provide a language for conceptualizing and evaluating other personality constructs and scales. With this in mind, we turn now to interpreting some case profiles.

The cases presented are of actual individuals that have been culled from several sources. Some are of actual clinical clients; others are from data files accumulated by the author over several years. Every effort was made to select individuals with particularly interesting psychosocial histories and profile interpretations.

CASE HISTORY: DEBBIE K.

The first profile is of a 17-year-old White female named Debbie K. At the time of testing she was a senior in an all-girl parochial high school. She was in the top of her class academically, having already received several academic scholarships to many large, well-known universities. Over the course of her high school experience, she had served in numerous leadership positions, including class president. Her profile is presented in Figure 3-1.

As can be seen, her overall Neuroticism score is very low, suggesting a young lady who is emotionally stable and well adjusted. All her facet scales for N are in the low to very low levels. She is portrayed here as being calm, amiable, seldom sad, secure, self-controlled, and hardy. If she does experience any negative affect, it may be around feelings of inadequacy (N4), which is her highest N facet.

On Extraversion, she again scores in the low range, suggesting a more formal, and reserved approach to others. On the facet scales there is great scatter. Debbie scores high on the E3 (Assertiveness) facet, suggesting that she is confident and dominant. In a group of people she would prefer to be the leader rather than a follower. She scores in the low range on E4 (Activity) and E5 (Excitement Seeking). This suggests that Debbie has a very measured and unhurried personal tempo. There would appear to be little pressure in her efforts at undertaking various tasks. Her low E5 score indicates someone who is cautious and uninterested in thrills. Her other E scores are in the average range, suggesting a more flexible orientation toward others. E1 (Warmth) indicates that Debbie can be talkative and outgoing, although there may be some sense of distance and aloofness experienced by those who may meet her for the first time. Her E2 (Gregariousness) score is on the average to high cusp, and would suggest a degree

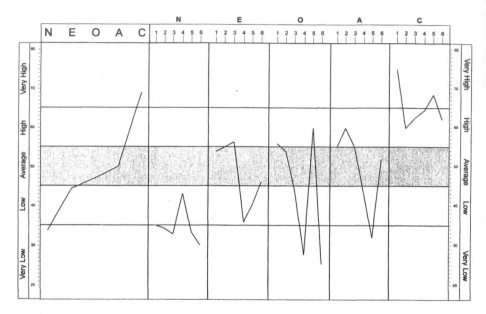

FIGURE 3-1. NEO PI–R profile of Debbie K.

of sociability and a desire for social contacts, although there is room for solitary pursuits as well. Her low average score on E6 (Positive Emotions) indicates a person who appears somewhat serious and may express happiness in a somewhat muted fashion.

The Openness to Experience domain score is average, suggesting an individual who has some inner needs for structure and direction as well as a capacity to explore new avenues of activity. Underlying this person is some degree of rigidity; there are limits to how much change or novelty Debbie would tolerate. Again, however, there is quite a degree of scatter among the facet scales for this domain.

She is high on O1 (Fantasy) and O5 (Ideas). Debbie has an active inner life composed of imagination and fantasy. No doubt this inner world contributes to and benefits from her fond desire for reading. The characters in her books are brought to life by her capacity to imagine. Her high score on O5 (Ideas) suggests that Debbie is very much interested in intellectual pursuits, theoretical arguments and discussions, and is willing to consider new and unconventional ideas. These characteristics certainly work well with her academic abilities and successes.

However, Debbie scores very low on O4 (Actions) and O6 (Values). The low Actions suggests that Debbie prefers a great deal of structure in her life.

There is a preference for the known and a dislike for change. As Debbie once told me, "I am pretty set in my ways." Her score on this scale indicates some degree of personal rigidity. Her low score on O6 (Values) indicates that Debbie also holds some very dear personal beliefs and values that are not open for discussion, evaluation, or change. Low scores here reflect a dogmatic orientation to a value network that may be difficult to penetrate or to change. She is accepting of authority and conforms to the dictates of her beliefs.

Debbie's average score on O2 (Aesthetics) represents some enjoyment and appreciation of the arts. This score reflects her interests in reading, although this scale also reflects interests in other aspects of the arts, such as theater, ballet, and opera, for which Debbie has far less interest. Her average score on O3 (Feelings) suggests an individual who has some receptivity to emotional information and may have some sensitivity to the feelings of others. However, given her low scores on the Neuroticism facets, Debbie may feel much more comfortable on a cognitive level than on an emotional one. Yet, her score is on the average to low cusp, suggesting that there may be some emotions that Debbie does not like to confront. Feelings may be less important to her than ideas.

Concerning Agreeableness, Debbie scores again in the average range. This indicates an individual who is generally warm and trusting, but has a degree of skepticism that will not allow her to take all people and events at face value. She scores high on the A1 (Trust), A2 (Straightforwardness), and A3 (Altruism) scales, suggesting an individual who presents herself to the world in a frank and "up front" manner and believes that others do the same. She has a desire to help others in distress and can be very generous and considerate. Debbie scored low on A5 (Modesty), indicating that she has no problems in talking about her achievements and may have a feeling of superiority because of them. This low score in conjunction with her low score on Values (O6) suggests that Debbie may come across to others as being arrogant or superior. She may project, in word and deed, a strong sense of righteousness that others may find off-putting.

She scored in the average range on A4 (Compliance) and A6 (Tender-Mindedness). A4 indicates that although Debbie can be deferential and compliant, she can also be competitive and confrontational; when pushed, she may push back. Her score on A6 indicates that she may not always be moved by emotional appeals from others. Although her A3 score says she is helpful, such assistance may not always be forthcoming, especially if she believes that the person may have brought the problem on him- or herself.

Finally, her Conscientiousness score is in the very high range, suggesting that Debbie is a very organized woman with a strong sense of personal organization and competency. She sets very high standards for herself and strives hard to reach them. All of her facet scores for this domain are in the high to very high range indicating that Conscientiousness is a broad-based definer of Debbie's personality. C1 (Competence) is very high, indicating that Debbie believes herself to be very capable and competent, and that this sense of self-efficacy generalizes to any context she may find herself in. C2 (Order) shows her to be very organized and methodical. C3 (Dutifulness) shows her to be dependable and organized; she will follow through on her commitments. C4 (Achievement Striving) shows that Debbie sets very high standards for herself and will work very hard to attain them. C5 (Self-Discipline) shows her to be focused in her efforts and not easily distracted from her goals. Finally, C6 (Deliberation) shows that Debbie is a thoughtful and careful young woman. She is not one to make spontaneous decisions; rather, she will weigh her options carefully and make measured responses.

These very high Conscientiousness facet scores, coupled with the low facets on Openness (e.g., Feelings and Actions) and the low A5 (Modesty) score may also suggest someone who has a high need for control over her environment and possibly the people in it. Given her low Neuroticism scores, this need for control is not defensive in nature (i.e., an attempt to protect herself against perceived emotional vulnerabilities). Rather, it stems from this young woman's clear sense of direction and purpose in life.

The overall impression that emerges from this profile is one of a young lady who is very ambitious and competent. Debbie has set some very high goals for herself (such as getting a full scholarship to college) and will do what it takes to reach them. What also emerges is a sense that Debbie may be perceived as somewhat aloof and distant from others. Although active in extracurricular activities at school, these endeavors may serve the purpose of obtaining recognition and success more than as a means of making friends and socializing. Her low Openness facets show Debbie to have some personal rigidity in terms of her belief and value systems which may serve to isolate her from others who may not conform to these personal ideals. Further energizing this rigidity is her high Dutifulness (C3) scores, which show her to have a committed sense of right and wrong. Whether she is involved with others is dependent on whether or not they conform to her values and goals; her average score on E shows that she can be comfortable with others or be alone. Her high Assertiveness (E3) and low average Compliance (A4) show her ability to be a leader and manage others in ways that will take her closer to her goals.

CASE HISTORY: JOE W.

The second case profile is for Joe W., a 45-year-old White male who is being seen in treatment for being a compulsive gambler. His profile is presented in Figure 3-2. At first glance, the profile seems to be rather "flat."

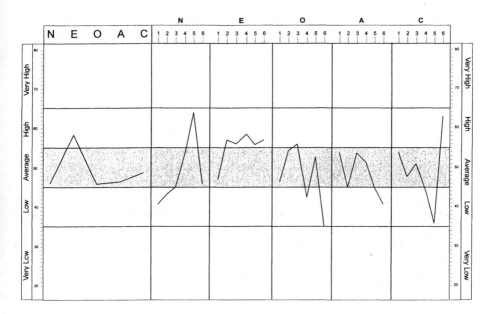

FIGURE 3-2.   NEO PI–R profile of Joe W.

However, this belies the many interesting features that are present in this case.

The overall N score shows an individual who experiences an average amount of negative affect in his life. He is as blue and distressed as most of us. An examination of his facet scales shows Joe to be low on N1 (Anxiety) and N2 (Hostility), suggesting that he is a rather calm and easygoing person. This low level of anxiety perhaps allows him to gamble without having to worry about the future. His high score is on N5 (Impulsiveness), indicating that Joe is frequently bothered by thoughts of doing things that he feels may not be appropriate. He experiences strong urges or temptations. His average score on N6 (Vulnerability) suggests that he can cope with these feelings relatively well, although there may be times when he feels overwhelmed.

A point of interest here. According to the NEO PI–R manual (Costa & McCrae, 1992c), high scores on N5 suggest that an individual will give in to their temptations. I have found from my own usage of the NEO PI–R that individuals high on Impulsiveness are indeed bothered by many urges, but whether they capitulate to them is a function of their scores on Conscientiousness, particularly the C5 (Self-Discipline) and C6 (Deliberation) facets. If an individual's scores are low on these facets, then it is likely that the person will give in to the urges. If scores are high, then the individual is unlikely to give in.

The domain score for Extraversion is in the high range, indicating that Joe is, overall, a sociable and engaging individual. He likes the company of others and is very spirited and engaging. E1 (Warmth) is in the average range, suggesting that Joe is discriminating in his approach to others; he can be formal and aloof or friendly and approaching, depending on the situation. A more consistent description is provided by the remaining E facets, which are all in the high range. Joe is certainly gregarious, wanting to be with others. When in the presence of others, he enjoys being the leader or center of attention. He wants others to look to him for direction. He is high on E4 (Activity), so Joe is energetic and active. He has a fast personal tempo to his life, always liking to be busy. High on E5 (Excitement-Seeking), he enjoys risks and thrills. He wants to be where the action is, preferably in the center of it. Finally, the high score on E6 (Positive Emotions) shows Joe to have a high degree of élan and spiritedness. He exudes much personal energy, and others may be attracted to his very upbeat and positive outlooks. People may consider him to be charismatic.

His average score on the Openness domain shows Joe to have some flexibility but also to have areas that need more structure. He is low on the O4 (Activity) and O6 (Values) facets. This, like Debbie, portrays an individual who is rigid and dogmatic. He has a clear structure that he likes to follow and a value system that clearly outlines what he needs to do. Joe scored high on O3 (Feelings), suggesting that he is open to his own feelings and those of others. He realizes the value of emotions in his life and is comfortable working with a wide range of them. Joe's average scores on O1 (Fantasy), O2 (Aesthetics), and O5 (Ideas) suggest that Joe does not have a developed inner world and may prefer to keep focused on tasks and people around him. His average Ideas score indicates that he may concern himself less with "the big picture" and more with the bottom line. He would appear direct and pragmatic.

Scores on Agreeableness are in the average range, suggesting that although caring and concerned about the welfare of others, there is a realization that people may not always be what they appear. As such, there is some caution in Joe's evaluation of others. Of note is his low score on A6 (Tender-Mindedness), reflecting a more hard-hearted, intolerant attitude toward others. Joe is not moved by emotional appeals from others, tending to interpret situational distress in more rational, cognitive ways. It would be of interest to evaluate this low A6 with his low O6 score. Perhaps this insensitivity may work out of his own value network. Given his high O3 (Feelings) score, it can be concluded that this coldness does not originate from some avoidance of emotions or fear of them.

Finally, scores on Conscientiousness are also average, indicating that Joe has some degree of personal organization and reliability that enables him to work successfully at goals and to aspire toward socially approved ideals. However, his Conscientiousness score is not so high as to indicate a narrow focusing on success that may filter out other endeavors (as noted with Debbie). He works hard, but may not bring his work home with him. His low Achievement (C4) score, coupled with his low Anxiety (N1) score suggests that he is unlikely to worry that the time and money spent on gambling will hurt or take away from his career status. Of note in this profile is the high C6 (Deliberation) score, which shows Joe to be thoughtful and cautious. Although he is high on this facet, his low C5 (Self-Discipline) suggests that Joe may not have the discipline and motivation to follow through on those tasks he knows he should. He can be easily distracted because he may lack the motivation to accomplish some of his goals.

Overall, there are some interesting points to be noted. First, as stated previously, Joe is a compulsive gambler. Compulsive behaviors, whether gambling, drug usage, or sexual, are all noted by scores on three facets: high on N5 (Impulsiveness) and E5 (Excitement-Seeking) and low on C5 (Self-Discipline) and/or C6 (Deliberation). Individuals high on N5, E5, and low on C5 and/or C6 all present some type of compulsive behavior. This pattern of scores represents an individual who craves excitement and thrills, is plagued by recurring thoughts to give in to those urges and who lacks the personal discipline necessary to control the urges.

The average scores on Neuroticism and Conscientiousness, as well as the high score on O3 (Feelings) indicates a good therapeutic prognosis for Joe. Unlike most psychotherapy patients, Joe does not have a lot of negative affect that can clutter and undermine therapeutic interventions. His scores on Conscientiousness indicate that Joe would work at therapy and follow through on the therapy interventions. His openness to feelings provides a doorway into his inner world; Joe is aware of his feelings and comfortable in discussing them. His levels of Extraversion make Joe a suitable candidate for group therapy. He would enjoy working with others and would certainly blend in well.

It is interesting to note that Joe is employed as a police officer. This would explain his lower scores on Tender-Mindedness (A6), Actions (O4), and Values (O6). As a police officer he has a clear set of values that guide his behavior. His clear sense of right and wrong, respect for authority, and appreciation for structure are all coincident with a career in law enforcement, where the legal system provides a clear sense of structure and organization. The lower A6 makes adaptive sense in this circumstance. Joe is a man who encounters a wide range of individuals in his daily work, most of whom may have broken the law. His low Tender-Mindedness may provide a healthy skepticism and degree of objectivity in evaluating the circumstances surrounding the events in which he is involved in.

CASE HISTORY: FRANK AND JUDY V.

In the beginning of this chapter I talked about the usefulness of self-report data. Although much effort has gone into (and continues to be invested in) developing scales to evaluate the validity of self-report information, the data to date suggest that self-reports are relatively free from deliberate distortions. However, there are limitations to self-report data. Even in good circumstances, there is always some level of distortion present because no one has a perfect view of him- or herself. That is why the use of observer ratings is encouraged. Observers can provide a very different perspective on a client; at a minimum, an observer rating indicates how the client is perceived by others and the kinds of impressions that the client makes on others. Certainly, observer ratings have their own limitations, but a comparison of a rating with a self-report can provide a broader assessment context for evaluating a client. Points of convergence between the two sets of assessments can provide greater confidence in the accuracy of the self-report. Areas of divergence may indicate blind spots or a lack of insight on the part of the client in terms of how they are perceived by others in their environment. Chapter 5 provides more details for observer data, particularly with couples.

The current case example involves a self-report by Frank V., a 35-year-old White male employed in the family business which is sales-based. He has a college degree. He is married to Judy V., a 38-year-old White female who is employed in the mental health field. She provides an observer report. They had been married for five years at the time of the assessment. This is the first marriage for him and the second for her. They have two children from the current union, and she brings two additional children from her past marriage. The two profiles are presented together in Figure 3-3 in order to facilitate comparison. For purposes of illustration, I interpret the self-report first, and then evaluate the wife's responses in relation to the self-report.

As can be seen in Figure 3-3, Frank scores high on the Neuroticism domain. This indicates an individual who is experiencing some degree of negative affect in his life. Worried and anxious, he may be unable to manage the stresses of his life. Individuals who score high on Neuroticism experience many somatic complaints and have a tendency to burn out when their jobs become stressful. In evaluating Frank's facet scores for this domain, he scores high on N1 (Anxiety), N2 (Hostility), and N4 (Self-Consciousness). Frank worries a lot about his life and finds himself easily frustrated by events. His high N4 score indicates that Frank has low self-esteem and may feel inadequate and inferior to others. The high score on Hostility indicates Frank's tendency to become easily frustrated and upset.

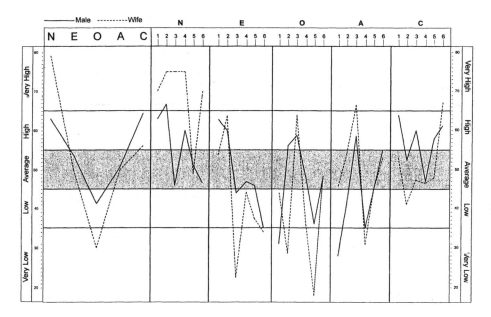

FIGURE 3-3. NEO PI–R profile of Frank V. along with his spouse's rating.

Determining whether this score represents a potential for Frank to strike out at others requires an examination of his Agreeableness and Conscientiousness scores. Low Agreeableness and low Conscientiousness would argue for the potential of Frank to act out his anger and aggress on others. However, in this case, his average level of Agreeableness and high level of Conscientiousness would suggest a good amount of impulse control.

The average score on N6 (Vulnerability) suggests that despite the presence of ongoing distress, Frank claims to be able to manage it appropriately. Although he does admit to having his "bad" days, overall his capacity to cope is commensurate with most other people's. His average score on N3 (Depression) and N5 (Impulsiveness) suggest that these qualities are less defining of his overall distress. It should be pointed out here again that high scores on the Neuroticism facets are *not*, in and of themselves, indicative of any type of psychopathology. An individual can score high on the Depression facet and not have a diagnosable condition. All these affects are within the *normal* range of functioning; they represent areas of distress and discomfort, not areas of psychosocial impairment and dysfunction.

Frank's score on Extraversion is in the high average range, suggesting that he enjoys the company of others. An examination of the facets shows

Frank high on E1 (Warmth) and E2 (Gregariousness), indicating that he is a very personable individual who enjoys the company of others. Interpersonal activities are very much valued by Frank and reflect an adaptive aspect of his vocational endeavor: sales. Frank scores low on E3 (Assertiveness) and E6 (Positive Emotions), indicating that among people he is not very assertive or "pushy"; rather, he will tend to follow the lead of others. His low E6 indicates a lack of spiritedness about him; he does not radiate energy or ebullience. Instead, he has a more serious demeanor.

His Openness domain score is in the low range, suggesting a lack of permeability between his inner and outer worlds. The low Openness suggests a need for structure and clarity as well as a desire to follow routine. Frank scores low on O1 (Fantasy), showing a very limited inner world; he is more concerned with what is going on outside of him than on responding to inner issues. His low O5 (Ideas) score shows Frank to be a very "bottom-line" type of person, not concerned with large theoretical issues but focusing on more immediate, practical concerns. He scores high on O2 (Aesthetics), indicating an interest in and appreciation of art and beauty. His high score on O3 (Feelings) indicates an openness to a wide range of feelings. High O3 indicates an empathic orientation as well. Frank's average score on O6 (Values) indicates that there are some values that are important to him and are not available for debate or modification. However, other values are more flexible and amenable to change and development.

On the Agreeableness domain Frank scores average, suggesting a somewhat positive orientation toward others that may be conditional. He likes others, but believes that some people may not be as trustworthy as others. An examination of his facet scales shows Frank to be very high on A3 (Altruism). He sees himself as being considerate and generous, certainly very willing to help others in need. He also scored in the very low range on A4 (Compliance). This suggests that Frank is willing to compete with others rather than cooperate and is capable of expressing anger when necessary. Scores on this scale indicate a desire to do things one's own way rather than acquiesce to the wishes of others. All the other facet scores on this domain are in the average range, suggesting that Frank is as trusting and straightforward as most people, and has a certain skepticism about the motives of others.

Frank rates himself high on overall Conscientiousness, suggesting that he sees himself as an organized, reliable, and hard-working individual who can be counted on to follow through on his commitments. An examination of his facet scores supports this broad-based interpretation. He is high on C1 (Competence), indicating a general sense of personal self-efficacy. The high score on C3 (Dutifulness) reflects that Frank strictly adheres to his own ethical principles and can be counted on to fulfill all his moral obligations. High C5 (Self-Discipline) and C6 (Deliberation) scores reflect an individual who is premeditative and focused. He carefully prepares his course of action and will find the motivation to pursue it until completion. His average score on C4 (Achievement Striving) shows that Frank has some degree of personal aspiration and will strive for his career goals. However, he has the capacity to step back from these job-related goals and indulge in more leisurely pursuits. In short, it is not likely that Frank would become a "workaholic"; he can set limits on the demands of his job so that they do not interfere with other aspects of his life, such as family. His average C2 (Order) score reflects some degree of personal organization.

From a larger, profile perspective, there are some points of interpretive interest in this self-report. First, low scores on E3 (Assertiveness) and A4 (Compliance) indicate possible passive-aggressive qualities. Here is an individual who, in a group, prefers more the follower role than the leader role. Yet, the low Compliance score indicates a preference to do things his own way. Thus, Frank may find himself caught in many conflicting situations, wanting to follow along with the group, but feeling that they may not be responding to his needs and desires to move in another direction. His high score on N2 (Hostility) shows that Frank may frequently wind up frustrated and angry. Although his A4 (Compliance) score shows him likely to express anger directly, high C5 (Self-Discipline) and C6 (Deliberation) scores suggest that any expression of anger may be very controlled and not fully convey the depth of frustration he may be experiencing.

Another point of interest is the apparent contrast between the N4 (Self-Consciousness) and C1 (Competence) scores. One may question how a person can feel both inadequate and efficacious at the same time. The presence of this type of profile pattern underscores the reality that these dimensions are indeed *independent* of one another. They are capturing very distinct types of dispositions. In this case, the high N4 suggests that Frank has some internal feelings of inadequacy. These feelings may make him appear defensive and he may shy away from some challenges because the real potential for failure may exacerbate his self-consciousness. The high C1 score suggests that within certain limited circumstances, Frank has developed a good sense of competence and ability at performing defined tasks. High scores on both scales suggests that Frank may not have the ability to generalize readily his developed competencies from one circumstance to another. Each new performance situation may find Frank anxious, worried, and insecure. He may need much reassurance and support in order to succeed. Once he does reach a level of success, feelings of self-efficacy will emerge and he will feel increasingly secure. However, movement to another performance situation will begin this process again.

Frank's high scores on E1 (Warmth) and E2 (Gregariousness) indicate a person who likes being with people, and others are attracted to him because of his easy demeanor and approachability. Because of his high scores on N1 (Anxiety) and N2 (Hostility), he may become dependent on others in order to find solace for his distressing feelings. He may look to others to provide solutions to his problems or to take the lead in addressing his issues. Yet, given his low E3 (Assertiveness) and high N4 (Self-Consciousness), he may not be sufficiently direct or forthcoming with others about his own needs and inadequacies. Thus, they miss his indirect and oblique attempts at sharing and he may wind up becoming frustrated with the relationship. As a result, there may be much turnover in Frank's relationships with others.

In evaluating the wife's (Judy's) ratings of Frank, it is clear that there is much convergence between the two profiles. Thus, one can be confident in the accuracy of the information provided by Frank. However, there are some areas of disagreement that provide useful interpretive material. Keep in mind that disagreements do *not* represent areas where Frank may be deliberately lying or distorting, or mean that the self-report is invalid. Rather, areas of disagreement may indicate that the respondent has blind spots in self-evaluation, or is not aware of the kinds of impressions he or she generates in others (Chapter 5 discusses the fact that when dealing with a married couple such distortions may reflect areas of conflict or dissatisfaction that the rater may be experiencing). Of course, the context of the rating needs to be appreciated as well. A rater may encounter the target only in a specific environment, or see the subject from a particular perspective. In such circumstances, more confidence should be given to areas of agreement than disagreement. However, a spouse's report can provide information that may not be available from other types of raters, such as friends or acquaintances. In this case, disagreements may be as revealing as areas of convergence.

For this couple, the one salient difference between the two reports is the magnitude of the ratings. This is most pronounced on the Neuroticism and Conscientiousness domains. Yes, Frank's wife sees him as experiencing negative affect, but much more than he admitted to himself. Yes, the wife sees Frank as ambitious, organized, and reliable, but not to the same degree as Frank perceives. Overall, Frank sees himself as rather closed, but not as impermeable and dogmatic as Judy sees him. From this, one may hypothesize that Frank may tend to minimize his weaknesses and maximize his strengths. Given his high score on N4 (Self-Consciousness), this may be a real possibility. However, it is equally possible that his wife tends to exaggerate Frank's weaknesses and play down his strengths. Observers do not have a "lock" on the truth and should not be seen as the ultimate criterion.

There are some specific areas of disagreement that are noteworthy. First, the difference on N6 (Vulnerability) indicates that Judy does not believe that Frank is coping as well with his negative affects as he indicates. Frank believes that he is able to cope with his difficulties as well as the average person. Judy believes that Frank is frequently overwhelmed by these stressors. In fact, Judy believes that Frank is more depressed (N4) than he admits. The difference on the E3 (Assertiveness) facet suggests that Judy sees Frank as much more passive and nonassuming. On the Openness domain, Judy rates Frank much lower on O2 (Aesthetics) and O5 (Ideas). Judy sees Frank as not at all concerned about artistic issues and very much concerned with the immediate implications of events. Frank is seen as having a very focused, narrow, and unimaginative orientation toward the world. On Agreeableness, Judy rates Frank much lower on A1 (Trust), suggesting there are real issues around intimacy and closeness with others. Finally, on Conscientiousness, Frank is rated lower on all of the facets except C6 (Deliberation). Most notable are the C2 (Order) and C3 (Dutifulness) facets. Here Judy believes Frank to be less organized and reliable than he contends.

PROVIDING FEEDBACK

The NEO PI–R provides a wealth of information about an individual. The information that is available is intended for interpretation by a professional trained in psychological testing. Thus, providing test takers with their interpretive reports would be inappropriate. However, there are times when it may be useful therapeutically to share the results of testing with a client. Feedback from the NEO PI–R may help provide a paradigm for clients to understand their presenting problems and issues. Sometimes clients suffer from distress that they are unable to articulate. The five-factor model can provide a framework for thinking about these personal issues and can facilitate personal insight. Second, the five-factor model can be used as a common language for both therapist and client in discussing therapeutic issues. The NEO PI–R may help frame the clinical dialogue in ways that the patient can comprehend and that are meaningful for the therapist.

To make such a disclosure would require a method of presentation that, while accurate, would be nonthreatening to the client and understandable. The NEO PI–R comes with two methods for sharing results with the client. The first is "Your NEO Summary," a standardized one-page form that provides a general overview of the client's standings on the domains. A reproduction of this form is presented in Figure 3-4. Each of

Your
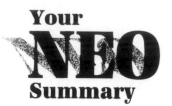
Summary

Paul T. Costa, Jr., Ph.D., and Robert R. McCrae, Ph.D.

The NEO inventory measures five broad domains, or dimensions, of personality. The responses that you gave to the statements about your thoughts, feelings, and goals can be compared with those of other adults to give a description of your personality.

For each of the five domains, descriptions are given below for different ranges of scores. The descriptions that are *checked* provide descriptions of *you*, based on your responses to the inventory items.

The NEO inventory measures differences among normal individuals. It is not a test of intelligence or ability, and it is not intended to diagnose problems of mental health or adjustment. It does, however, give you some idea about what makes you unique in your ways of thinking, feeling, and interacting with others.

This summary is intended to give you a general idea of how your personality might be described. It is not a detailed report. If you completed the inventory again, you might score somewhat differently. For most individuals, however, personality traits tend to be very stable in adulthood. Unless you experience major life changes or make deliberate efforts to change yourself, this summary should apply to you throughout your adult life.

Compared with the responses of other people, your responses suggest that you can be described as:

☐ Sensitive, emotional, and prone to experience feelings that are upsetting.	☐ Generally calm and able to deal with stress, but you sometimes experience feelings of guilt, anger, or sadness.	☐ Secure, hardy, and generally relaxed even under stressful conditions.
☐ Extraverted, outgoing, active, and high-spirited. You prefer to be around people most of the time.	☐ Moderate in activity and enthusiasm. You enjoy the company of others but you also value privacy.	☐ Introverted, reserved, and serious. You prefer to be alone or with a few close friends.
☐ Open to new experiences. You have broad interests and are very imaginative.	☐ Practical but willing to consider new ways of doing things. You seek a balance between the old and the new.	☐ Down-to-earth, practical, traditional, and pretty much set in your ways.
☐ Compassionate, good-natured, and eager to cooperate and avoid conflict.	☐ Generally warm, trusting, and agreeable, but you can sometimes be stubborn and competitive.	☐ Hardheaded, skeptical, proud, and competitive. You tend to express your anger directly.
☐ Conscientious and well-organized. You have high standards and always strive to achieve your goals.	☐ Dependable and moderately well-organized. You generally have clear goals but are able to set your work aside.	☐ Easygoing, not very well-organized, and sometimes careless. You prefer not to make plans.

FIGURE 3-4. An example of "Your NEO Summary"

---

the five rows corresponds to one of the major dimensions. When an individual scores in the high range for a domain (e.g., T-score from 55 and above), one simply checks the first box. Average-range T-scores (e.g., 45–55) are represented in the second box. Finally, the interpretation for low range T-scores (e.g., 0 to 45) are provided in the third column. These descriptions are clear and easily understood by individuals not familiar with psychological terminology. Further, the presentation is nonthreatening, especially for the more sensitive dimensions of high Neuroticism.

Another way that information can be shared with clients is through the computer scoring program. This flexible program provides many advantages for clinical use. First, individuals can complete the NEO PI–R at the computer itself. Information can then automatically be scored and profiles generated. If this is not possible, then responses can be manually entered. The computer program provides a number of interpretive options, including a section on clinical hypotheses. But for our current purposes, the computer scoring program produces a three-page summary report that can be given to the respondent. An example of this report is provided in the Appendix, where the results for Debbie K. are given. As can be seen, this report provides more information than the "Your NEO Summary" form. It can be generated easily when the computer scoring program is used.

Of course, for some clients feedback may be inappropriate, and it is the test user's ultimate responsibility to determine the suitability of the information for the client's consumption. However, this information can help reinforce the therapeutic alliance between client and therapist. For the therapist, the wide range of information provided by the NEO PI–R can help foster greater understanding and empathy for the client.

Particularly in the short-term therapy situation, NEO scores can be helpful in facilitating understanding by providing a wider personological context for evaluating the client's presenting problems. For the client, NEO scores can provide an opportunity for new insight and personal understanding. By being able to more succinctly voice personal issues, the client may come to feel better understood. Finally, the language of the five-factor model can provide a common bridge for client and therapist to use in discussing the issues that emerge over the course of treatment.

WHAT IF MY NEO PI–R PROFILE DOES NOT MATCH THE SELF-CONCEPT?

Whenever a test is given, there is always the possibility that the profile that emerges is inconsistent with the respondent's self-concept. There may be areas of agreement, but there may also be points of difference that seem very inconsistent with the person's apparent personality. When such disagreements arise, there are several points to consider.

There is always the possibility that the test is in error. Remember, error is everywhere! No personality instrument is infallible and there is always the chance that the test failed to capture the person accurately. If it seems likely that the test is incorrect, then you should consider accessing a different source of information about the client, such as an observer rating. Observer ratings provide a different perspective on the client that may be revealing. But before concluding that the test is in error, consider the following two possibilities.

ERROR IN TEST COMPLETION

First, there could have been an error made in completing the test, not so much that the respondent was distorting or "lying," but that the individual may have made clerical errors in filling out the forms. For example, responses on the NEO PI–R are arranged from strongly disagree to strongly agree. It is possible that a respondent may have reversed that ordering accidentally. Instead of indicating agreement, the respondent may have circled the disagreement response. One way of detecting this problem is to refer to the three simple "validity checks" at the end of the self-report answer sheet. Individuals are asked if they have completed each of the items correctly. Someone who answers "Disagree" or "Strongly Disagree" to this item may have made a mistake in responding.

Another possibility is that the person may have inadvertently shifted answers on the answer sheet, so that the response to question 15 was placed in the response space for question 16. Therefore, all remaining answers are moved down one. This would serve to skew the entire scoring process.

However, if such clerical errors can be dismissed, then an examination of the item content with the respondent may be in order. It may be that the client filled in the wrong response to several items. However, if this can be ruled out, then test score variation from one's self-concept may be an indication that the test has captured something new about the respondent.

RECONTEXTUALIZING THE CLIENT'S MOTIVATION

Once clerical errors can be ruled out, it may be informative to sit down with the respondent and review their responses on the scale(s) that seem in error. It may be that the client does not have a good understanding of what a particular facet scale represents. Keep in mind that the five-factor model has very specific meanings for each of its measured constructs. The usage of these labels may not necessarily correspond to the way the client is using language. For example, I use the NEO PI–R in a number of religious and pastoral contexts. Frequently I give the instrument to clergy members who usually score average to low on the Values (O6) facet. Frequently they are taken back by this score, believing that this means they have few, if any, values; that they are amoral or immoral. I am frequently told that they certainly *do* have values! What they may not understand at first is that the Values facet does not speak to whether one is moral or not. Rather, it examines the degree to which an individual has made some fundamental commitments to a worldview that he or she is not willing to compromise. Certainly clergy have made some decisions about how the world operates, and they feel strongly about those values. Thus the low to average score on Values makes more sense for this group when it is properly understood.

Educating the client in the language of the five-factor model is very important. It can not only clear up any misinterpretations of what scores represent, but it also provides a clear and concise language for discussing his or her own personality and the kinds of motivations that influence his or her behavior. Both client and therapist can use the same language for communicating.

Another advantage to reviewing the items is that it allows you to discern the context the client was using in responding to the items. At times, clients will say that they were evaluating their behavior in terms of their work personae, or how they are at home. Or they may have understood the item differently from how it was intended. In a study looking at disagreements between spouses on their NEO PI–R ratings, McCrae, Costa, Stone, and Fagan (1996) found that the context and referent behaviors used for interpreting the items were the most frequent reasons for lack of agreement.

A final reason for discrepancy may be that the respondent is doing things for reasons different than they think. It has been my experience that when you can rule out all clerical and interpretive reasons for a discrepancy, the most likely explanation is that the individual may not be truly aware of his or her motivations. The systematic evaluation of a person's behavior that is afforded by a standardized personality instrument may provide a different interpretation. For example, a client does very well in college, always in the top 10% of her class, always excelling in each class, always wanting to do more and learn more. She may believe that she is highly achievement motivated, and as such, high on Conscientiousness. Although Conscientiousness is related to academic achievement, there are many motivational reasons for excelling in school. If this woman scores low on Conscientiousness, then it may be that her success can be attributed to other sources of motivation, such as her high level of Openness to Ideas (O5) and Openness to Actions (O4). Such individuals are very theoretically oriented, like new and different adventures, and enjoy new experiences and new knowledge. So, her success may be due less to her ambitiousness than to her innate curiosity and enjoyment of novelty. Or she may be high on Compliance (A4) and does well in school because of the high expectations her parents have set for her.

Although certain behaviors may be thought of as prototypical of particular dispositions (e.g., Buss & Craik 1980, 1983), the reality is that any given behavior can express any number of traits, and a given trait can be expressed through any number of behaviors. We should never take behavior at face value. The merit of a personality assessment instrument is that it can provide insights into the individual that are unobtainable from other sources. If a test told us only what an individual can verify, then there would be no reason to give a test. It is exactly this type of discrepancy that lies at the heart of evaluation—the opportunity to gain an enhanced understanding of the individual.

APPENDIX   NEO PI–R feedback report for Debbie K.

——YOUR NEO PI–R SUMMARY——

Results For : Debbie K
Age : 17
Sex : Female
Test Form : S
Test Date : 03/28/96
Test Administrator : Ralph L. Piedmont, Ph.D.

The Revised NEO Personality Inventory measures five broad domains or factors of personality, and six more specific traits or factors within each domain. The responses that you gave to the statements about your thoughts, feelings, and goals can be compared to those of other college-age respondents to give a description of your personality.

The NEO Personality Inventory measures differences in personality traits. It is not a test of intelligence or ability, and is not intended to diagnose psychiatric disorders. It does, however, give you some idea about what makes you unique in your ways of thinking, feeling, and interacting with others. This summary is intended to give you a general idea of how your personality might be described. If you completed the inventory again, you might score somewhat differently, and other people might have different views of what you are like.

If you have any questions or concerns about this summary, please feel free to discuss them with the professional who administered the inventory.

A Description of Your Personality

The N Domain

Traits in the N domain reflect different ways of reacting emotionally to distressing circumstances. Low scorers are resilient, rarely experiencing negative emotions; high scorers often have strong emotional reactions. Overall, your responses suggest that you are very low on this factor. Specifically, you are calm, relaxed, and generally free of worry. You seldom feel frustrated, irritable, and angry at others and you rarely experience lasting feelings of sadness or depression. Embarrassment or shyness when dealing with people, especially strangers is not a problem for you. You report being good at controlling your impulses and desires and you are able to cope well with stress.

The E Domain

The E Domain measures traits related to energy and enthusiasm, especially when dealing with people. Low scorers are serious and introverted; high scorers are outgoing extroverts. Your total score puts you in the low range on this factor. You are average in your level of warmth toward others, but you sometimes enjoy large and noisy crowds or parties. You are as assertive as most women when the circumstances require. You have a low level of energy and prefer a slow and steady pace. Excitement, stimulation, and thrills have little appeal to you and you are less prone to experience feelings of joy and happiness than most women.

The O Domain

The facets of this domain measure responses to various kinds of experience. Low scorers are down-to-earth and conventional; they prefer the familiar and the tried-and-true. High scorers are imaginative and open-minded. You score in the average range. Your responses suggest that you are somewhat open. You have a vivid imagination and an active fantasy life. You are like most people in your appreciation of beauty in music, art, poetry, and nature, but your feelings and emotional reactions are muted and unimportant to you. You seldom enjoy new and different activities and have a low need for variety in your life. You are interested in intellectual challenges and in unusual ideas and perspectives, but you are conservative in your social, political, and moral beliefs.

The A Domain

This domain is concerned with styles of interpersonal interaction. Low scorers are hard-headed and competitive; high scores compassionate and cooperative. Across the six facets in this domain, you describe yourself as being generally average on this domain. In particular, you have moderate trust in others, but are not gullible, recognizing that people can some-times be deceptive. You are very candid and sincere and would find it difficult to deceive or manipulate others, and you are reasonably considerate of others and responsive to requests for help. You can be very competitive and are ready to fight for your views if necessary. You are quite proud of yourself and your accomplishments, and happy to take credit for them. Compared to other people, you are average in your concern for those in need, and your social and political attitudes balance compassion with realism.

The C Domain

Traits in this domain describe differences in motivation and persistence. Low scorers are easygoing and not inclined to make plans or schedules. High scorers are conscientious and well-organized. Compared to other college-aged respondents, your score falls in the very high range on this factor. You are rational, prudent, practical, resourceful, and well-prepared. You are very neat, punctual, and well-organized, and you are highly conscientious, adhering strictly to your ethical principles. You have a high aspiration level and strive for excellence in whatever you do. You are determined, persistent, and able to force yourself to do what is necessary. You are cautious and deliberate and think carefully before acting.

PROFILE ANALYSIS USING THE NEO PI-R

ORGANIZING NEO PI-R INFORMATION

GENERAL

The five domain scores and 30 facet scales found in the NEO PI-R provide a tremendous amount of information about a client that may appear overwhelming to the beginning NEO PI-R user. Keeping the names of the scales at one's fingertips can be difficult, and remembering the meaning of each scale even more challenging. It is always good practice to use this terminology as frequently as possible, not just when interpreting a profile. The language of the NEO PI-R is useful for conceptualizing the motivations of people, and you should try to use these labels for describing the behaviors of others. The more you use the terminology, the more adept you will become at both remembering and understanding the constructs.

No doubt when a scale provides a great deal of information, it is helpful to organize that information into meaningful, interpretive chunks. Such aggregation appreciates the naturally occurring covariance among scales, and enables a broader interpretation of the individual. Rather than focusing on specific traits and qualities, the test interpreter can discern larger trends and patterns in the respondent's life. Such "chunking" is referred to as either profile or typological analysis.

A typology is the flip side of the taxonomic coin (Bailey, 1994). A taxonomy enumerates the fundamental elements that describe some set of objects, while a typology identifies constellations of these elements that co-occur. For example, we can talk about an individual's desire to compete, high activity level, and proneness to anger; each construct tells us something about the person and begins to provide a sketching of their personality. Or we can see each of these traits as being part of some larger psychological organization that, as a whole, may reflect patterns of behavior and life outcomes that may not be discernible from an examination of each of the individual traits—say, the Type A personality (Friedman & Rosenman, 1959). This well-known typology represents an aggregation of traits that naturally occur and are easily identified. Most important, though, are the behavioral and health consequences associated with this pattern of behavior. These outcomes are not readily inferred from the individual traits that comprise this typology.

The typological approach is not uncommon in assessment. Perhaps the best-known measure of type is the Myers–Briggs Type Indicator (Myers & McCaulley, 1985). Here responses to questions are used to find a person's standing on four separate dimensions, which are then used to classify the individual into one of 16 different "types." Each type provides information about the person that goes beyond what each of the four scales reflect. The MMPI is another example. The information provided from the 10 clinical scales is frequently reported in terms of a "two-point" or "three-point" code, which reflects the highest two or three scales. These codes have been developed to provide an expanded clinical picture of the respondent (Butcher, Dahlstrom, Graham, Tellegen, & Kaemmer, 1989; Graham, 1990).

Similar research has been done with the five-factor model. Lorr and Strack (1993) cluster analyzed the NEO PI responses of a group of college students (cluster analysis is a multivariate procedure that identifies homogeneous subgroups of individuals based on similarities across a set of attributes, in this case NEO PI scores. For an expanded discussion of this technique see Aldenderfer & Blashfield, 1984; L. Kaufman & Rousseeuw, 1990). Lorr and Strack found six orthogonal sets of profiles. Each cluster contained a different combination of the five domains. For example, Cluster 1 contained emotionally stable, extraverted, and agreeable individuals. Cluster 2 included high neuroticism, low agreeableness, and high openness scores. The presence of such cluster types sets the stage for identifying NEO PI–based typologies; each may have their own psychosocial sequelae.

Hofstee, de Raad, and Goldberg (1992) provided a different approach to organizing and presenting five-factor data. They combined the five dimensions into their 10 nonredundant pairs (e.g., Neuroticism and Extraversion, Openness and Agreeableness, Extraversion and Conscientiousness) and constructed them as circumplexes. A circumplex is a circular ordering of traits around two independent, bipolar dimensions. This type of organization permits an evaluation of how the two dimensions blend together personologically. For example, we can discuss the meaning of high Extraversion or high Agreeableness; each has its own established construct validity, and high scores on these domains represent clear psychological dynamics. However, what does being high on *both* Extraversion and Agreeableness mean? What kind of person reflects high levels of each simultaneously?

Using self- and observer reports, Hofstee and colleagues (1992) provided descriptive labels for the entire circumference of the circumplexes. They referred to this as the Abridged Big Five Dimensional Circumplex (AB5C). In some ways, the AB5C model is the five-factor model equivalent of the two-point codes found with the MMPI. The value of the AB5C is that it provides a methodology for aggregating information from the five-factor model into brief typological-like sketches, which may have their own psychological significance. A portion of this information infuses the interpretive presentations in later sections. Readers are encouraged to obtain a copy of the descriptors for each of the 10 circumplexes for use with their interpretation of NEO PI–R profiles.

In the discussion that follows, the interpretive strategy presented is based on the circumplex approach of Hofstee and colleagues (1992), but not all 10 models are used. Rather, 5 particular two-dimensional models have been selected because of their theoretical and practical importance in applied contexts. As we saw in Chapter 2, research has been done linking the five-factor model to other theoretical and empirical personality models (see Table 2-3), and the results of these studies have indicated that some personality systems can be efficiently located within the two-factor space defined by various five-factor domains. The five particular two-dimensional models that are presented in the following sections are Interpersonal Functioning, Emotional Well-Being, Competitive Capacities, Character, and Psychotherapeutic Treatment Response.

Profiling NEO PI–R Scores

The interpretive models presented here are not circumplexes in the true sense of the term. As noted earlier, a circumplex is a circular ordering of traits around two independent dimensions. A summarization of such a circumplex is presented here: a simple 2 × 2 matrix that contains the personological descriptions of that area of the circumplex that blends the two factors together. Imagine a circle bisected by two axes, one running north to south, the other east to west (these axes represent the two independent dimensions contained in the circumplex and form a 90-degree angle to each other). The ends of these two axes represent the poles of one of the personality domains. The descriptive labels found here have already been presented in Chapter 2 in describing each of the domain scores. However, the interpretive descriptions presented here are taken from the part of the circle that is located 45 degrees from these two axes.

The two personality domains that are involved in these matrices are listed. An individual is considered high on a domain if his or her T-score is above 55, and considered low if the T-score is below 45. Of course, the higher (or lower) the scores, the more clearly an individual can be assigned a category, and the more characteristic the description is of the client's personality.

Individuals with scores in the mid-range on one or both of the domains are more problematic. If an individual has a single T-score in the average range (e.g., T-score between 45 and 55), classification is still possible although the description may be less accurate. If the respondent's other score is in the high range, then consider the average score to be low. Conversely, if the extreme score is in the low range, then the average score should be considered high. For individuals whose scores are *both* in the average range, no real classification is possible for the particular model. For such respondents, it may be more useful to place emphasis on the facets for each of the domains.

Interpersonal Functioning

Perhaps one of the most influential modern theories of personality is the Interpersonal Circumplex (Leary, 1957). Interest in interpersonal relations has a long history (see Wiggins, 1996, for a brief history), and current researchers have done much to extend this conception of personality to a wide range of psychological phenomena, including abnormal behavior, problems of living, and human social interaction (Horowitz, 1996; Lorr, 1996; Pincus, 1994; Pincus & Wiggins, 1990; Wiggins, 1980).

The circular ordering of interpersonal behaviors is anchored by the constructs of Dominance versus Submission and Love versus Hate. All of our interpersonal strivings are a combination of these two motivations. Given our social nature, these qualities cut across much of human endeavor. Wiggins and Trapnell (1996) showed persuasively the utility of these two dimensions across a wide range of perspectives, including evolutionary psychology, sociology, and anthropology. They argued that Dominance and Love are expressions of the higher-order constructs of Agency and Communion (Bakan, 1966).

Given the value of this model, it is not surprising that the two constructs that define this circumplex also define the first two factors of the five-factor model (in factor analytic studies the order in which these dimensions emerge is Extraversion, Agreeableness, Conscientiousness, Neuroticism, and Openness). McCrae and Costa (1989c) jointly analyzed measures of interpersonal behavior and the NEO PI and found that the domains of Extraversion and Agreeableness corresponded well to Status and Love, respectively. Domain scores from the NEO PI–R for Extraversion and Agreeableness can be used to evaluate the interpersonal style of a respondent. Definitions of the quadrants defined by these two domains are presented in Table 4-1.

The four "types" presented here speak for themselves. They describe very clear styles of interacting. Each has its strengths and weaknesses; no one style should be considered superior. Again, the more extreme a respondent's scores are on the Extraversion and Agreeableness domains, the better these brief snapshots define the person's style. Finally, this table, like the others to be presented, provides only broad descriptions of the respondent. If more specific information about interpersonal style is needed, then one should rely on inspection of the facet scales for these two domains. In any event, these tables are best considered as hypotheses about a client's interpersonal style that are in need of substantiation through the

TABLE 4-1. Interpersonal Styles Matrix

| | | EXTRAVERSION | |
		Low	High
A G R E E A B L E N E S S	Low	These individuals may experience difficulties in expressing affection toward others and may appear detached and unconcerned. They may tend to hold grudges. Such individuals may enjoy more solitary pursuits and pride themselves on their self-reliance. Some descriptors for this category are aloof, skeptical, unfriendly, joyless, cynical, and impersonal.	These individuals are dominant and self-assured. They tend to be assertive, forceful, firm, persistent, and self-confident. In a group they tend toward the leadership positions: They certainly enjoy directing and managing others.
	High	These individuals tend to be unassuming and self-effacing. In a group setting, they may feel uncomfortable with leadership roles. They are easily involved in worthy projects, but their support is given without much fanfare. Descriptors for this category include humble, modest, naive, lenient, and obliging. They are usually accommodating of requests made of them for assistance.	These individuals are warm and agreeable type people. They are accommodating, kind, charitable, and sympathetic. They enjoy being with others and interact with them in a very nonthreatening, compassionate manner.

use of additional, relevant material (e.g., observer reports, responses from other instruments, clinical evaluation).

Emotional Well-Being

Psychological or emotional well-being is an important aspect of psychological functioning that researchers have been interested in examining for decades (Andrews & Withey, 1976; Cantril, 1965). Many important questions revolve around this issue: What makes people happy? How does illness and disease impact levels of well-being? Do good things improve our emotional well-being, while traumatic events reduce it? Does well-being decrease over the life span? All of these questions speak to central issues of concern for all of us. Research in this area has provided several important insights into how our sense of well-being emerges. First, subjective well-being is very different from our objective life situations (Costa & McCrae, 1984). One would think that poorer health, less money, loss of sexual vigor and physical attractiveness would all contribute to making our lives less "happy," but this is not substantiated in the literature. Increasing age is not associated with lower levels of well-being (Costa, McCrae, & Zonderman, 1987; Larson, 1978). What the research literature does show is that levels of well-being seem to be quite stable over the adult life span (Costa, McCrae, & Zonderman, 1987), and that life's ups and downs, although impacting us in the short run, have little to do with our long-term levels of happiness (Costa, McCrae, & Norris, 1981; McCrae & Costa, 1988).

Given the stability of our levels of well-being, it is not surprising that this life view is strongly linked to personality. Research has shown that subjective well-being is a function of levels of Neuroticism and Extraversion (Costa & McCrae, 1980a; McCrae & Costa, 1983a). These two dimensions play the major role in how we perceive the world we live in and cope with the stressors we face. In short, Neuroticism reflects the amount of negative affect we experience in life, while Extraversion is linked to levels of positive affect. Note that positive and negative feelings are not opposite ends of the same continuum. Rather, they define independent affective experiences (see Watson & Clark, 1992). Although at any given moment one or the other affect can dominate our feelings, over the course of life we can certainly experience strong negative and positive emotions simultaneously.

The domains of Extraversion and Neuroticism also influence our experience of stress and our ability to cope with it (Costa & McCrae, 1980b, 1987, 1989b). Specifically, individuals high on Neuroticism tend to experience more somatic complaints although they do not experience higher levels of disease (e.g., S. Cohen et al., 1995; Costa & McCrae, 1987; Zon-

TABLE 4-2. Emotional Well-Being Matrix

		NEUROTICISM	
		Low	High
E X T R A V E R S I O N	Low	These are individuals who may not experience much negative or positive affect. They may appear always to be on an even keel, appearing unflappable and perhaps emotionally detached. Descriptors for this category include tranquil, placid, and unexcitable. These individuals may not respond to situations with much emotionality.	These individuals have a low sense of well-being. They can be easily distressed and overwhelmed by the pressures of the situation. Life may be perceived as subjectively difficult and they may feel unprepared for the pressures of life. Descriptors include self-critical, insecure, negativistic, fearful, self-pitying, nervous, and fretful.
	High	These individuals have a strong sense of well-being. They are hardy and adaptive, look forward to what life has to offer. Adjective descriptors for this category are courageous, strong, assured, confident, hearty, buoyant, uninhibited, and bold.	These individuals experience a wide range of affects. There are high levels of BOTH positive and negative affect. Life may be experienced as a series of emotional ups and downs. Sometimes their outgoingness may mask their own inner pain. Descriptors for this category include explosive, extravagant, excitable, and volatile.

derman, Costa, & McCrae, 1989). Individuals who are high on Extraversion appear to be quite hardy and happy and are able to cope well with stress. The combination of these two domains and their psychological significance are presented in Table 4-2.

A client's standing on these two domains can provide insights into the general happiness of the respondent, his or her levels of subjective well-being, and his or her ability to cope with stress. Clinical clients tend to have very high levels of Neuroticism. This makes sense; individuals who are experiencing a great level of psychological distress tend to seek out counseling for relief of symptoms. Interestingly, individuals high on both Neuroticism and Extraversion may not appear in need of treatment; the positive emotions characteristic of the extraverted individual may mask his or her need for treatment. Nonetheless, therapists with clients high on Neuroticism need to keep in mind that their efforts with such clients may impact only current stress levels. More intense, long-term therapy may be needed to bring about a more broad-based impact on the client's overall sense of well-being and to improve his or her ability to manage stressful events more effectively.

Competitive Orientation

With the publication of their seminal work on achievement motivation, McClelland, Atkinson, Clark, and Lowell (1953) provided a new perspective on individuals and their aspirations. The construct of need for achievement was found to have great heuristic and empirical value for understanding why some individuals and societies succeed and others fail (Bendig, 1958; Edwards & Waters, 1983; H. B. Gough & Hall, 1975; Piedmont, 1988b; Piedmont & Weinstein, 1994; Schmeck & Grove, 1979; Steers, 1975). Need for achievement is clearly located on the Conscientiousness domain, where personal organization and reliability reflect a capacity of the individual to delay immediate gratification so that larger, long-range goals can be met (Digman, 1989: Digman & Takemoto-Chock, 1981).

However, with time, research began to show that achievement motivation alone was insufficient to explain or anticipate competitive performance, especially for women (e.g., Horner, 1968, 1972; see Tresemer, 1976, for a review). New constructs were added in order to enhance predictability, for example, Fear of Success, Fear of Failure, and Test Anxiety. These variables addressed the ability of the individual to manage the inevitable stressors that any competitive situation involves and the sense of personal confidence and esteem necessary to support any failure that is encountered. This ability to manage threats to self-confidence and negative affective arousal is the domain of personality named Neuroticism. Both of these constructs were seen as essential for understanding competitive performance (Piedmont, 1988a, 1995). The Neuroticism by Conscientiousness matrix is presented in Table 4-3.

Adding the domain of Neuroticism (specifically, the facet scale N4: Self-Consciousness) to predicting competitive outcomes provides a new window for understanding how individuals approach and interpret achievement situations. It helps to explain why some individuals who are capable and have high aspirations fail, while others who are capable succeed. In the former situation there is the individual who is high on both Neuroticism (N4) and Conscientiousness. These individuals may aspire in an attempt to compensate for actual or perceived personal weaknesses. Their competitive endeavors are characterized as being very intense and focused. Although ambitious, their inability to manage their own feelings of inadequacy may undermine their ability to reach long-range goals, or to function well under circumstances of close observation.

In the latter situation are those who are low on Neuroticism (N4) and high on Conscientiousness (particularly the facet C4: Achievement Striv-

TABLE 4-3. Competitive Performance Matrix

		NEUROTICISM (N4: Self- Consciousness)	
		Low	High
CONSCIENTIOUSNESS	Low	These are individuals who may appear to have rejected conventional or socially approved definitions of success. These individuals are not competitive or ambitious, and are quite comfortable following their more "live for today" philosophy. They prefer to follow their own inner needs and may eschew notions of materialism. Descriptors include informal, noncompetitive, easy-going, and relaxed.	These are individuals who actively avoid competitive situations because the potential for failing may exacerbate internal feelings of inadequacy and poor self-esteem. These individuals are likely to experience fear of success, fear of failure, and test anxiety in response to achievement-related situations or tasks. Descriptors include impulsive, frivolous, self-indulgent, hypocritical, inconsistent, and fidgety.
	High	These are the prototypical achievers: Emotionally stable, capable with a heightened sense of competence and a drive to succeed. They set high standards for themselves and have the personal organization to attain those goals. They may appear to be overly dispassionate. Some descriptive adjectives for this category are: robotic, objective, poised, concise, mechanical, methodical, and self-disciplined.	These are individuals who are ambitious and competitive, but worry about the outcome of their efforts. They set high standards for themselves because they may believe that reaching them will be an outward sign that they are not as inadequate as they feel on the inside. Obstacles to obtaining their goals are responded to with anger and hostility. Adjective descriptors include particular, competitive, sore losers, intense, and highly focused.

ing). These are the prototypical achievers—those who set goals and work hard to attain high, socially meaningful standards of success. The effort these individuals bring to achievement situations can oftentimes compensate for weaknesses in ability. Their lower levels of Neuroticism (N4) indicate that they have high levels of self-esteem and can cope well with whatever setbacks they may encounter. Thus, failure may not be perceived as much of a discouragement, but rather as a barometer of how far they have progressed. They persist until they are able to overcome their challenges.

Scores on these two dimensions can be useful in assessing clients with job selection issues. Challenging environments attract those who have high aspiration levels. To succeed in such a context necessitates a temperament that can withstand the many stressors that arise, whether they are time constraints, task demands, or managing the inevitable failures that occur. Therefore addressing self-esteem issues, or working to improve this quality, would have tremendous benefits to high Conscientious people: It would help them remove obstacles to their own success. The more general domain of Neuroticism has important implications for a wide range of work-related outcomes and therefore needs to be considered in any performance context. Individuals high on Neuroticism tend to burn out (Piedmont, 1993), are rated poorly by supervisors on various aspects of their job performance (Piedmont & Weinstein, 1994), have a low level of reliability (Hogan & Hogan, 1989), and will tend to perform poorly on employer-given integrity tests (Mount & Barrick, 1995; Ones, 1993).

Character

Perhaps one of the more established terms in personality is the concept of "character." In one of the first textbooks on personality (Stagner, 1937), character is described as a subset of the entire personality that relates to moral or ethical activity. Allport (1937) captured this idea of ethical admirability in his review of the concept: "character is the aspect of personality that engenders stability and dependability, that is responsible for sustained effort in the face of obstacles, or works for remote ends rather than those that are nearer in time but of less worth. . . . *Character enters the situation only when this personal effort is judged from the standpoint of some code*" (p. 51; italics in original).

There are two components of this definition. The first is the effort to work toward long-range, socially valued and respected goals that have higher "payoffs," to delay gratification, and to overcome immediate obstacles. This quality certainly describes the personality domain of Conscientiousness. This dimension reflects an individual's personal organization and reliability, his or her capacity to delay gratification and aspire toward socially valued goals. Individuals high on Conscientiousness can be counted on to follow through on their obligations and commitments.

The second element centers on the notion of social evaluation of efforts. The struggle and the means by which the individual pursues the goal are marked by ethical and moral features. Such qualities may include a respect for others and a belief in higher principles of justice (either of a religious or patriotic nature). Such personal features usually constitute what is referred to as a philosophy of life. The five-factor domain relevant to these qualities is Agreeableness, which impacts our social attitudes and values (Costa, McCrae, & Dye, 1991).

One may have thought that Openness would be the relevant domain; after all, it has a facet scale for Values (O6). But an important distinction needs to be drawn here. Openness refers to our inner permeability, the degree to which outer events impact our inner lives and the ability of our inner dynamics to find expression in our outer behavior. Individuals high on Openness have value systems that are available for evaluation and modification; the inner world is always being "updated" as new information becomes available. Closed individuals have a system that is more rigid and fixed; the commitment to tradition and respect for authority restricts oppor-

TABLE 4-4   Character Matrix

		AGREEABLENESS	
		Low	High
CONSCIENTIOUSNESS	Low	These are individuals who are self-seeking and controlling. They are interested in gratifying their own needs in the here and now. They seek hedonistic fulfillment and may see others as objects to satisfy these physical needs. They may engage in subterfuge to gain their ends. They may be slow to recognize and respond to the needs of others. Descriptors include eogtistical, impolite, inconsiderate, thoughtless, rash, disrespectful, self-absorbed, and rebellious.	These individuals project a nurturing orientation toward the world; they will tend to see the best in others and the potential they may offer. Although they may involve themselves in social justice causes, they may lack the stamina and discipline to follow through on these involvements. Their efforts may be casual and appear self-indulgent. The flower children of the 1960s may provide the prototype here. Descriptive adjectives include tolerant, accepting, socially aware, sensuous, indulgent, and superficial.
	High	These are individuals who have set high standards for themselves and are ambitious. These individuals may have internalized positive values and are willing to fight for what they believe. They can be very determined and focused on reaching their goals. There is much passion in their efforts and they may be confrontative and direct when resistance is encountered in reaching their goals. Such individuals may love humankind, but distrust specific humans. Descriptive adjectives for this category include strict, deliberate, stern, and rigid.	This category represents individuals who are very concerned and involved in the plight of others. They are responsive to the needs of others, and will respond in helpful ways. When moved to action, this group may not respond in confrontative ways. Rather, they are willing and able to "work through the system" in order to reach their goals. They have the persistence and discipline to see their efforts bear fruit. Adjectives that describe this category include moral, respectful, reverent, polite, considerate, sincere, and understanding.

tunities for change. However, regardless of the amount of flexibility, the Openness domain does not speak to the *kinds* of values one possesses. Agreeableness, on the other hand, reflects a style or philosophy of life. Agreeableness reflects one's orientation toward others, an evaluation of how one comes to perceive the motives, intentions, and goals of others. Agreeable people tend to see the best in others and wish to reach out to them. People with low Agreeableness tend to see others as being disingenuous and self-oriented, and therefore view others with suspicion and distrust.

The combination of the Agreeableness and Conscientiousness domains is presented in Table 4-4. As can be seen, quite a wide range of character styles is represented. Low Agreeableness and Low Conscientiousness represents a selfish, manipulative style that tries to find immediate gratification for personal needs. Others are valued only in terms of what they can offer the individual. This combination is frequently found with the Antisocial and Passive-Aggressive Personality disorders (see Table 2-6). On the other hand, there is the high Agreeable–high Conscientious individual, who may be described as the antithesis of the psychopath. There is a strength of purpose and a compassion of action in these types of individuals.

Psychotherapeutic Treatment Response

The real value of clinical assessment is that it provides information about a client that the therapist can use for determining intervention strategies. Although the nature of the problem primarily dictates the type of intervention, to the extent to which there is room for choice (i.e., directive versus nondirective, group versus individual treatment, etc.), personality traits of the individual have important implications for both treatment selection and outcome (Costa & McCrae, 1992a, 1992c). Miller (1991) provided an interesting analysis of the five-factor dimensions and how clients evidence these qualities in the therapy session. This study provides the basis for the information presented in this section.

Although Miller (1991) noted that all five domains have something important to tell about a client's response to psychotherapy, he noted that Extraversion and Openness were most useful in terms of selecting treatment method. Those high on Extraversion may appear eager for therapy because they may value the interpersonal opportunities it presents. High Extraversion individuals have energy and enthusiasm as well as an ability to translate mental events into language. Openness, on the other hand, considers the patient's ability to consider novel solutions to their current problems. Individuals high on Openness can appreciate learning new things about themselves, can accept a wide range of their emotional experiences, and can respond well to the active imagination techniques that are part of many therapies. Low Openness individuals may not respond well

TABLE 4-5. Psychotherapy Treatment Matrix

		OPENNESS TO EXPERIENCE	
		Low	High
E X T R A V E R S I O N	Low	These are individuals who may be reticent in talking with others about inner feelings and emotions. They may not be responsive to a wide range of feelings, most of which remain diffuse and nonspecific. Descriptive adjectives for this category include passive, bland, apathetic, uninquisitive, inarticulate, and unimaginative. Such individuals may respond well to a direct, nonemotional approach, such as a cognitive-behavioral regimen.	These are individuals who have a wide, developed inner world They are curious about feelings and emotions, and may spend time naturally inquiring into their own feelings and motives. Their low Extraversion suggests that they may be somewhat focused on their own inner experiences. Adjective descriptors for this category are inner-directed, contemplative, introspective, and meditative. These individuals may value therapies that focus on inner dynamics, such as Freudian or Jungian analysis, Gestalt therapies, or hypnotherapy.
	High	These are individuals who enjoy the company of others, but may not be comfortable with expressing inner feelings, or difficult emotional topics, such as anger and sex. There may be a moralistic or self-righteous quality about these individuals. Adjective descriptors include verbose and pompous. Such individuals may benefit from a more goal-directed, problem-focused approach to treatment. Group therapy may be useful, but more as a support network than any type of encounter group.	These individuals also have a developed inner world, and are focused on ideas, feelings, and emotions. However, they also bring a strong need for socialization. They like talking about these feelings with others. They are into sharing and working with others. Descriptive adjectives include Inquisitive, eloquent, worldly, witty, dramatic, expressive, spontaneous, and adventurous. Group environments that are oriented toward personal revelation such as encounter groups or even psychodramas may provide an ideal therapeutic medium.

to efforts at exploring their emotions, and may want "therapy to be a reassuring, practical experience" (p. 426).

The matrix of these two domains is presented in Table 4-5. As can be seen, different combinations of these qualities may respond to vastly different kinds of therapeutic modalities, if available. The closed introvert, for example, may need a very direct, functional therapy that does not focus on emotions, ideas, or novelty. Conversely, the open extravert may enjoy a wide range of imaginative, creative therapies that combine interpersonal contact with fantasy-based exploration (e.g., psychodrama or Imago therapy). Assessing clients on these five personality dimensions may help increase the impact of therapy by matching clients to therapies that they are prepared to accept. In closing, it is sad to note that there are not that many treatments available to match with patient characteristics. However, our understanding of personality can give form and direction to efforts at developing new interventions that may be differentially sensitive to these personality issues.

Caveats and Conclusions

The matrices just described are provided to facilitate interpretation of the NEO PI–R by enabling one to evaluate various facet scales and domains in relation to one another rather than in isolation. This more configural process has much to commend it. However, these are only a few of the possible matrices that can be created. In a new adaptation of the NEO PI–R, the NEO-4, six different configural "styles" are identified and their interpretive significance highlighted. With increased experience and proficiency in using the NEO PI–R, users are encouraged to identify new interpretive patterns that are of significance in particular assessment situations.

The heuristic value of these matrices is found in their ability to outline the personological implications of NEO PI–R scores. They certainly provide a broader interpretive context to the scores. However, their ultimate benefit is for the NEO PI–R user who can integrate the important psychological aspects of their own unique assessment context into these frameworks. As they stand now, these matrices provide broad descriptions; it is up to you, the user, to provide the nuances and subtleties. In no instance, though, should these descriptions fill in for, or supersede, good clinical insight and judgment.

Finally, keep in mind that each of these matrices is, by definition, an incomplete description of personality. There are five major dimensions of personality, and any complete portrayal needs to include information from each of these areas. The interpretations offered for each matrix can certainly be meaningfully expanded by including information from the other domains. For example, with regard to the Treatment matrix, certainly Extraversion and Openness are important, but Neuroticism also plays an important role. As Miller (1991) noted, Neuroticism was an important predictor of treatment outcome; those with lower levels of negative affect responded better to any intervention than those with higher levels. Conscientiousness will also have much to contribute to deciding on the appropriate treatment. Those high on Conscientiousness will certainly work harder toward their treatment goals, and can be relied on to follow through on any assignments they are given. Thus, these matrixes are useful for highlighting important psychological issues, but do not forget that they do not provide *all* relevant information. Any interpretation of the NEO PI–R must include all five domains as well as an evaluation of the facet scales.

The following sections present a variety of case histories for interpretation. The reader is encouraged to consult the definitions presented in Chapter 3 as you follow along with the personality descriptions provided. Eventually, the reader should be able to form interpretations from the profiles directly without having to refer to the definitions presented in Chapter 3. Every effort is made to apply each of the matrices to the case, although such applications are not always relevant (e.g., using the Psychotherapy Treatment matrix with an individual who is not in therapy). It is important to keep in mind that the matrix descriptors are more characteristic of clients with extreme scores on the relevant dimensions than for those with scores nearer the mean.

SELECTED CASE HISTORIES

In this section, several case histories are presented along with their NEO PI–R results. Before turning to the text interpretation provided, I encourage you to try to evaluate the profile. In this way, you can apply and stretch your own interpretive skills and then compare your results with mine. Of course, you may find insights into these cases that are not discussed in the interpretations; the evaluations provided here should not be seen as exhaustive. Rather, every effort was made to capture only the most salient features. In making the interpretations, we start with a consideration of scores in each domain, always moving from the domain score to the facets for Neuroticism, Extraversion, Openness, Agreeableness, and Conscientiousness, in that order. Then we proceed to interpreting the individual's scores on each of the five matrics noted earlier.

CASE HISTORY: ROBERT R.

Robert R. is a 35-year-old White, married academic. He has a doctorate in the sciences and enjoys teaching and research in his area of expertise. His NEO PI–R results are presented in Figure 4-1.

As can be seen, his overall level of Neuroticism is average, with particularly low scores on N5 (Impulsiveness) and N6 (Vulnerability). In general, he experiences some negative affect but no more or less than most

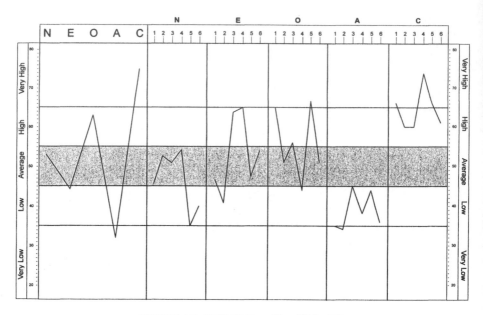

FIGURE 4-1. NEO PI–R profile of Robert R.

people. His low score on N6 shows that he copes very well with whatever stressors he encounters, both from within himself and in his environment. His low N6 score shows that he can tolerate frustration well.

Levels of Extraversion are just in the low range, suggesting that Robert prefers small social circles and may prize his solitude. His high scores on E3 (Assertiveness) and E4 (Activity) show that he exhibits much energy, having a quick personal tempo and being in the forefront of any group activities: He likes to lead and has the energy to invest in leadership. He scores lower on the affiliative aspects of this domain: E1 (Warmth) and E2 (Gregariousness). He may appear to others to be formal and distant, and he prefers to do things either alone or with small groups. He would not consider himself to be a "people person," although he may do well in social circles and be seen as quite surgent and charming. However, Robert would find such social endeavors to be difficult or energy expending activities. After much interpersonal contact he may seek quiet time in order to "recharge" himself.

Robert scores quite high on Openness overall, although there is some important scatter on the facets for this domain. High scores on O1 (Fantasy), O3 (Feelings), and O5 (Ideas) show an active inner world, both emotionally and intellectually. The high O5 is not uncommon among individuals with advanced degrees: These individuals enjoy dealing and working with ideas and intellectual interests. The high O1 score may provide additional resonance for his attraction for ideas. Robert has a well-developed inner world, which may provide a medium for creative discourse. The noticeably lower score on O4 (Actions) suggests that his Openness is less expressed in the outer world of actions than in his inner world of ideas and fantasies. The facets of O2 (Aesthetics), O4 (Actions), and O6 (Values) focus on the outer world of the person, while the facets of O1 (Fantasy), O3 (Feelings), and O5 (Ideas) focus on inner events. Notice that Robert's scores are much higher on the latter set than the former. The average score on O6 (Values) suggests that Robert, although tolerant of diverse value systems and willing to reexamine some of his own values, has a core set of beliefs that are "nonnegotiable."

Robert's Agreeableness domain score is in the very low range, and all the related facets are uniformly in this range. Therefore, Robert may be perceived as skeptical of the intentions and motivations of others, egocentric, and ready to fight for his own interests. Skeptical and critical: these qualities may nicely suit someone who is a researcher by trade. However, being hardnosed and suspicious may restrict the number of close meaningful relationships Robert has with others. Coupled with his low Warmth (E1) and Gregariousness (E2), Robert may find himself very much alone, which is where he may want to be. His low Compliance (A4), coupled with high Assertiveness (E3), suggests a high amount of dominance and independence, and he may use bullying tactics to get into that dominant position. Robert may not take well to being supervised by others, especially if such oversight involves the need for making changes (see O4). Robert may be confrontational and argumentative when provoked, as well as guileful and manipulative. These characteristics may work well for an individual researcher, but if thrust into a leadership position that requires a more collaborative approach, this reliance on aggression and dominance may become a liability.

Finally, the overall level of Conscientiousness is very high and all the facets are also in the high to very high range. Such scores portray Robert as being very ambitious, strong-willed and determined. He has a high degree of competence and goal aspiration. He is well organized and capable of following through on his commitments. This high degree of focus and direction in conjunction with a strong personal tempo (E4) suggests an individual who can project considerable personal energy and strength. This persona may not have the cheerful optimism of someone who is high on Positive Emotions (E6), a quality that others may find attractive and infectious. Rather, Robert exhibits a strong personal presence that more reticent and retiring individuals may find abrasive, and more insecure individuals may experience as intimidating.

The most salient aspect of Robert's profile is his low Agreeableness and high Conscientiousness. This combination reflects an individual who has a general wariness and suspicion of others as well as strong ambitions to reach his own goals. In an individual context these traits may work well, especially given his low sociability needs. However, if he were to move into a more interdependent, nurturing environment, he may be found quite abrasive.

Overall, Robert R. is a very energetic and ambitious individual who has no doubt developed clear goals for himself which he pursues in a determined and vigorous manner. He has many qualities that make him well suited for a research career. He certainly prefers more solitary pursuits and enjoys thinking abstractly. He is a natural skeptic, never accepting anything at face value. However, he may be perceived as overpowering and abrasive by others, not by intention, but because of the tremendous amount of energy he possesses. However, when provoked, Robert can be confrontational and may overreact to perceived threats. He may not always capture the interpersonal subtleties of the situation. Once injured, Robert may not seek opportunities for reconciliation.

Within the Interpersonal Matrix presented in Table 4-1, it is clear that Robert is in the Low Agreeableness/Low Extraversion vector. Robert has a rough, curmudgeon-like interpersonal style that may make establishing meaningful interpersonal relationships difficult. He may appear brusque and uncaring, finding it difficult to express much tenderness and compassion. Concerning the Well-Being matrix of Table 4-2, Robert falls into the low Extraversion, high Neuroticism vector. Although Robert may experience many successes in his life, there is an underlying sense of lowered well-being. Life may be seen as a struggle, filled with hurdles to be cleared. Although energetic and confident, there may be times when Robert feels that events have worn him down. Keep in mind that Robert's scores on Neuroticism and Extraversion are mostly in the average range, so that his experiences are not as negative as those of someone who has more extreme scores on these dimensions. Very rarely would one expect him to be overwhelmed by events and self-pitying. Rather, Robert may experience life as a struggle, but one that he feels he can still win.

Concerning his Competitive Matrix status, he is high on Conscientiousness and in the average to high range on Neuroticism. This pattern is characteristic of an individual who is very competitive and ambitious. At times Robert may take his competitive strivings personally, so that a given setback may be experienced as evidence of personal failure or inadequacy. In general, though, Robert is a strong achiever, capable of setting high goals and reaching them. He can become very absorbed in his work, and may lose sight of his interpersonal commitments. On the Character Matrix, Robert falls into the high Conscientiousness–low Agreeableness vector. Here we see an individual who has set high, socially valued goals for himself, and who may pursue them in a guileful manner. Given the drive and focus of Robert's life, as well as the importance he has attached to his own goals, reaching them becomes important. He is willing to do what it takes to reach these ideals even if it means cutting some corners along the way. Finally, if Robert were a candidate for psychotherapy, his high levels of Openness and low levels of Extraversion would make him an appropriate candidate for some type of insight-oriented therapy. He would certainly enjoy the experience of sounding his inner world. The inner-directed, introspective nature of these types of therapy are very consistent with his temperament.

CASE HISTORY: ANGELA W. ✓

Angela W. is a 42-year-old, White, married female who is diagnosed with a Borderline Personality Disorder. She presents with many problems, including suicidal ideations. She has repeatedly injured herself in a number of ways, including cutting and burning herself. She has been on drugs for 10 years and abused alcohol for at least 5 years. She is also a compulsive spender, having spent her husband's credit cards to their limits several times. Even when everything is confiscated, she continually opens new credit card accounts and then proceeds to "max them out." She reports being a victim of child sexual abuse. Her profile is presented in Figure 4-2.

Evaluating her NEO PI–R profile shows much variability over the domains and facets. Most noticeably, her Neuroticism domain score is off the chart. She is experiencing an extremely high level of negative affect which, as can be seen from her facet scores, spans the entire spectrum of this dimension. She is highly anxious, depressed, hostile, with strong feelings of inadequacy, she is impulsive, and does not cope well with any types of stress. Such individuals find themselves unable to deal with any type of emotional difficulty.

With such a high level of distress, I consider it important to evaluate scores on Conscientiousness, which serves as a type of "control" dimension. Conscientiousness assesses the ability of the individual to manage and organize his or her worlds, despite the presence of any emotional distress or dysphoria. Angela's very low levels of Conscientiousness suggest that she will seek immediate gratification and succorance for her needs. Her behavior will appear erratic, undirected, and impulsive. When she is in pain, she seeks *any* outlet for relief, whether it is spending money, attempting to hurt or kill herself, or abusing controlled substances. For Angela, there needs to be relief, now. It is not uncommon to find this pattern of high Neuroticism and low Conscientiousness among people diagnosed

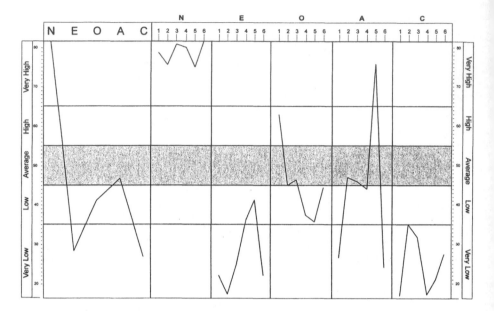

FIGURE 4-2. NEO PI–R profile of Angela W.

with Borderline Personality Disorder. But note the extreme level of functioning on these two dimensions; facet scores on these two domains are all
in either the "very high" or "very low" range.

Overall her levels of Extraversion are quite low, suggesting that Angela prefers to be alone. She has few social contacts and may feel isolated
and detached from others. She has no one to turn to for help, and therefore
seeks more solitary pursuits for self-gratification (e.g., going on spending
sprees). Note that the very low levels found with the facet scales reflect a
defect in her ability to establish social relationships and bonds. Scores in
this extreme high or low range are indicative of an aberrant level of functioning, especially when *all* the facets in the domain are extreme. Such ex-
tremity reflects more than just a strong tendency to express a particular
trait; there are real defects in functioning.

Concerning Openness, she again scores in the low range. Interestingly,
she scores high on O1 (Fantasy), suggesting that she has an active inner
life. This inner world may serve as an escape for her from the pain she experiences. It may be here that she is able to strike back at those whom she
feels have injured her in the past by acting out her anger on her mind's
stage. Her low scores on O4 (Actions), O5 (Ideas), and O6 (Values) shows

her to possess a high degree of rigidity. She prefers structure and familiarity. She is concrete in her thinking with a strong set of values which she adheres to strongly.

Agreeableness is in the low average range, but this score may be due to the very high A5 (Modesty) facet score. She is certainly not trusting of others (A1: Trust) and does not think warmly of others (A6. Tender-Mindedness). She is also just in the low range on A4 (Compliance), indicating that she likes to do things her own way. The combination of low Compliance and low Assertiveness (E3) presents the possibility of some type of passive-aggressive behavior. Individuals with this combination like to follow their own lead and have things done their way. However, being low on Assertiveness means that the individual may not have the capacity to speak up for herself in the presence of others. Because the unassertive person likes to take a back seat to others, when the group moves in a direction that the individual does not like, there is little recourse but to resist in nonconfrontational ways.

Angela's high Modesty (A5) score suggests that she may present herself in a nonassuming manner. Given her high scores on Neuroticism, such modesty may be used to protect her already impaired sense of self-esteem and value. Her modesty may help to keep others from looking critically at her and protect her from any additional psychological insults.

Angela's Conscientiousness was discussed previously. Such very low scores over the entire domain suggest a high degree of impulsiveness and self-seeking behavior. Individuals low on this domain jump at any opportunity that is convenient and holds the promise of gratification.

In examining Angela's scores in the context of the matrices, many additional insights emerge. Concerning the Interpersonal Matrix, she would certain fall in the low Extraversion quadrants, but given her average level of Agreeableness I would assign her to the "high" category. In many ways this category captures her behavior. She is certainly passive and shy. She may present as being timid and bashful. In a group situation she would prefer to have a very peripheral role. Although outwardly she may acquiesce to requests made of her, her low Compliance indicates that if she does not want to move in that direction, she will resist in nonconfrontational ways. The likelihood is that Angela would oppose trying new experiences given her low scores on the Openness facets (e.g., O4, O5, and O6). This pattern of results shows that Angela has a highly structured world with clear preferences. She is not likely to modify them or experiment with other options. Unless one approaches her through her narrow confines, it is unlikely that she would be cooperative.

On the Emotional Well-Being Matrix she can unambiguously be classified in the high Neuroticism and low Extraversion category. These are individuals with a very poor sense of well-being. Easily overwhelmed and distressed, these individuals may feel unprepared to manage the pressures of life. Angela certainly is negativistic, insecure, and self-critical. She experiences a profound sense of emptiness that is reflected in her many suicidal attempts. Her extreme scores on these domains, and across their respective facets, suggests a very dynamic profile in need of close clinical scrutiny.

In the clinical setting Neuroticism and Conscientiousness are key domains for evaluating the potential of an individual to act out their issues. Angela's high Neuroticism and low Conscientiousness signal a person quite likely to strike out unpredictably. Individuals with this pattern are very self-indulgent and impulsive. As I noted earlier, Conscientiousness serves as a control mechanism, evidencing the ability of a person to manage and direct their inner turmoil. For me, in many ways Conscientiousness is very similar to the Blocks' notion of Ego-Control (J. H. Block & Block, 1980). High levels of Conscientiousness reflects someone who is ego-controlled, that is, an individual who is constrained and inhibited, manifests needs relatively indirectly, and can delay gratification. Low Conscientiousness corresponds to the ego-undercontroller and reflects someone who can "manifest needs and impulses relatively directly in to behavior . . . to readily manifest feelings and emotional fluctuations, . . . to be distractible . . . and to live life on an ad hoc, impromptu basis" (p. 44).

When levels of Neuroticism are high, it is important to consider levels of Conscientiousness. When this latter construct is high, then one can have confidence that the respondent is not likely to act out inappropriately. This person would have internal mechanisms of control capable of keeping impulses internalized. Low levels of Conscientiousness should raise the concern about impulsive thoughts becoming expressed. If there are self-injurious ideas, then one must seriously consider the likelihood that the individual will act on them. If levels of Agreeableness are also low, physically assaultive behavior is possible. The extremeness of Angela's scores on these domains strongly indicates the likelihood of her striking out when under stress, towards either herself or others.

Evaluating Angela on the Character Matrix requires some subtlety. Clearly she is low on Conscientiousness, but her Agreeableness domain score is low average. It is likely that her average score is a result of the very high A5 (Modesty) facet score. All her other scores are in the low average to very low range. Because of this, I would place her in the low Agreeableness category. Her placement in this category certainly provides a useful description of her behavior: very self-centered and careless. Such individuals see things only in terms of what it means to them. There are some antisocial-type features in this category. This is typified in Angela's ongoing deceit and manipulativeness in acquiring credit cards and then consistently exceeding her limits.

Finally, on the Treatment Outcome Matrix, Angela falls squarely into the low Openness, low Extraversion category. She may respond well to a direct, nonemotional approach. However, given her emotional dysphoria and self-centered approach, she will certainly be a therapeutic challenge. In measuring therapeutic success, one may need to use a very modest measure. At one point in her treatment, she came in actively hallucinating and delusional. She went into a psychiatric hospital, but treatment there was not working well. She was transferred to a substance abuse program for about 3 weeks. She nearly died during withdrawal. When she came out of this program she was reasonably stable for about 1 to 2 weeks, but then reverted to her initial behavior.

Another interesting point about this profile centers on the substance abuse. As noted in the previous chapter with Joe W., compulsive substance abusers usually score high on N5, E5, and low on either C5 or C6, or both. This pattern was not found for Angela; she was high on N5 and low on both C5 and C6. Her E5 score was very low (although it was much higher than her other facet scores for this domain). That she does not conform to the typical substance abuse pattern casts some interesting light on the role drugs have played in Angela's life.

The N5, E5, C5/C6 pattern represents an individual who is impulsive and uses drugs as a thrill-seeking adventure. The drugs provide a "charge" for the person, a source of stimulation that offers a distraction from the more mundane qualities of the person's world as well as a source of pleasure and sensual gratification. Angela's personality pattern lacked the excitement-seeking aspect of this profile. Rather than a distraction or source of adventure, drugs may have been used as a tool for self-medication, an attempt to soothe and anesthetize the high levels of emotional pain she felt inside. The drugs may also have served as an immediate outlet for her self-destructive impulses. Despite heavy drug use and addiction, Angela may not be like the typical drug abuser.

Case History: Brian M.

Brian M. is a 40-year-old White male, father of three young children. He works in a white-collar management position and does not have much work ambition. Presenting symptoms are chronic depression with extreme pessimistic thinking. He is preoccupied with dying although he is not suicidal. He stays alive for his children. From an Axis II framework he was given the diagnosis of Schizotypal Personality Disorder by this therapist. Such individuals are characterized as having odd or eccentric speech and/or beliefs. As we saw in Chapter 2, Table 2-6, such individuals tend to have high scores on Neuroticism and low scores on Extraversion and Agreeableness. We want to see whether this pattern is present with Brian.

Completely enraged with his family of origin, he sees his parents as very horrible people, imbued with evil. In reality, they are very average people. According to his spouse he interacts with them very well, although he maintains these very bizarre thoughts and fantasies about them. He has been on a variety of antidepressants, but does not respond well to them. He took the NEO PI-R toward the end of treatment when he was being seen for marital counseling. His profile is presented in Figure 4-3.

As can be seen, Brian scores very high on Neuroticism, with all scales elevated except N5 (Impulsiveness). He clearly experiences a high level of negative affect, including anxiety, anger, depression, and low self-esteem. He does not cope well with these feelings, easily feeling overwhelmed by both environmental stress and the strong negative affects he experiences.

His overall Extraversion score is very low, suggesting a very restricted interpersonal circle. He is reticent, desiring to avoid group activities, and when in the presence of others would prefer to have a low profile, being very passive. He has a very slow personal tempo; he likes to take the course of events at a leisurely pace.

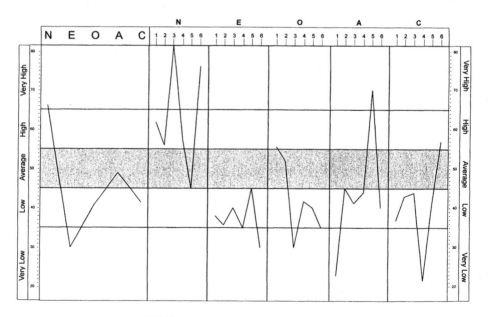

FIGURE 4-3. NEO PI-R profile of Brian M.

His overall Openness score is low, suggesting a closed, emotionally rigid individual. His very low O3 (Feelings) score shows that he has very restricted affect. There are many types of emotions that he does not like to deal with or express. This accounts for the noticeable degree of flat affect that characterizes him. Not very empathic, he is unable to resonate with the feelings of others. The low O4 (Actions), O5 (Ideas), and O6 (Values) suggests a very rigid individual who prefers much structure and routine. He is oriented to the bottom line, and tends to focus on a limited number of topics. Curiously, his O1 (Fantasy) score is in the high range. This suggests a well-developed and active inner life. This is consistent with the idiosyncratic and bizarre thoughts he maintains about his family of origin. All of the fantasies that he has about them are certainly well developed and reflect this capacity to elaborate and enhance daily experiences.

Brian's overall Agreeableness score is in the average range, although there is a high level of intertest scatter on the facets. Modesty (A5) is his highest score. He presents himself as very nonassuming and humble; he appears very nonthreatening. However, he is very low on Trust (A1), Tender-Mindedness (A6), and Altruism (A2). This pattern portrays an individual who is very suspicious of others and their motives. He does not care much for people in general and would not exert himself to reach out to help if called on. People may be seen as very threatening and hurtful.

Finally, Brian's overall Conscientiousness is low, suggesting an individual with a lackadaisical attitude, who may seek immediate gratification for his needs, and who may have a tendency to act out. His lowest facet scale is C4 (Achievement). He certainly is not a competitive individual, does not set high standards for himself, and may not have a sense of direction. This is consistent with his very unconcerned attitudes about work and career. He really does not care much for work and is not driven to succeed there. He is low in Competence (C1) and Order (C2), suggesting that he feels worthless and unable to successfully meet the challenges he may encounter. He is not fastidious or well organized. His low Dutifulness (C3) score suggests that he does not follow through on his commitments and obligations. Interestingly, he scores high on Deliberation (C6). Brian certainly will not act without thinking things through; he tries to be careful. Coupled with his low Impulsiveness (N5) score, one can be confident that Brian has some control over his impulses. Although it cannot be ruled out that at some point Brian may act against his parents or himself, such an outburst will not be a situationally provoked event. Rather, Brian will spend some time thinking through his actions.

Overall, the profile here matches the kinds of symptoms and issues Brian presents. The bizarre fantasies about his family and the idiosyncratic ideation he presents when discussing them may be working out of his high

Fantasy (O1) score. The flat affect or anhedonia is certainly characteristic of someone low on Feelings (O3). The pattern of high Neuroticism and low Extraversion is indicative of someone who is experiencing much distress and dissatisfaction in his or her life. There is little positive feeling or sense of well-being. Interpersonally, Brian has a Scrooge-like attitude toward people. He is untrusting and uncaring, perhaps perceiving others as potential threats. His high Modesty (A5) score coupled with his low facet scores on Extraversion would suggest that he presents himself in a very nonthreatening manner. He tends to keep to himself and takes a back seat in group activities. His nonassuming demeanor belies the churning emotions that exist below the surface.

From a Character perspective, Brian takes a selfish orientation toward life, concerned more with his own issues than with those who surround him. His low O6 (Values) facet score suggests that Brian has a very clear ideological framework from which he operates, although his low C3 (Dutifulness) score suggests that he may not be consistent in how he applies these values. Still, it would be important to try to understand his value network and its related imperatives. This would be important in understanding how he orients himself to the world.

From a therapeutic perspective, Brian presents numerous challenges. He is very concrete and emotionally limited. Although his fantasy world is rich, Brian may not be able to fully express the emotions that play themselves out in his mind's eye. A therapist would need to take a very focused and directed approach to Brian. His high levels of Neuroticism certainly complicate whatever treatment is employed. There is tremendous dysphoria indicated, and this may not improve greatly over the course of therapy. It may be possible to tactically manage issues with Brian's family of origin and his current marital issues. However, on a strategic level, there may always be a strong sense of inadequacy, anger, depression, and distrust.

His detached interpersonal style is another factor that undermines improvement. Brian's preference to form few relationships deprives him of important opportunities to draw on coping resources. The presence of others can help provide an additional sense of support and succorance for Brian's negative feelings and hostile attitudes toward his family. His reluctance to make such contacts isolates him and encourages his further retreat into his overpersonalized inner world.

It is interesting to note that the overall profile matches what one would expect for a Schizotypal Disorder. He scores very high on the Neuroticism facets, low on all the Extraversion facets, and low on all but one of the Agreeableness facets. The high Modesty (A5) score is interesting here because it is so distinct from the other facets on this domain and it also serves to give him an overall average level on the domain. In evaluating the high A5 score, one should turn to the N4 (Self-Consciousness) score, which is in the high range. His desire not to speak out about himself may be due to his perceived negative self-image. Thus his modesty may be a consequence of his belief that he has nothing of value to share with others. The low Trust (A1) and Tender-Mindedness (A6) scores are certainly characteristic of the Schizotypal, who may fear others and seek punishment for those who may be threateaning.

The high Fantasy (O1) and low Ideas (O5) scores are also relevant here to the Axis II issues. Certainly Brian has an active inner world where issues, people, and experiences are all elaborated on. These internal explorations may lead to the development of bizarre ideas and feelings, but the internal rigidity characterized by the low scores on the other facets suggests that such ideas may be difficult to remove.

Case History: Barbara W. ✓

Barbara is a 35-year-old married woman who is very depressed and resentful. She came into therapy to deal with sexual harassment in the workplace. She is very unhappy with her marriage and her life. She is employed as an office worker, and is very well organized and successful in this position. She is appreciated by her superiors and well thought of by her colleagues. She took the NEO PI–R prior to revealing the sexual issues at work. Her response to therapy (which was cognitive-behavioral) has been successful, and she is able to manage her issues of despair and feelings of sexual abuse. She is now moving toward dealing with more long-term issues concerning her ongoing feelings of emptiness. She is very duty-driven and lives her life by obligation. She needs to learn how to take time for herself. When she was very depressed, the only thing that kept her alive was her responsibility for her children. Marital therapy is effective in helping to obtain more emotional support from her husband. Her profile is presented in Figure 4-4.

As can be seen, Barbara has an extremely high level of Neuroticism, suggesting a tremendous amount of negative affect covering a broad range of dysphoric feelings. All of her facets are in the high to very high range, indicating that her negative feelings are indeed pervasive. She is depressed and anxious, easily angered, possesses low self-esteem and certainly is being bothered by recurring negative thoughts. Most important, though, is the fact that her Vulnerability score is off the chart; she certainly feels that she cannot manage the stresses that she confronts. She is easily overwhelmed by the pressures of her life as well as her inner turmoil.

On Extraversion Barbara scores very low, indicating a solitary orientation. She prefers to keep to herself, having few friends and social con-

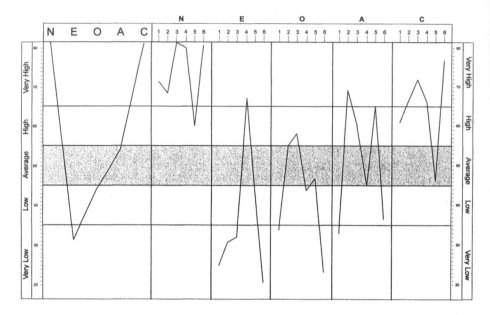

FIGURE 4-4. NEO PI–R profile of Barbara W.

tacts. She projects a stoical image to others, having few positive feelings or emotions. Interestingly, Barbara scores very high on E4 (Activity), indicating a rapid personal tempo. She likes to stay on the move doing things. The combination of very high Neuroticism and very low Extraversion indicates an individual with a rather poor sense of well-being. She feels insecure and vulnerable; she finds little support and comfort from her life. No doubt there is a strong feeling of emptiness and despair.

Scores on Openness are also low overall, suggesting a degree of personal rigidity. Barbara scores low on Fantasy (O1), Actions (O4), and Values (O6). This indicates an individual who very much desires structure and form. She has a clear sense of right and wrong, possibly appearing to others as conventional and conservative. There is little imagination, but more of a down-to-earth, black-and-white orientation. It is interesting to note her high score on Activity (E4). She likes to stay busy, but the low score on Actions (O4) indicates that she invests that energy in a very circumscribed routine. Such a restricted range of activity may help bind the high levels of negative affect that she experiences.

Barbara scores in the high range on Aesthetics (O2) and Feelings (O3). The latter score indicates that Barbara is open to a wide range of feelings, and would suggest that she experiences her negative affect with a greater level of sensitivity than someone who is low on this facet. The Aesthetics score suggests a further ability to be emotionally moved by artistic experiences. The imagination and creativity suggested by a high score on this facet stand in contrast to her low scores on Values and Actions. This combination of scores suggests that Barbara, although appearing formal and staid, can be moved by certain imagery, perhaps of a religious nature.

Barbara's score on Agreeableness is in the high average range, indicating that she does feel some compassion for others, but these feelings of care are certainly guarded. She scores low on Trust (A1) and Tender-Mindedness (A6), indicating a suspiciousness of the motives of others. She believes that the pain others may experience is likely to be a product of their own misplaced efforts. She scores high on Straightforwardness (A2), indicating that Barbara tends to be frank and sincere toward others. It is interesting that her Assertiveness (E3) score is so low. This suggests that Barbara is not proactive in sharing her thoughts. She is rather shy and reticent in social situations; one may have to directly query her to find out what her feelings are. Once asked, she would be forthcoming, but an invitation needs to be offered.

The combination of high scores on Straightforwardness (A2) and Altruism (A3) and the low score on Assertiveness (E3) may mean that Barbara is vulnerable to exploitation. She may wish to reach out to others less out of a sense of social responsibility than out of compassion. She may feel compelled to reach out altruistically to others, even though she knows that they may take advantage. Perhaps her high levels of Neuroticism may prevent her from appropriately establishing boundaries to her helping behavior. She may be seeking her own personal sense of solace from helping others, and the strength of her needs for reassurance and comfort may override her natural suspiciousness.

Barbara also scores high on Modesty (A5), indicating that she is modest and unassuming. Again, the picture that is emerging of Barbara is of a woman who is quiet and reticent. She prefers to stay in the background and not attract any attention to herself. If offended, she may not respond directly. Instead, she may wait for some invitation to speak. Then she may voice her issues. In short, one should not mistake her outward quiet and calm for assent. There may be many issues percolating within her that are not readily apparent. This is evidenced in the therapeutic situation where the most pressing issue for her was the apparent sexual discrimination she experienced at her job. These events distressed her greatly, yet it was some time into the treatment process before she brought it up. Some of this reticence may be a function of her low Trust; she needs to feel safe and secure before she shares her intimate feelings.

Her low average score on Compliance (A4) suggests that Barbara would prefer to do things her own way. Given her strong commitment to her value system and her high need for structure and routine, it may be very important that events proceed in ways that are consistent with her expectations. A relatively low Compliance score in conjunction with a low Assertiveness score may indicate passive-aggressive tendencies as well. The strong need to follow her routine coupled with an equally strong need to shrink from social leadership roles creates a conflict for Barbara when events begin to move in directions that are inconsistent with her values. Rather than initiating some response, she is prone to acquiesce, not wanting to create a "situation." She may therefore try to sabotage the process in an oblique manner.

Barbara scored high on Altruism (A3), indicating an active concern for the welfare of others. This is interesting given her very low scores on Trust (A1) and Tender-Mindedness (A6). This may be indicative of Barbara's commitment to "duty," an acute awareness of social responsibilities that are defined by her value system. She helps others not out of a feeling of deep compassion or empathic concern (even though she does score high on O3—Openness to Feelings). Rather, she has a sense of obligation that needs to be fulfilled. Her assistance is more perfunctory than compassionate.

On Conscientiousness Barbara scores extremely high, suggesting some serious psychological issues. She has a high degree of personal responsibility and organization. She sets very high standards for herself and strives hard to attain them. Although she may experience a number of impulsive ideas, her high level of Conscientiousness argues against her acting on them without due consideration of their consequences. She has a high degree of personal competence and is well organized. Interestingly, her lowest score on this domain is C5, Self-Discipline. She believes that at times she is distracted from her obligations and indulges herself. This may be a source of guilt in her life, given her high levels of Depression, Impulsiveness, and Vulnerability, as well as her strong attachment to her value system. Given her high score on Achievement Striving (C4), she no doubt sets very high, perhaps unrealistically high, standards for herself to attain. She may not feel that she is able to reach these goals all the time and one may want to evaluate to what degree she may be self-punishing.

Her high score on Dutifulness (C3) fits well into the developing picture of this client. Individuals high on this scale follow through on their commitments. This scale represents the "superego" function; individuals scrupulously adhere to their moral principles. The combination of low O6 (Values), low O4 (Actions), high A3 (Altruism), high C3 (Dutifulness) and high C4 (Achievement) all portray a moralistic, rigid, determined individual who aspires to very high, perhaps unrealistic, standards. There may be an unrelenting quality to her endeavors, given the high E4 (Activity) and high C4 (Achievement Striving) scores. As noted in the description of her case, she is very duty-bound, leaving little or no room for her own needs and desires. She was able to thwart her suicidal issues by thinking of her children. No doubt, she was reminded of what a "good mother" should be like.

An interesting combination in this profile is the high score on N4 (Self-Consciousness) and the high score on C1 (Competence). The former indicates a low level of self-esteem and feelings of inferiority. Yet she scores high on Competence, suggesting a good sense of self-efficacy. Such a combination of scores usually suggests an individual who has found a particular niche in which they feel very comfortable and competent, often receiving much recognition for his or her performance. However, these individuals may be very reluctant to move from this environment to another, new one. Increased responsibilities, new job reporting structures, and so on, can all induce a high degree of anxiety and feelings of inadequacy. Expertise in one situation is not perceived as generalizable to new situations. These individuals feel very uncomfortable with the change, but over time will recapture their feelings of competence in this new niche, until the next time they have to move (the Impostor Phenomenon is a related construct; see Clance, 1985; Clance & Imes, 1978).

Another point of interest in this profile is the combination of high Self-Consciousness and high Achievement. This is a very powerful combination of constructs. High achievement is associated with individuals setting higher personal standards for themselves. They aspire to reach goals that are socially valued. High achievers can become quite absorbed in their efforts and ambitions and find success to be quite satisfying and rewarding. However, a corresponding high score on Self-Consciousness adds another dimension to these aspirations. Because of the underlying feelings of inadequacy, the competitive strivings become an attempt by the individual to find redemption for their perceived inadequacies. The very high standards such individuals set for themselves are in compensation for the weaknesses they feel.

As was noted in the "Competitive Performance" section, individuals with high N4 and high C4 perceive success as bringing relief from their inner pangs of deficiency, but this respite is only temporary. Soon the need for new successes rises and the quest to achieve begins again. In this process, failure becomes an awful experience to be avoided because it provides some external confirmation of the weaknesses kept hidden within. This is similar to Horney's (1950) notions of the "search for glory" (p. 23), the neurotic's attempt to reach the comprehensive neurotic solution—that fantasied image that, when attained, will solve all the problems. But this image of success is unattainable. So the individual high on these two facets pursues his or her goals with the affective intensity of a desperate individual. Barbara may be looking for validation and approval through her efforts to live up to high, socially commendable criteria of success. Being "the best" is more than just personal development; it is an effort to find personal justification. Her successes provide an emotional high point, her failures an affective nadir.

From a therapeutic standpoint, treatment needs to consider that such high levels of affective dysphoria may not be entirely ameliorated. There may always be high levels of negative affect, whether depression, anxiety, self-consciousness, or anger. These feelings are characteristic of Barbara, and treatment should focus on techniques that can help her deal better with her internal distress. The high levels of Conscientiousness are an asset for the therapist. Barbara will work hard toward her therapeutic goals and can be counted on to follow through with the treatments on her own time. Her lower levels of Openness suggest that a more focused, behavioral path may be most effective. Although she is open to experiencing her emotions, whether she feels comfortable speaking about them may be a function of her values and level of trust and comfort with the therapist. Marital therapy may be ideal for Barbara because it gives her a much needed interpersonal context with an individual with whom she should have some level of trust and comfort.

It should be pointed out that despite the presence of so much affective and personal distress, Barbara is able to function in her environment. Although one may be tempted to see much more impairment in such extreme scores, it is important to remember that the NEO PI–R is a measure of *normal* personality dynamics. High scores on these domains are not direct indicators of psychopathological functioning. Although most of the cases presented here are clinically oriented and therefore such high scores are not surprising, it must be remembered that one can have high scores on these domains and *not* have any type of discernible pathology.

CASE HISTORY: BEVERLY N.

Beverly N. is a 38-year-old woman seen in treatment for social phobia. She has been diagnosed by her therapists as having a severe Avoidant Personality Disorder. When she first entered treatment, her avoidance behaviors were so severe she would vomit before going to her part-time job several times each week. She was terrified of facing the public, even though she was a receptionist. Beverly dropped out of college because she was unable to stand up and give presentations in class. She is a religious individual who is very conscientious. She is a good wife and mother. Behavioral therapy and cognitive work was effective for the avoidance behavior. Her NEO PI–R profile is presented in Figure 4-5.

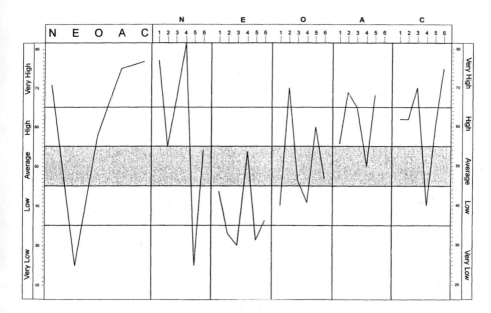

FIGURE 4-5. NEO PI–R profile of Beverly N.

As can be seen, Beverly scores very high on Neuroticism, indicating a large amount of negative affect. The facet scores indicate that this negativity is centered around issues of Anxiety, Depression, and Self-Consciousness. Interestingly, she scores in the average range on Vulnerability, indicating some capacity to cope with the stressors she encounters. Thus, although suffering from a severe social phobia (high N4: Self-Consciousness), she is able to manage these profound feelings sufficiently to obtain and keep her part-time job.

On Extraversion Beverly scores very low, suggesting a very detached, socially isolated world. She prefers to have very few interpersonal contacts, and would not be considered very "approachable" (low scores on E1, Warmth and E6, Positive Emotions). She is very passive, although she has an average level of personal energy (E4, Activity). Like Angela W., Beverly does not experience much personal well-being; there is not much perceived quality of life.

Overall Openness is in the high range, suggesting a degree of personal flexibility and originality. Beverly is particularly high on Aesthetics, easily moved by the arts. She is also high on Ideas (O5), suggesting that she likes to look at the "big picture"; she is theoretically oriented and broad based in her thinking. Her average score on O6 (Values) suggests that Beverly has some values that are important to her and toward which she is firmly committed. However, there are other aspects of her belief system that are much more flexible and open to evaluation and change. She is low on O4 (Actions), indicating a desire for structure and clarity. She prefers to follow an established routine and does not do well in unstructured situations. She is also low on O1 (Fantasy), which indicates that Beverly prefers to keep her mind on the tasks at hand.

She scores in the very high range on Agreeableness, indicating a very prosocial, compassionate orientation toward others. She is very trusting of others, tending to see the best in them. She is direct and honest in revealing information about herself; she tends to tell others how she feels. However, like Angela, her low Assertiveness score indicates that she may not be very proactive in making her ideas or wishes known to others. She would prefer to wait to be asked rather than to take the lead and initiate a conversation. She is very Altruistic, ready to help others when called upon. The key term here is "called upon." She may not initiate a response. High on Modesty and Tender-Mindedness, Beverly is self-effacing and easily moved by emotional appeals. She is friendly, soft-hearted, and gentle, never overbearing or arrogant. She scores in the average range on Compliance, suggesting that at times she likes to have things done her own way. Given her low score on Assertiveness, she may resort to passive-aggressive strategies.

The domain score on Conscientiousness is in the very high range, indicating an individual who is very ambitious, organized, reliable, and self-controlled. She is high on all facets except Achievement (C4). She has a good sense of Competence (C1), although given her N4 score, these feelings may be experienced within a certain well-defined niche. She may have difficulty in generalizing these feelings to other situations. She is Orderly (C2) and Dutiful (C3); she is efficient and organized, and can follow through on commitments that she makes. Scores on the C5 (Self-Discipline) and C6 (Deliberation) scales, along with an average N6 score, show that Beverly is not likely to act out impulsively on any of the negative feelings she experiences. She has enough personal control and discipline to manage these dysphoric feelings in appropriate ways.

It is interesting to note that Beverly's avoidant personality exists despite her very high Agreeableness score. Although she is afraid of being with others, she sees them as basically good. Her fears of interpersonal contact may stem from very deep feelings of inadequacy and real fear of social ridicule. She may feel truly conflicted, liking people and possibly wanting to be with them, but afraid that she may not live up to their standards or may falter interpersonally. The high level of Neuroticism is consistent with the Avoidant Personality Disorder diagnosis and *not* with the Schizoid Disorder.

Therapeutically, Beverly's high Openness and Conscientiousness scores augur well for treatment. She is capable of thinking in new ways about herself and will work hard at reaching the treatment goals. Given her scores on the Agreeableness facets, it should be relatively easy to establish a therapeutic alliance with her. Her relatively low N6 score is an additional resource that Angela W. does not have. Beverly already has developed an important sense of being able to cope with the difficulties that confront her. Despite her fear about being with others, she was still able to take on, and perform well, a position as, of all things, a receptionist. This job certainly puts her in a position to meet and work with others, a natural outlet for someone high on Agreeableness. Yet she is able to manage the terror this position provokes in her. This is an important foundation on which therapy can build.

Case History: Tom S. ✓

Tom S. is a 34-year-old, born-again Christian fundamentalist. He has a severe gambling disorder which led to the breakup of one relationship. He is working as a salesperson. He presents as a very likable person, a very good conversationalist. He came to therapy because he is engaged to be married and his fiancée was curious to know how trustworthy he was. He was abstinent from gambling for about 60 days before coming to therapy. He was in treatment 4 weeks before taking the NEO PI–R. His results are presented in Figure 4-6.

Tom's overall domain score on Neuroticism is in the high range, showing a broad range of negative affect. He claims to be anxious, easily frustrated, depressed, having low self-esteem, and distressed by thoughts about doing things that he knows he should not. The only Neuroticism facet in the average range is N6 (Vulnerability), suggesting that Tom can manage his distress to some degree.

His domain score on Extraversion is in the average range, indicating that Tom can do well in groups, although he appreciates his privacy. His lowest facet score is on E3 (Assertiveness), indicating a desire to let others provide initiative in group situations. He scores in the high range on the E5 (Excitement-Seeking) and E6 (Positive Emotions) facets. He exudes a cheerful and optimistic persona; others may perceive him as being humorous, enthusiastic, and jolly. People may seek out his company to enjoy the positive energy he radiates. His high score on Excitement-Seeking indicates an enjoyment of thrill-seeking activities and being where "the action is." He may be perceived as being charming and spunky. Some may even consider

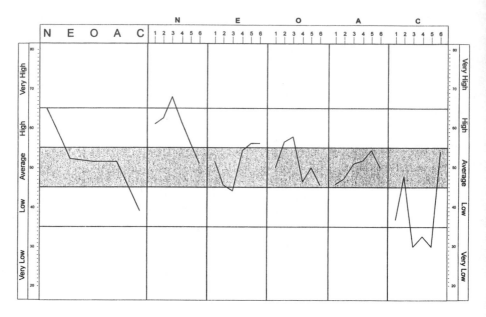

FIGURE 4-6. NEO PI–R profile of Tom S.

him to have some degree of charisma. However, despite this personal "energy," Tom may lack a good sense of personal well-being. His levels of negative affect may overwhelm any positive feelings he may have.

Openness to Experience is in the average range, suggesting some degree of personal flexibility, creativity, and spontaneity, although there are aspects that call for some need for structure and conventionality. His highest scores are on the facets O2 (Aesthetics) and O3 (Feelings). The Aesthetics facet relates to one's interest in art and beauty. Tom certainly can be emotionally and physically moved by theater, poetry, and music. His high Feelings score indicates an individual who is open to a wide range of emotions within himself, and is capable of responding empathically to the affective needs of others.

It is interesting to note that although he is a born-again Christian fundamentalist, he does not have the low O6 (Values) score that one may expect from someone who adheres to such a conservative ideology. Tom's average level score on this facet suggests that the type of clarity and structure he wants in his religious values does not generalize to other aspects of his life (e.g., political views). In some areas he may be very tolerant of divergent viewpoints, and even enjoy some philosophical debates on those topics. However, there are issues, possibly religious, where he needs to have a strong sense of tradition.

Concerning Agreeableness, Tom scores overall, and on all of the facets, in the average range. Such a pattern of scores indicates an individual who has a basically "pro-person" attitude toward others, but who may not be uncritically accepting. He may initially approach others in a friendly, accepting way, but may need some period of evaluation before becoming fully welcoming.

Finally, overall Conscientiousness is in the low range, indicating that Tom may not always be as reliable as he needs to be. He enjoys his free time, may feel encumbered by commitments and responsibilities, and may not always follow through on them (low C3, Dutifulness). There is also a degree of distractibility (low C5, Self-Discipline); other, more enticing events (especially those with an adventurous or thrill component—see his E5 score) may lure him away from the "drudgery" of his work. The low Conscientiousness also speaks to a degree of selfishness and a preference for the immediate gratification of needs. He also experiences an impaired sense of self-efficacy; therefore he may give up on tasks if he finds them too difficult or demanding.

Tom's profile evidences the classic impulsive triad—high N5, high E5, and low C5 and/or C6. This is consistent with his gambling problem, which is certainly of an impulsive nature. He likes the "action" and excitement that gambling brings. Even though he has been "clean" for more than 60 days, his profile continues to manifest this triad, suggesting that he may be likely to recidivate. Whatever treatment he has received for this problem has not been effective in changing its underlying motivation.

CASE HISTORY: ERICA J.

Erica J. is a 38-year-old single female. She is the mother of a teenage daughter and works part-time as a hair stylist. She is not presenting for treatment. Interpersonally, Erica is an outgoing, engaging woman. She enjoys the "club scene," going out frequently to meet new people. She has never been married, although she was in a committed relationship for a 5-year period. She found this relationship to be unfulfilling and eventually broke it off. Since that time she has had a string of mostly superficial relationships and is hoping to meet that "special someone." Her sole source of support is from her part-time stylist position, so money is always "tight." She is able to make ends meet with the support of her mother. The results of her NEO PI–R are presented in the Appendix, which provides her computerized report. This information was obtained from the computer scoring software that is available for processing NEO PI–R responses.

The first page of the computer-scored document provides the basic copyright information. Page 2 of this report contains a profile plot of the client's scores. The third page of the report lists the T-scores for each of the 35 scales. These values have been standardized by gender and age. It should be pointed out that the T-scores for the domain scores are based on the validimax factors. (Keep in mind that T-scores have a mean of 50 and a standard deviation of 10). These factors optimize the independence of the domains and provide assessments of each domain based on all 35 facets.

The overall interpretation of Erica's NEO PI–R profile begins on page 4 of the report. The first step in interpretation focuses on domain scores. As can be seen, she scores very low on Conscientiousness and high on Extraversion. Scores on the remaining domains are in the average range. Global interpretations of what these scores mean are provided.

On the fifth page of the report, a more detailed evaluation is given based on facet scores. It should be pointed out that at times there may appear to be contradictions within the report between the overall and detailed interpretations. The overall interpretations are based exclusively on the overall domain score, without considering the facets. Thus, someone may score low on say Conscientiousness and would be interpreted as having low levels of order, competence, dutifulness, achievement orientation, self-discipline, and responsibility—an across-the-board evaluation. However, it is possible that on some of those facet scales the individual scored in the *high* range. Therefore, in the later section of the report, the printout will say that the person *is* competent, or achievement oriented, or responsible—the opposite of what was said earlier.

Although this may appear confusing, one has to keep in mind that personality is hierarchically organized. As one moves from the broad to the specific, more information becomes available and nuances can be detected. High, or low, domain scores provide overall assessments of the respondent, but do not argue for uniform facet scores; there can be tremendous interfacet scatter within a domain. In Erica's case, we see examples of this. On Extraversion, she scores in the high range, suggesting that she is very other-oriented, enjoys social contacts, and has a very upbeat personal style and tempo. For the most part, her facet scales mirror this pattern; all are in the high range *except* for Assertiveness (E4). Despite such surgency, Erica tends to be passive in the presence of others.

Similar outcomes are found with Conscientiousness, where her domain score was in the very low range. Erica has low levels of Competence, Achievement Orientation, Self-Discipline, and Responsibility. In contrast to that, she evidences average levels of Order and Dutifulness. Although she may not be competitive and focused, she has a sense of personal organization and can be counted on, to some degree, to follow through on her obligations. In working with the interpretive report, keep in mind that the process of evaluation is working from the broad to the specific. If there are any apparent inconsistencies, rely on the facet interpretations to be more accurate than the domain evaluations.

Some of the psychosocial implications of the scores are on page 7 of the computer report. Included in this discussion are sections on Coping and Defense styles, Somatic Complaints, Psychological Well-Being, and Interpersonal Characteristics, Needs and Motives, and Cognitive Style. All of this information was taken from the extensive construct validity research that has been done using the NEO PI-R. Also included in this report is a section concerning Axis II clinical hypotheses. Although the NEO PI-R is a measure of *normal* personality, as shown in Chapter 2, there are strong linkages between these dimensions and abnormal personality functioning. What these associations mean is that high (or low) scores on any of the NEO PI-R scales do not indicate pathology, but individuals with various characterological disorders have distinct NEO PI-R profiles.

When dealing with a clinical client, this section may be useful for diagnostic formulations. When dealing with a nonclinical client, this section may help outline salient characterological styles of a nonpathological nature. Erica's profile is similar to those characteristic of the Histrionic and Dependent Personality Disorders. This does not mean that Erica can be diagnosed as having either or both of these disorders. Rather, it should be interpreted that she has an interpersonal style that seeks attention and succorance from others. The final section provides some treatment implications for this profile, how the individual is likely to appear in therapy, and issues that are likely to emerge.

The last page of the report (not reproduced here) provides a statement of the answers recorded for each item. This is useful in case there is a disagreement between the stated interpretation and any perceptions, either by the interpreter or the client. When such disagreements arise, the first thing to do is check the accuracy of the responses. Either the client made a mistake in recording his or her answer, or the person entering the data into the computer made a mistake. Another strategy is to examine the response summary at the bottom of the page. This tells the percentage of scores for each response category. Someone who answers "Strongly Agree" or "Agree" to all or most of the items (an acquiescence effect) can be easily identified. The number of items not responded to is also presented. A high percentage here may invalidate the profile (no more than 40 items, 17%, should be missing). In the case of Erica, the response summary suggests a valid protocol, with no items left blank.

CASE HISTORY: SALLY INES ✓

Our final case history for this section is for Sally Ines, a 36-year-old married female. She has two young children and is employed full-time in the banking industry. She has an MBA degree and is currently a mid-level manager for a large financial institution. She is not seeking treatment for any problems. Her profile is presented in Figure 4.7.

As can be seen, Sally has a low level of Neuroticism, suggesting a calm, emotionally secure, and hardy disposition. If there is any type of negative affect in her life, it is likely to be either Anxiety (N1) or Self-Consciousness (N4). She is certainly not very Impulsive (N5) and copes very well with the stressors she encounters in her world (low N6).

Overall she is average on Extraversion, suggesting a more flexible need for interpersonal interaction. Her low Excitement-Seeking score (E5) shows that she does not like thrills or risks. Sally scores in the high range on both the Gregariousness (E2) and Assertiveness (E3) facets. This suggests that Sally enjoys the company of others, and may prefer doing things in groups. Her high E3 score shows that when with others she prefers to be the one moving the group. She likes to be the leader rather than a follower. The combination of low Neuroticism and relatively higher Extraversion

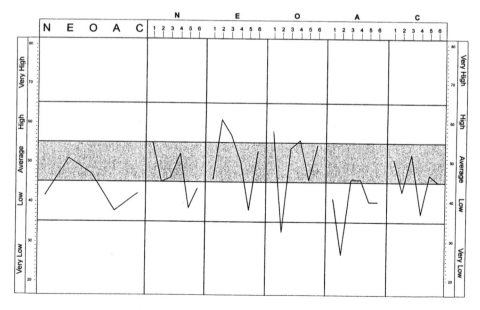

FIGURE 4-7. NEO PI–R profile of Sally Ines.

domain scores suggests that Sally feels a sense of personal well-being and overall life satisfaction.

Interestingly, although Sally sees herself as being gregarious, she indicates that she may have a more formal style in dealing with others (low average Warmth score, E1). People may not always find her to be easily approachable, and this may at times lead Sally to experience a sense of distance from others. She may enjoy being with people, but finds it difficult that others may not immediately "warm up" to her.

On Openness Sally scores in the average range overall. This suggests that although capable of being flexible and receptive to ideas, feelings, and activities, Sally may evidence some degree of conventionality. An examination of her facets shows that the Aesthetics facet (O2), is very low; that is responsible for the average overall score. A score on O2 at this level suggests an individual who is not concerned with art and beauty.

Sally scores high on O1 (Fantasy) and O4 (Actions). The former suggests a developed inner world and an active fantasy life. This is consistent with her strong interest in reading romance novels, which she feels provides her with a way of relieving tension and finding solace and enjoyment. Her high Actions score indicates an ability to work in unstructured situations and a desire for novelty and variety. As she likes to tell others at her work, "Justifying doing something on the basis that it is the way we have always done it is not acceptable."

Sally's score on O5 (Ideas) is in the low average range, suggesting a bottom-line–oriented attitude. Although on one level this seems consistent with someone who is employed as an accountant (and even adaptive), usually individuals with advanced degrees score higher on this facet. Sally may not be a "big-picture" thinker, but she is certainly concerned with the nuts and bolts of any process, and focuses her energies on creating tangible results.

Sally's score on Agreeableness is in the low range, suggesting a more suspicious, competitive orientation toward others. Sally can be skeptical and critical of the intentions and motivations of others. Most of her facet scales are also in the low to very low ranges. A1 (Trust) is low, indicating that Sally does not always see others as being honest or helpful. The low A2 (Straightforwardness) score indicates someone who is guarded in expressing her feelings. She may use flattery and craftiness to manipulate others. In some ways this is an adaptive quality for a manager to have. Managers need to be able to motivate individuals to reach established goals. Some people may need a pat on the back, others may need to be patted a little lower; some need cajoling, others confrontation. A good manager is able to look past his or her own feelings about an individual and provide the kind of feedback and incentives that will be useful to the other person.

Sally scored low on the A5 (Modesty) and A6 (Tender-Mindedness) facets, indicating that she is quite able to talk about her accomplishments and can promote herself when necessary. Her low A6 score indicates an individual who is not moved by emotional appeals and instead focuses on rationality and logic. She scores in the average range on the Compliance (A4) and Altruism (A3) facets. Sally may prefer to do things her own way, and certainly can be interpersonally adept at developing support for her agenda, but she can also take direction. Her A3 score shows that she can be generous and willing to help when a request appeals to her rationality. Overall, Sally's Agreeableness scores seem to be well suited for someone in a management position.

Finally, Sally's overall level of Conscientiousness is in the low range, indicating an individual who may be lackadaisical in moving toward goals. Individuals low in Conscientiousness are not very ambitious, organized, or focused. Sally's lowest facet scale is Achievement Orientation (C4), suggesting that she is not driven to succeed; she may not have her eyes on attaining any type of upper management position, and may be quite content with her current level. She prefers not to work excessive overtime and tries not to bring any of her office work home with her. She also scores low on Order (C2), indicating a tendency to be unmethodical. Her highest facet scores are on the Competence (C1) and Dutifulness (C3) scales. Sally maintains an average sense of her value and worth, feeling that she can accomplish those tasks that are assigned her. She can be counted on to follow through on commitments that she makes, although she may strive to do only what is minimally required. Levels of Self-Discipline (C5) and Deliberation (C6) are in the average range and show Sally to have some degree of personal organization and control.

Sally's configuration of scores on this domain show her not to be necessarily sloppy and disorganized. She has other priorities and goals for herself that may not necessarily be consistent with those of the competitive business world, but may be concerned with her family life and other recreational commitments. Nonetheless, she is very successful in her professional career. Mid-level management is the place in which she feels the most comfortable. She can interact with others and manage them through setting their goals, delegating tasks, and mobilizing others into cooperative undertakings. At the end of the day, though, she can leave this all behind and go home to devote her attentions to her family. Her Competitive Style (see Table 4-3) is relaxed, informal, and easygoing.

Sally's Character Style (Table 4-4) reflects a more self-seeking and manipulative orientation. She enjoys getting other people to move toward goals that she has selected. However, the descriptions in the low Agreeableness–low Conscientiousness category appear too extreme to describe Sally. Her scores on the C3 (Dutifulness) and O6 (Values) facets indicate someone who may be more conventional than the prototype suggests. Again, this underscores the importance of looking at *all* the facets in making any interpretation. Certainly Sally can manipulate, but her efforts may not have the same brazen, self-indulgent qualities that are found with a sociopathic-type individual.

The Interpersonal Style Matrix (Table 4-1) provides a more accurate portrait of Sally. Her high Extraversion–low Agreeableness placement is quite accurate. She is dominant with a degree of self-assurance; Sally is certainly assertive and firm. She gravitates toward leadership positions and is quite successful in managing groups of people.

What I find of interest in Sally's profile is that it contains elements that some may consider socially undesirable. For example, low Agreeableness is usually not seen as a positive value. However, one needs always to keep in mind that there are adaptive and maladaptive aspects to each of these five domains. Being low in Agreeableness may not be an asset in someone wanting to be in a religious ministry, but for someone in the corporate environment, this can be adaptive. In Sally's case, her lower levels of Agreeableness are probably instrumental in creating the level of success she experiences in managing others. Leadership is inherently a manipulative endeavor; one needs to persuade, threaten, encourage, force, and appease. Low Agreeable individuals can assume not only a supportive role, but can also be confrontive when the situation requires. They are also able to look beyond the immediate needs of the individual toward larger goals.

Another interesting aspect of Sally's profile is her lower levels of Conscientiousness. Levels of Conscientiousness have been shown to be a strong predictor of work success (Barrick & Mount, 1991; Piedmont & Weinstein, 1994). Despite such a low score, Sally has been quite successful in her career. Again, there are many factors that predict job success, depending on the specific qualities of the position itself. Leadership ability is important for management, and Sally certainly has this quality. What can be anticipated from Sally's profile, though, is that she most likely has reached the highest level of management she is capable of attaining. Moving into upper management may require the kinds of focus, dedication, and time commitment that Sally may not be comfortable in making. Her aspiration levels do not take her in such a competitive direction. Nonetheless, even her relatively modest amounts of Conscientiousness can provide her with a degree of success.

CONCLUSIONS

The eight case histories described should provide the reader with some exposure to the kinds of issues and concerns involved in making NEO PI–R interpretations. There are, no doubt, many nuances involved in making any interpretation, and only practice and experience can provide that level of expertise. However, there are a few issues that one needs to keep in mind about making interpretations.

First, never assume pathology in the profile, especially when dealing with clinical clients. The NEO PI-R is a measure of *normal* personality; it highlights personological issues that are characteristic of everyday levels of functioning. Extreme scores are not necessarily indicators of pathology. The only way to determine whether pathology is present is to employ an instrument designed to measure such. It is important to develop an interpretive skill that enables you to appreciate what various levels of a construct represent personologically. How does a low Openness individual appear and what type of environment do they gravitate toward? Being able to appreciate how these constructs are expressed in everyday living will provide you with a better interpretive sense of the instrument.

Second, remember that there are adaptive and maladaptive aspects of each pole of the five factors. Do not immediately assume that it is inherently better to be Agreeable or Conscientious. Personality is an adaptive structure that individuals develop to help them manage their environments. So the question is never whether a personality is "good" or "bad"; rather the issue is whether someone with a certain disposition would function well in a new environment. Always appreciate the context within which the respondent functions. Then, personality assessment can be useful for highlighting potential issues the person may experience and identifying resources that can be drawn on.

Finally, always strive to incorporate multiple sources of information in your assessment battery, and look for convergence over these diverse instruments. Never rely on a single scale or test to provide definitive answers. Rather, psychological tests are designed to generate hypotheses (about a client) that are in need of further experimentation. Evidence can be gleaned from other instruments, clinical interviews, and observer reports. Finding convergence for a hypothesis over diverse information sources provides a high degree of confidence in its accuracy. There is no substitution for good information and no test is perfect—error is everywhere!

APPENDIX   NEO PI–R Computerized Report for Erica J.

—— REVISED NEO PERSONALITY INVENTORY ——
Interpretive Report

Developed By

Paul T. Costa, Jr., Ph.D.
Robert R. McCrae, Ph.D.
and PAR Staff

—— CLIENT INFORMATION ——

Results For	:	Erica J.
Age	:	38
Sex	:	Female
Test Form	:	S
Test Date	:	07/31/96
Prepared For	:	Ralph L. Piedmont, Ph.D.

The following report is based on research using normal adult samples and is intended to provide information on the basic dimensions of personality. The interpretive information contained in this report should be viewed as only one source of hypotheses about the individual being evaluated. No decisions should be based solely on the information contained in this report. This material should be integrated with all other sources of information in reaching professional decisions about this individual. This report is confidential and intended for use by qualified professionals only; it should not be released to the individual being evaluated. "Your NEO PI–R Summary" provides a report in lay terms that may be appropriate for feedback to the client.

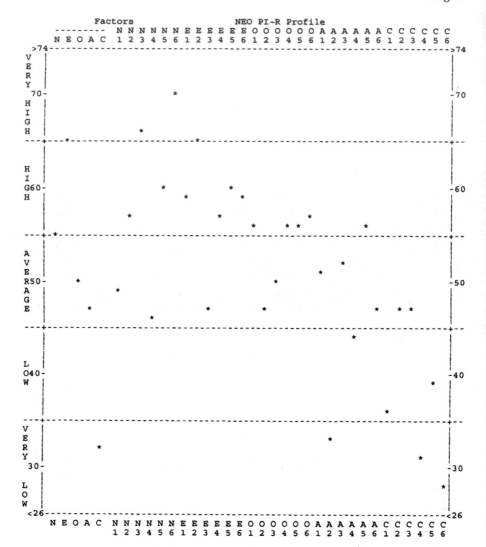

—— NEO PI–R DATA TABLE ——

Scale	Raw Score	T Score	Range
Factors			
(N) Neuroticism	—	55	AVERAGE
(E) Extraversion	—	65	HIGH
(O) Openness	—	50	AVERAGE
(A) Agreeableness	—	47	AVERAGE
(C) Conscientiousness	—	32	VERY LOW
Neuroticism Facets			
(N1) Anxiety	15	49	AVERAGE
(N2) Angry Hostility	16	57	HIGH
(N3) Depression	22	66	VERY HIGH
(N4) Self-Consciousness	13	46	AVERAGE
(N5) Impulsiveness	21	60	HIGH
(N6) Vulnerability	19	70	VERY HIGH
Extraversion Facets			
(E1) Warmth	27	59	HIGH
(E2) Gregariousness	24	65	HIGH
(E3) Assertiveness	14	47	AVERAGE
(E4) Activity	21	57	HIGH
(E5) Excitement-Seeking	21	60	HIGH
(E6) Positive Emotions	25	59	HIGH
Openness Facets			
(O1) Fantasy	19	56	HIGH
(O2) Aesthetics	17	47	AVERAGE
(O3) Feelings	21	50	AVERAGE
(O4) Actions	19	56	HIGH
(O5) Ideas	21	56	HIGH
(O6) Values	23	57	HIGH
Agreeableness Facets			
(A1) Trust	22	51	AVERAGE
(A2) Straightforwardness	15	33	VERY LOW
(A3) Altruism	25	52	AVERAGE
(A4) Compliance	17	44	LOW
(A5) Modesty	22	56	HIGH
(A6) Tender-Mindedness	20	47	AVERAGE
Conscientiousness Facets			
(C1) Competence	17	36	LOW
(C2) Order	18	47	AVERAGE
(C3) Dutifulness	22	47	AVERAGE
(C4) Achievement Striving	12	31	VERY LOW
(C5) Self-Discipline	17	39	LOW
(C6) Deliberation	8	28	VERY LOW

TM

Client Name : Erica J.NEO PI–R
Test Date   : 07/31/96 INTERPRETIVE REPORT

——Validity Indices——

Validity indices (i.e., A and C questions, total number of items missing, and response set) are within normal limits.

——Basis of Interpretation——

This report compares the respondent to other adult women. It is based on self-reports of the respondent.

At the broadest level, personality can be described in terms of five basic dimensions or factors. NEO PI–R domain scores provide good estimates of these five factors by summing the six facets in each domain. Domain scores can be calculated easily by hand and are therefore used on the (hand-scored) Profile Form. More precise estimates of standing on the five factors, however, are provided by factor scores, which are a weighted combination of scores on all 30 facets (see Table 2 in the NEO PI–R Professional Manual). Factor scores are best calculated by computer.

Because factor scores have somewhat higher convergent and discriminant validity, they are used as the basis of this report. In general, domain T scores and factor T scores are very similar; occasionally, however, they differ. In these cases, the factor T score, which incorporates information from all 30 facets, is usually a more accurate description of the individual.

Factor scores are used to describe the individual at a global level, based on a composite of facet scale scores. To the extent that there is wide scatter among facet scores within a domain, interpretation of that domain and factor becomes more complex. Interpretive statements at the factor level may occasionally conflict with interpretive statements at the facet level. In these cases, particular attention should be focused on the facet scales and their interpretations.

——Global Description of Personality: The Five Factors——

The most distinctive feature of this individual's personality is her standing on the factor of Conscientiousness. Women who score in this range have little need for achievement, putting personal interests or pleasure before business. They prefer not to make schedules, are often late for meetings and appointments, and have difficulty in finishing tasks. Their work is typically accomplished in a haphazard and disorganized fashion. They lack self-discipline, prefer play to work, and may seem aimless in setting goals for their lives. They have a relaxed attitude toward duties and obligations, and typically prefer not to make commitments. Raters describe such people as careless, neglectful, unreliable, and negligent.

This person is high in Extraversion. Such people enjoy the company of others and the stimulation of social interaction. They like parties and may be group leaders. They have a fairly high level of energy and tend to be cheerful and optimistic. Those who know such people would describe them as active and sociable.

Next, consider the individual's level of Neuroticism. Individuals scoring in this range are average in terms of their emotional stability. They experience a normal amount of psychological distress and have a typical balance of satisfactions and dissatisfactions with life. They are neither high nor low in self-esteem. Their ability to deal with stress is as good as the average person's.

TM

Client Name : Erica J.NEO PI–R
Test Date   : 07/31/96 INTERPRETIVE REPORT

This person is average in Agreeableness. People who score in this range are about as good-natured as the average person. They can be sympathetic, but can also be firm. They are trusting but not gullible, and ready to compete as well as to cooperate with others.

Finally, the individual scores in the average range in Openness. Average scorers like her value both the new and the familiar, and have an average degree of sensitivity to inner feelings. They are willing to consider new ideas on occasion, but they do not seek out novelty for its own sake.

——Detailed Interpretation: Facets of N, E, O, A, and C——

Each of the five factors encompasses a number of more specific traits, or facets. The NEO PI–R measures six facets in each of the five factors. An examination of the facet scores provides a more detailed picture of the distinctive way that these factors are seen in this person.

Neuroticism

This individual is occasionally nervous or apprehensive, but no more so than the average individual. She often feels frustrated, irritable, and angry at others and she is prone to feeling sad, lonely, and dejected. Embarrassment or shyness when dealing with people, especially strangers, is only occasionally a problem for her. She reports being poor at controlling her impulses and desires and she is unable to handle stress well.

Extraversion

This person is very warm and affectionate toward others and she usually enjoys large and noisy crowds or parties. She is as assertive as most women when the circumstances require. The individual has a high level of energy and likes to keep active and busy. Excitement, stimulation, and thrills have great appeal to her and she frequently experiences strong feelings of happiness and joy.

Openness

In experiential style, this individual is somewhat open. She has a vivid imagination and an active fantasy life. She is like most people in her appreciation of beauty in music, art, poetry, and nature, and her feelings and emotional reactions are normal in variety and intensity. She enjoys new and different activities and has a high need for variety in her life. She is interested in intellectual challenges and in unusual ideas and perspectives and she is generally liberal in her social, political, and moral beliefs.

Agreeableness

This person has moderate trust in others, but is not gullible, recognizing that people can sometimes be deceptive. She is willing at times to flatter or trick people into doing what she wants, but she is reasonably considerate of others and responsive to requests for help. This individual can be very competitive and is ready to fight for her views if necessary. She is humble, unassuming, and uncomfortable talking about her achievements. Compared to other

TM

Client Name : Erica J.NEO PI–R
Test Date   : 07/31/96 INTERPRETIVE REPORT

people, she is average in her concern for those in need, and her social and political attitudes balance compassion with realism.

Conscientiousness

This individual is sometimes inefficient or unprepared, and has not developed her skills and talents fully. She is moderately neat, punctual, and well-organized, and she is reasonably dependable and reliable in meeting her obligations. She has limited aspirations and might be considered somewhat lackadaisical or lazy. She sometimes finds it difficult to make herself do what she should, and tends to quit when tasks become too difficult. She is occasionally hasty or impetuous and sometimes acts without considering all the consequences.

——Personality Correlates: Some Possible Implications——

Research has shown that the scales of the NEO PI–R are related to a wide variety of psychosocial variables. These correlates suggest possible implications of the personality profile, because individuals who score high on a trait are also likely to score high on measures of the trait's correlates.

The following information is intended to give a sense of how this individual might function in a number of areas. It is not, however, a substitute for direct measurement. If, for example, there is a primary interest in medical complaints, an inventory of medical complaints should be administered in addition to the NEO PI–R.

Coping and Defenses

In coping with the stresses of everyday life, this individual is not very likely to react with ineffective responses, such as hostile reactions toward others, self-blame, or escapist fantasies. She is likely to use both faith and humor in responding to threats, losses, and challenges. In addition, she is somewhat more likely to use positive thinking and direct action in dealing with problems.

Somatic Complaints

This person likely responds in a normal fashion to physical problems and illness. She is prone neither to exaggerate nor to minimize physical symptoms and is fairly objective in assessing the seriousness of any medical problems that she might have.

Psychological Well-Being

Although her mood and satisfaction with various aspects of her life will vary with the circumstances, in the long run this individual is likely to experience the normal course of positive and negative feelings and generally be happy.

Cognitive Processes

This individual is likely to be about average in the complexity and differentiation of her thoughts, values, and moral judgments as compared to others of her level of intelligence and

TM

education. She would also probably score in the average range on measures of ego development.

Inperpersonal Characteristics

Many theories propose a circular arrangement of interpersonal traits around the axes of Love and Status. Within such systems, this person would likely be described as dominant, assured, warm, loving, and especially gregarious and sociable. Her traits are associated with high standing on the interpersonal dimensions of Love and Status.

Needs and Motives

Research in personality has identified a widely used list of psychological needs. Individuals differ in the degree to which these needs characterize their motivational structure. The respondent is likely to show high levels of the following needs: abasement, affiliation, aggression, change, dominance, nurturance, play, succorance (support and sympathy), and understanding (intellectual stimulation). The respondent is likely to show low levels of the following needs: achievement, cognitive structure, and harm avoidance (avoiding danger).

——Clinical Hypotheses: Axis II Disorders and Treatment Implications——

The NEO PI–R is a measure of personality traits, not psychopathology symptoms, but it is useful in clinical practice because personality profiles can suggest hypotheses about the disorders to which patients are prone and their responses to various kinds of therapy. This section of the NEO PI–R Interpretive Report is intended for use in clinical populations only. The hypotheses it offers should be accepted only when they are supported by other corroborating evidence.

Psychiatric diagnoses occur in men and women with different frequencies, and diagnoses are given according to uniform criteria. For that reason, information in this section of the Interpretive Report is based on Combined Sex norms.

Since Same Sex Norms were used for the Interpretive Report, there may be some apparent inconsistencies in score levels and interpretations.

Axis II Disorders

Personality traits are most directly relevant to the assessment of personality disorders coded on Axis II of the *DSM-IV*. A patient may have a personality disorder in addition to an Axis I disorder, and may meet criteria for more than one personality disorder. Certain diagnoses are more common among individuals with particular personality profiles; this section calls attention to diagnoses that are likely (or unlikely) to apply.

Borderline Personality Disorder. The most common personality disorder in clinical practice is Borderline, and the mean NEO PI profile of a group of patients diagnosed as having Borderline Personality Disorder provides a basis for evaluating the patient. Profile agreement between the patient and this mean profile neither suggests nor rules out a diagnosis of Borderline Personality Disorder; it is comparable to agreement seen in normal individuals.

TM

Client Name : Erica J.NEO PI–R
Test Date   : 07/31/96 INTERPRETIVE REPORT

Other Personality Disorders. Personality disorders can be conceptually characterized by a prototypic profile of NEO PI–R facets that are consistent with the definition of the disorder and its associated features. The coefficient of profile agreement can be used to assess the overall similarity of the patient's personality to each of the nine other *DSM-IV* personality disorder prototypes.

The patient's scores on N2: Angry Hostility, N4: Self-Consciousness, N6: Vulnerability, E1: Warmth, E2: Gregariousness, E4: Activity, E5: Excitement-Seeking, E6: Positive Emotions, O1: Fantasy, O3: Feelings, O4: Actions, O5: Ideas, A1: Trust, A2: Straightforwardness, A3: Altruism, C1: Competence, and C5: Self-Discipline suggest the possibility of a Histrionic Personality Disorder. Histrionic Personality Disorder is relatively common in clinical practice; the patient's coefficient of profile agreement is higher than 90% of subjects in the normative sample.

The patient's scores on N1: Anxiety, N3: Depression, N4: Self-Consciousness, N6: Vulnerability, E3: Assertiveness, A3: Altruism, A4: Compliance, A5: Modesty, and C4: Achievement Striving suggest the possibility of a Dependent Personality Disorder. Dependent Personality Disorder is relatively common in clinical practice; the patient's coefficient of profile agreement is higher than 90% of subjects in the normative sample.

It is unlikely that the patient has Paranoid Personality Disorder, Schizoid Personality Disorder, Schizotypal Personality Disorder, Avoidant Personality Disorder, or Obsessive-Compulsive Personality Disorder because the patient's coefficients of profile agreement are lower than 50% of the subjects in the normative sample.

Treatment Implications

Like most individuals in psychotherapy, this patient is high in Neuroticism. She is likely to experience a variety of negative emotions and to be distressed by many problems, and mood regulation may be an important treatment focus. Very high Neuroticism scores are associated with a poor prognosis and treatment goals should be appropriately modest.

Because she is extraverted, this patient finds it easy to talk about her problems, and enjoys interacting with others. She is likely to respond well to forms of psychotherapy that emphasize verbal and social interactions, such as psychoanalysis and group therapy.

Because the patient is low in Conscientiousness, she may lack the determination to work on the task of psychotherapy. She may be late for appointments and may have excuses for not having completed homework assignments. Some evidence suggests that individuals low in Conscientiousness have poorer treatment outcomes, and the therapist may need to make extra efforts to motivate the patient and structure the process of psychotherapy.

————Stability of Profile————

Research suggests that the individual's personality profile is likely to be stable throughout adulthood. Barring catastrophic stress, major illness, or therapeutic intervention, this description will probably serve as a fair guide even in old age.

END OF REPORT

APPLICATIONS OF THE RATER VERSION OF THE NEO PI-R

Self-reports are perhaps the most frequently employed method of assessment. Doubtless this is because of their ease of administration, scoring, and interpretation. However, as was noted in Chapter 3, there are issues surrounding the use of self-report measures in applied settings. The issues of concern center on whether individuals are able to be straightforward in responding to the items, or, whether they distort their responses, either deliberately or unconsciously. Such concerns have motivated many to develop "validity scales," indices designed to detect the presence of both random (e.g., capricious response to items) and systematic (e.g., acquiescence) error. As noted in Chapter 3, much more energy needs to be invested in establishing the ability of these validity scales to detect such errors. Piedmont and McCrae (1998) noted that validity scales seem to possess little validity themselves. They argued that test users need to be sensitive to the dynamics of any assessment situation and to present the testing materials in such a way as to enhance candidness and cooperation from the test respondent. But even in the best of cases, there is always some possibility that distortion may be present. In such circumstances, Piedmont and McCrae argued that one should include other, nonself-report measures as part of the testing battery. Of particular relevance are observer ratings.

Observer ratings provide a counterpoint to self-reports (e.g., McCrae, 1994a). Individuals providing ratings rarely have the same motivations to distort their responses as the target him- or herself. Raters are not necessarily committed to making the target appear "good" or socially desirable. Further, raters can provide another perspective on the individual, such as the type of social impressions he or she generates. Thus, observer ratings provide fresh insights into a person that may not be obtainable from a self-report and are an alternative source of information when a self-report may be of questionable validity.

As noted in Chapter 2, the NEO PI–R is unusual among personality measures in that it has its own established observer rating form (Form R). Statements in this version are identical to Form S (the self-report) except that they are phrased in the third person; one format is for individuals rating women, the other for rating men. Separate norms have been developed for Form R, allowing one to directly compare a rating with a self-report. Research has shown that among volunteer, nonclinical groups there is substantial cross-observer convergence: Scores on the self-reports agree very well with observer ratings (see Table 2-5).

This chapter focuses on the utility of observer ratings, how they can both complement and extend self-report data. Of particular interest is the use of self- and observer-ratings with married couples. Systematic comparisons of self-reports with spouse ratings may provide insights into the kinds of issues and problems a couple may be facing. Such an analysis outlines the underlying sources of personal motivation that may be fueling conflict in the relationship. It also provides an opportunity to explore the perceptions each member of the relationship has of the other and the resulting expectations such perceptions may entail.

USING OBSERVER RATINGS

The NEO PI–R computer scoring program provides a very useful platform for evaluating observer ratings and offers a number of advantages. First, not only does the program carry the normative data for a rating, it also allows one to directly compare a self-report with a corresponding rating within the same report. The program lists, side by side, results from the two assessments. The program also highlights the location of significant differences between any given pair of ratings. Second, it is possible to simultaneously plot the results of such tests on a graph. One can, therefore, see areas of convergence and divergence between the two profiles. Finally, the computer-generated report provides an empirical index of profile similarity, allowing one to determine how congruent the two ratings are. These values have also been normed, permitting one to assess the likelihood of finding a particular level of agreement.

As noted earlier, ratings provide an independent source of information about an individual that is not contaminated by response distortions characteristic of a self-report. Therefore, when scores from a self-report converge with observer ratings, one can have confidence that the results are not the product of any type of response distortion. Such agreement can have important therapeutic consequences. For example, a college student presents herself to the counseling center because she is experiencing erratic school performance. The student rates herself high on Conscientiousness. Personality ratings provided by the parents also rate her high on this domain. This agreement would alert the counselor that the problematic academic performance represents a recent change rather than a long-standing habit and would influence the direction of further assessment.

Areas of disagreement can also be interpretively valuable, depending on the context. For example, a client in treatment may see herself as being very low on Neuroticism, while her family members may see her as being quite high. Such a disagreement can alert the therapist to a number of possibilities. The client may be unaware of the level of her emotional distress or there could be significant family dysfunction. The client could be deliberately attempting to hide her issues from the therapist, or she may be in denial. In either case, the therapist has important information that can be employed in the therapeutic context.

Observer ratings can also be used to help validate a self-report that may be questionable for any number of reasons. In Chapter 3 I brought up the issue of validity scales in assessment. Validity scales are indices developed by test makers to determine whether some response pattern evidences any type of distortion or bias. Such biases include, but are not limited to, denial of problems, random responding, trying to create a positive image of self, trying to create a negative image of self, and acquiescence. Such biases tell us nothing about the individual and therefore a profile contaminated by such distortions cannot be trusted. Numerous scales have been developed to detect the presence of such errors.

All too often, however, high scores on these validity scales are used to reject a test protocol. On the one hand, a test interpreter does not want to make an erroneous conclusion about a respondent, especially when the stakes are quite high (as they may be in a forensic or job selection environment). Yet, to reject the protocol out of hand because of a high score on one or more validity indices may waste resources. Time, energy, and money were invested in having the assessment completed and scored; there is a real financial cost to discarding a protocol. Further, asking the individual about who they are is the most direct and intuitively appealing approach to doing assessment. To reject what a person has told us undermines many aspects of the assessment process. For example, do we rely on a structured interview? If the person distorted information on a assessment questionnaire, what confidence do we have that they will not distort responses in the interview? After all, interviews are less reliable than self-report measures. Do we turn to letters of recommendation? Well, the same issue applies here. If the respondent is not forthcoming with us, either directly in an interview or indirectly through the questionnaire, then what assurances do we have that they are not being manipulative with certain others whom they elected to write letters of support?

Observer ratings can be helpful in this type of situation. Of course, ratings are not perfect indices; they, too, have their own sources of error and bias. And, as previously noted, the individual selected to provide the rating may have an impact on the result. However, the value of ratings is threefold. First, a rating enables an individual to do a more nuanced and precise assessment of a target in a standardized format. Unlike a recommendation where a rater can provide broad generalizations within a self-selected range of convenience, a questionnaire rating outlines the personological issues of interest. Second, the level of assessment requires a degree of precision and depth that is not necessarily required or found in a recommendation. Finally, the results of a personality rating are evaluated normatively, making possible a broader interpretive perspective not available with either an interview or recommendation.

Thus, observer ratings provide a robust alternative to self-reports and have advantages that may not be paralleled by other types of assessment. Further, the more raters one has providing information, the more confidence one can have in conclusions based on areas of convergence. An illustrative example may help here. Piedmont and McCrae (1998) evaluated the efficacy of a number of validity scales and were interested in determining whether scores on such indices really were able to identify invalid protocols. The criterion for these analyses were observer ratings of the person. If a validity scale was truly "valid," then self-report protocols that had high scores on these indices (indicating the presence of some type of distortion) would not show good convergence with observer ratings (which were based on the combined scores of *two* independent raters). If, however, good convergence was found, that would question the efficacy of the validity scales. The results of our study provided strong evidence that validity scales (we evaluated 13 different indices) do *not* do a good job in identifying invalid protocols. The profile in Figure 5-1 shows why.

The person represented here (Barbara Nettle, a fictitious name) is one of the subjects from this study. In looking at each subject's scores on the 13 validity indices, this 20-year-old college student was found to have a high score (indicating an invalid protocol) on 4 of them. That means, according to 4 different measures of test validity, this profile should be considered invalid. No one in our sample had high scores on more than 4 of these indices. In Figure 5-1 her self-reported profile (the solid line) is presented along with a composite rater evaluation based on two observers (the dotted line). This figure is the graph generated by the computer software scoring program.

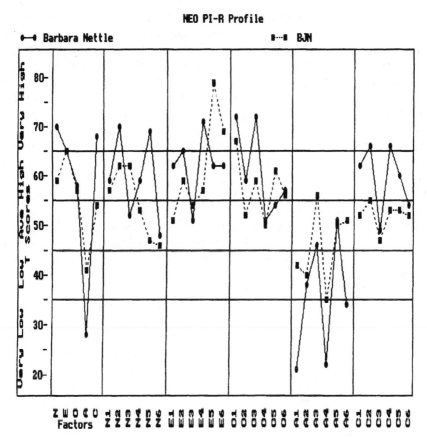

FIGURE 5-1. NEO PI–R self-reported and composite observer rating for Barbara Nettle.

A visual inspection shows that the two profiles agree quite well. Ratings on the Extraversion, Openness, and Agreeableness domains are all similar. On the Neuroticism domain both she and the composite rating see her as high, although there is a difference in magnitude. A noticeable difference is observed on the Conscientiousness domain, where she rates herself in the Very High range while the rating is in the high Average range. Consistent with this visual similarity, the profile agreement index (which is generated by the scoring software) between the two sets of ratings is .81, suggesting an overall agreement that is very high in comparison with the level of agreement seen among research volunteer couples. A statistical evaluation of the differences between the self and rating scores indicates a significant difference on only two of the 35 scales: Impulsiveness (N5) and Tender-Mindedness (A6). All other differences are nonsignificant.

Interpreting this profile provides much valuable information. Clearly Barbara sees herself as being more emotionally distressed than do the individuals who provided the composite rating, particularly when it comes to levels of Hostility (N2) and Impulsiveness (N5). Given her ability to cope with distress (average score on Vulnerability, N6) her internal distress may not spill out into her relationships with others; this may explain why the ratings are lower on these two domains. Also, given her low score on Straightforwardness (A2), Barbara may do well in concealing her negative feelings from onlookers. Interestingly, the raters see Barbara as having much more Trust (A1) and being more Tender-Minded (A6) than she sees herself. Clearly, others see endearing capacities in Barbara that she may not be able to recognize in herself, particularly given her high self-rated score on Self-Consciousness (N4). She may feel inadequate and unworthy as a person; therefore, she may undervalue her own abilities to reach out and touch the lives of others. The high rating on Altruism (A3) shows that Barbara is perceived as being much more caring and helpful than she recognizes. Others see her as greatly extending of herself; yet as reflected in Barbara's high Self-Consciousness score, she, again, will tend to undervalue her gifts.

Barbara's slightly higher self-ratings on the Conscientiousness facets may reflect her own efforts at compensating for these perceived inadequacies. By having a strong aspiration to control and master her environment, Barbara may believe that she can win for herself the personal value she does not feel she currently has. Her raters do not see these aspirational strivings as strongly, suggesting that Barbara may restrict her ambitions for very select environments (e.g., doing well in school). These discrepancies in scores may also reflect some of Barbara's unique interpretations of situations; interpretations of which others may be unaware.

This profile is interesting because of the high degree of convergence that is found although the protocol would have been considered invalid. Relying exclusively on those validity indices would have led a test interpreter to reject this profile, even though it does indeed have much validity to it. Certainly, the most immediate lesson here is never to rely exclusively on validity indices to determine profile adequacy. Such measures should never preempt good assessment practice, which should endeavor to include multiple sources of information (such as observer ratings). Throwing away this protocol would have been wasteful: wasteful of Barbara's time and effort and wasteful of the test materials that would have been unnecessarily consumed. Also wasted would be the opportunity to help Barbara. The observer rating shows that this self-report is indeed quite valid and has some important insights into Barbara.

It is also interesting that we get additional interpretive mileage obtained by including an observer report. It is comforting to see such strong convergence between the two sets of ratings. It reinforces our belief in the accuracy of our interpretations. However, within this context of agreement, the areas of disagreement also become of interest. As we saw with Barbara's profiles, there may be issues occurring within her that are not available to those who are close to her. This may be due to her reluctance to share some of her own inadequacies, because she herself is quite sensitive to this issue. Therefore, she may not always be straightforward in expressing her feelings. In a therapeutic context one would want to carefully explore her inner world. Her feelings of inadequacy may lead her to devalue the gifts she has to offer others, but she may compensate for these feelings by trying to achieve high goals for herself.

The value of observer ratings is that they enable us to look at a given person from two different angles. The focus of these views is slightly different, providing greater interpretive clarity where the focus overlaps and generating additional hypotheses in reconciling the differences. However, disagreements between a self-report and a rating do not always cast doubt on the accuracy of the self-report. Such disagreements may speak more to the distorted perceptions of the rater than to any inaccuracies in the self-report. The next section amplifies the issues that arise when using such multimodal assessments within the marital context. Observer ratings can be used to great advantage when dealing with couples and attempting to evaluate and manage their issues and conflicts. Here, discrepancies between observer ratings and self-reports can be used to highlight the possible motivational bases of ongoing conflict in the relationship.

OBSERVER RATINGS WITH MARRIED COUPLES

Understanding couples seems to be a most appropriate application of the NEO PI-R. The availability of a standardized and normed observer version is well suited to the task of understanding the quality of a relationship as well as exploring those personological qualities that may be operating to disrupt or undermine the level of satisfaction that each member may be experiencing.

Researchers have long been interested in understanding committed relationships (see Karney & Bradbury, 1995, for a review) and have found that personal dispositions significantly impact the relationship in many ways. Levels of neuroticism have consistently been shown to correlate negatively with the amount of marital satisfaction experienced by the couple (Kosek, 1996b; Lester, Haig, & Monello, 1989; Russell & Wells, 1994). Individuals with high levels of neuroticism experienced less satisfaction with the relationship, although neuroticism was not linked with decreasing satisfaction over time (Karney & Bradbury, 1997).

Personal temperaments also have been linked to the kinds of problems individuals confront in their relationships. For example, Buss (1991a) showed that submissive men (low Extraversion) complained about their wives being condescending; low Conscientious males complained that their wives were moody and self-centered; men low on Openness complained that their wives were possessive, abusive, unfaithful, and physically self-absorbed. The pattern of personality correlates with complaints was very different for women. Wives low on Agreeableness complained that their husbands were possessive, neglecting, abusive, unfaithful, moody, sexually withholding, and inconsiderate.

In a separate study, Buss (1992) showed that the five major dimensions of personality were differentially linked to the kinds of manipulation tactics individuals employed in their relationships. Interestingly, all five personality domains were linked to a variety of tactics, and the patterns were similar for both genders. For example, those scoring high on Agreeableness tended to use Pleasure Induction as a tactic of influence; those low on Extraversion tended to use self-debasement tactics (e.g., allowing themselves to be debased so that their spouses would do what they wanted); those high on Openness and Conscientiousness would use reason as a major tactic; those high on Neuroticism would use coercion and monetary reward to get their way.

These two studies show that one's personality has a profound impact on both the quality and tempo of one's relationships with intimate others. Our personal dispositions bring with them tendencies to enact certain predictable behavior patterns in order to fulfill our basic needs. These actions, which are so much a part of ourselves, may be found objectionable by spouses. Buss (1991a) showed that both husbands and wives who were low in Agreeableness performed actions that created upset in their spouses, such as being condescending, unfaithful, moody, self-centered, and abusive. Husbands and wives high on Neuroticism provoked upset in their spouses through actions that were deemed possessive, dependent, and jealous in nature.

It is obvious that what an individual brings temperamentally to a relationship has a significant impact on levels of intimacy and satisfaction. There is no doubt that someone high on Neuroticism will experience a lower level of marital satisfaction. Such individuals find little succor in the world; they are unhappy at work, unhappy in play, and unhappy in love. Further, such individuals also behave in ways that may provoke negative reactions from spouses. But relationships are not static arenas in which a single individual attempts to find personal gratification. Rather, they are dynamic. There are two individuals working (or competing) to find satisfaction. Rather than merely imposing our will on the environment, the presence of an "other" represents a salient stimulus in our environment that must be attended to, responded to, and accommodated.

One of the limitations of the research mentioned previously is its reliance on self-report data. Self-reported behaviors are linked to self-reported personality characteristics or self-reported problems of one individual are correlated with the self-reported personality of the spouse. This type of research, although important for outlining how individuals act in a relationship, overlooks more of the dynamic aspects of the dyad. Specifically, I am referring to the kinds of internal representations individuals carry of their spouses, and how these images create expectations about the partner and the relationship itself. In order to capture this dimension, one needs to assess not only individuals, but their perceptions of their spouses, something that can be done only through an observer rating.

Observer ratings provide an opportunity to access an entirely new level of the relationship through comparisons of a person's ratings of his or her spouse with the spouse's self-report. Systematically comparing the degree of congruence between these two sets of images may provide a window into the degree of marital satisfaction experienced by the couple and the motivational sources contributing to their level of harmony or conflict.

SELF–OTHER CONGRUENCE IN COUPLES

Early research on marital happiness provided two theories of marital satisfaction. One theory, complementarity (Winch, 1958), suggested that individuals looked for mates who balanced their own personal needs. For example, a dominant male would search for, and be happy with, a wife who was submissive. Another theory, homogamy, asserts that individuals select as mates those who resemble themselves in temperament (Barry, 1970; Tharp, 1963). Research showed that the correlation between personality self-reports was higher among happily married couples, although the pattern of these results has been inconsistent. Some believe that happy couples become more similar over time (e.g, Gruber-Baldini, Shaie, & Willis, 1995), while other research shows that any similarity is a function of initial assortment (e.g., Keller, Thiessen, & Young, 1996). Overall, recent research shows that generally there is a low, positive relationship between the self-rated personalities of spouses (e.g., Buss, 1984, 1991a).

Other research has begun to evaluate the kinds of perceptions individuals hold of their spouses and the degree to which they correspond to spouses' self-perceptions. The driving hypothesis here is that the amount of congruence between a self-report and the spouse's rating would be revealing of the level of satisfaction experienced by the *rater*. This approach goes by different names, such as *insight analysis* (Megargee, 1972) or *criss-cross testing* (Taylor & Morrison, 1984). Whatever its label, the approach provides a new method of evaluating couples by focusing on the images each holds of the other and the role these expectations play in the unfolding process of marital adjustment.

What I find appealing about this process is that it addresses the heart of the relationship, which is how each partner perceives the motivations underlying the behavior of his or her spouse. When individuals get married, they have an inner image of the person they believe their spouse to be. These internal images generate certain expectations about their spouse's behavior both inside and outside the relationship. As the couple spends more time together, these expectations, or, better yet, hypotheses, are tested out. Behaviors are observed and the correspondence of these behaviors to the putative personality are evaluated. A good "fit" leads to more satisfaction in the relationship. After all, the spouse is acting in a way consistent with the images and expectations the person has. However, when these behaviors are not consistent with the assumed personality of the spouse, then dissatisfaction begins to set in. The spouse is acting in ways that are unexpected and unanticipated, leading to a general sense of discomfort. The reality of the spouse's personality does not match the images that were originally developed. This leads to a general decline in satisfaction.

Another reason that a lack of congruence would be related to dissatisfaction is that the individual misperceives the motivations of the spouse. For example, John may believe that his wife scores low on Neuroticism; she is an emotionally stable person who is not prone to emotional outburst and prolonged experiences of negative affect. If, however, his wife is indeed high on Neuroticism, then John will misperceive her many complaints, her nagging, and her yelling at him. Rather than seeing these behaviors as a sign of her need for succorance and reassurance, he will interpret these behaviors as attacks on him. He may see her as very antagonistic, leading him to withdraw from her or to retaliate in kind. This, in turn, only exacerbates her feelings of loneliness and abandonment. Thus, a negative cycle of conflict and disharmony is created because John does not accurately perceive the needs of his wife.

In either scenario, the nature and degree of cross-observer congruence between a rating and self-report can be a useful barometer of the levels of marital satisfaction, and can outline the motivational dynamics that may be precipitating and maintaining conflict. It is important to note here that disagreement between the rater and the self-report is diagnostic of the lack of satisfaction in the *rater*. If the rater has misperceived the spouse, then he or she will be unable to accurately anticipate the spouse's behavior or will be led to make incorrect attributions of the spouse's motivations. In either case, the individual has a tenuous grasp of the interpersonal context of the relationship and this leads to conflict and unhappiness.

There is not a large literature that evaluates cross-observer dynamics. Creamer and Campbell (1988) outlined a model of interpersonal perception in dyadic adjustment and found that the level of cross-observer agreement was positively correlated with levels of adjustment, although the relationship was stronger for women than men. Further, they noted that self-reported agreement in personality also predicted greater satisfaction (i.e., the homogamy hypothesis). Ptacek and Dodge (1995) showed that the correspondence between self-reported coping ability and spouse ratings of coping ability was positively related to relationship satisfaction. These authors noted that the perceived similarity in coping abilities was a stronger predictor than those based on self-reported "actual" similarities. As Ptacek and Dodge noted:

> This suggests the possibility that one's perceptions may be more important to relationship satisfaction than are "actual" coping similarities. Consistent with this possibility are the arguments of other authors that negative affect in relationships stems not from incompatibility but from misunderstandings and faulty interpretations of each other's behaviors. (p. 82).

Thus, evaluating cross-observer agreement provides an opportunity to evaluate the expectations individuals hold of their spouses' actual behaviors, and the interpretations made of those behaviors. This is why the analysis is taken from the vantage point of the observer. As we saw in Chapter 2, there is good cross-observer agreement in NEO PI–R scores among normal adults. Therefore, the lack of agreement between a rating and a self-report (particularly between individuals in a marital relationship), speaks more to the distorted perceptions of the perceiver than any inaccuracies in the self-report. This approach, I believe, leads to a more dynamic assessment of the relationship. It addresses the needs and expectations of both members of the dyad and the behavior patterns these forces may be following in order to find satisfaction.

The value of the NEO PI–R in this context is threefold. First, the NEO PI–R provides a useful language for talking about and describing personality. Second, it provides a medium for couples to express their own expectations about each other. Finally, it provides for clinicians' insights into the motivational forces that may be creating conflict and dissatisfaction for the couple. These patterns may suggest intervention strategies that would benefit the couple. Taylor and Morrison (1984) provide a good description of the value of cross-observer analysis:

> The test profiles can be effectively used to shift the focus from the immediate complaints to an examination of the influence of the two personalities; as well as to develop an understanding of the interpersonal dynamics involved. The test results can help the couple objectify their problems and focus more on the role played by their individual personalities and behavior in the overall situation. (p. 17)

The next section provides an overview of what is involved in performing cross-observer analyses of this type, as well as several case histories that outline the interpretive value of this approach.

CROSS-OBSERVER AGREEMENT ANALYSES

Overview

To conduct a cross-observer agreement (COA) analysis, one needs to have a couple complete the NEO PI–R for both themselves and their partner. This generates four separate profiles for each couple. The NEO PI–R works well in this scenario because it provides self-report and observer booklets as well as separate norms. Scores can also be readily translated into T-scores and the resulting profiles can be jointly plotted on the same profile sheet. In addition, the computer scoring program has the capacity to combine a self-report and an observer rating into a single report, and will statistically compare the two profiles as well as determine whether any facets are significantly different. The computer scoring program can also generate a simultaneous plotting of both profiles (as was demonstrated in Figure 5-1).

Given the four profiles, which ones should be compared? Any combination would be of interest and value. One can directly compare the two self-reports. This would provide information about how well the two individuals complement each other temperamentally. For example, if one individual is high on Assertiveness (E3) and low on Compliance (A4) and the other is just the opposite, then this couple may find themselves a good "fit." However, such comparisons could also indicate potential areas of conflict. For example, if both individuals score high on Neuroticism, then one could expect a great deal of emotional controversy and contentiousness in the relationship. Finally, a comparison of the two self-report scores could be the foundation of a discussion of the kinds of life directions each person is likely to follow and how the life trajectories of the spouse may fit with the expectations or needs of the self-reporter.

A similar type of analysis could be performed on the two observer ratings. These scores reflect the perceptions each person has of the other. To some extent, these observer ratings reflect expectations each holds of the other. For example, he may see her as being passive while she may see him as being dominant. Although there may be a complemetarity to these ratings, one needs to determine whether they reflect "real" dispositions on the part of the ratee. Because he sees her as passive, the man believes that he must act in a dominant way. But there are two important questions to be evaluated here. First, is the woman really passive? Second, does the man really prefer to act in a dominant manner? Thus, comparing the two ratings allows for couples to discuss the images they hold of each other and the latent expectations that may coincide with these perceptions. They can then determine whether they are trying to live up to these expectations or acting in a more genuine manner, consistent with their own personal dispositions.

Finally, one can compare an individual's ratings of his or her spouse with the partner's self-report. For our purposes, this is the focus of our work. As we noted earlier, such a COA (cross-observer agreement) profile speaks to the needs and issues of the person doing the rating. Areas of disagreement should be diagnostically revealing of the kinds of issues and problems the rater is experiencing with the partner. Differences are determined by subtracting the self-report T-score from the observer rating T-score (i.e., Rating minus Self-Report). Differences of 15 points or more should be considered statistically significant. Significant differences on the domains indicate a general class of problems that the rater is experiencing. For example, a higher rating on Extraversion in comparison to a self-report may suggest that the rater finds the spouse to be too dominant, overly involved with friends and acquaintances, overcontrolling, and taking too many risks. A lower rating on Extraversion may suggest that the rater finds the spouse to be unaffectionate, passive, unassertive, and not communicating in the relationship. Significant differences on the facet scales may suggest more specific issues and areas of contention.

Overall, the more discrepancies between the two profiles, the more dissatisfaction the rater is experiencing. Given the interpretive pedigree of the NEO PI–R, it would be relatively straightforward to derive hypotheses for interpreting cross-observer differences for each domain and facet scale. Because of the paucity of research in this area, clinicians will need to rely on their understandings of the personological content of each NEO PI–R scale to use fully COA analysis with couples. However, I have conducted some basic research that may help to provide a framework for using the NEO PI–R in this manner. The next section outlines some of these findings.

Cross-Observer Differences and Marital Problems

In order to evaluate the validity of COA analysis it was first necessary to have a criterion measure that could empirically document the interpretive value of the process. Such a measure would need to have a number of specific, behaviorally oriented items that would be relevant to interpersonal conflict in a relationship. These particular behaviors would also have to be theoretically relevant to the personality dimensions of the five-factor model. In this way it could be demonstrated that discrepancies between observer ratings of the spouse and his or her self-report results on each of the five personality factors could be linked with specific interpersonal issues. To address this need, the *Couples Critical Incidents Check List* was created (CCICL; Piedmont & Piedmont, 1996).

The CCICL was developed with specific emphasis on content validity. To this end a number of clinicians who work with couples in crisis were asked to generate a list of specific behaviors that have been raised as issues of conflict among their clients. Further, we also developed a list of specific behaviors that we believed would reflect the behavioral tendencies of someone very high (or very low) on each of the five factors. This list was reviewed by another group of clinicians to determine the appropriateness of each behavioral item. Then the items were sorted into one of six categories. The first five, *Emotional, Interpersonal, Flexibility, Cooperativeness,* and *Personal Reliability* were designed to parallel the five major personality dimensions, respectively. Items included reflected potential problems that someone either high or low on that personality dimension would be likely to have. The final category, *Relationship Context,* contained behaviors that were seen as being particularly relevant to understanding conflict and dissatisfaction but could not be classified unambiguously into one of the other categories (e.g., physically abusive, sexual difficulties, gambler, mocks me in front of others). Table 5-1 provides examples of items for each category.

As can be seen, individuals high on Neuroticism are more likely to be perceived by their spouse as being moody and whiny, while those low on Neuroticism would be seen as exhibiting too much emotional control and never showing any weaknesses. Those high on Extraversion would be perceived by their spouses as being too dominant and too bossy, while those low on Extraversion would be seen as aloof and passive. These categories reflect the "dark side" of each of these personality domains; the dimensions of the five-factor model have their adaptive *and* maladaptive aspects. As we have noted, individuals with certain personality characteristics tend to exhibit certain types of behaviors likely to be found upsetting to a spouse (Buss, 1991a). From the perspective of COA analysis, it is hy-

TABLE 5-1   Prototype Items for Each of the Six CCICL Categories

Couples Critical Incidents Check List Domain	CCICL Items	
	High end of domain	Low end of domain
Emotional	is whiny, easily panics, obsessive, moody	never shows weakness, too calm, too much emotional control
Interpersonal	too dominant, has too many friends, always wants to be boss	loner, very passive, aloof, poor social skills
Flexibility	dreamer, nonconformist, untraditional	rigid, intolerant of diversity, unimaginative, uncultured
Cooperativeness	naive, gullible unable to set limits, easily manipulated	cynical, stubborn, selfish, conceited, arrogant, manipulative
Personal responsibility	too regimented, miserly, lets work interfere with family time	sloppy/messy, lazy, unfaithful, unorganized, self-centered
Unassigned items	gambler, sexual difficulties, physically abusive, substance abuser, mocks me in front of others	

Note. Items from Couples Critical Incidents Check List, by R. L. Piedmont and R. I. Piedmont, 1996, Baltimore: Author. Copyright 1996 by R. L. Piedmont and R. I. Piedmont. Reproduced with permission.

pothesized that rating a spouse higher (or lower) on a given personality domain than the spouse's self-rating makes it likely that the rater would identify problems noted in the high end (or low end) for that domain as sources of dissatisfaction in the relationship.

The CCICL is a simple check list of 133 items that cover a wide range of interpersonal issues. Individuals check off those behaviors that they find problematic in their *spouse*. Individuals also rate, on a 7-point Likert scale, the amount of dissatisfaction they are currently experiencing in their relationship. In collaboration with a student, we evaluated the validity of the CCICL and its utility for COA analysis (see Kosek, 1996a, for a more complete listing of the study's details).

One hundred and seven married couples (average length of marriage 22 years; range 1 to 58 years) were given the NEO PI–R to complete for themselves and to rate their spouse. They also completed the CCICL and the Locke–Wallace Marital Adjustment Test (LWMAT; Locke & Wallace, 1959). The CCICL was scored so that high scores for each section represented the high end of the personality domain putatively assigned to that category. (It should be noted that scoring for the CCICL is complex; scores need to be adjusted statistically for the total numbers of adjectives checked and for gender.) The first order of business was to show that scores on the CCICL have no correlation with self-rated personality. In other words, how an individual rates his or her spouse should have nothing to do with the individual's personality. There were no significant correlations between the CCICL and self-rated NEO PI–R scores.

The next step was to show that ratings on the CCICL are correlated with both NEO PI–R observer ratings of the spouse and with the spouse's self-reported NEO PI–R scores. Table 5-2 presents these results. These results provide some preliminary validity evidence to the CCICL. First, they show that an individual's ratings on the CCICL (which indicate the types of problems the person is having with the spouse) correlate with the person's ratings of the spouse on the NEO PI–R. The pattern of correlations is consistent with our hypotheses, in that the categories of the CCICL converge with their appropriate dimensional relative on the NEO PI–R. For example, individuals who are rated as evidencing many emotional problems on the CCICL are rated as being high on NEO PI–R Neuroticism. A second interesting piece of validity evidence is that this pattern of convergence between the CCICL and the NEO PI–R extends to the self-report scores as well, indicating that the behavioral issues people are finding problematic in their spouses correspond with temperamental dispositions acknowledged by the spouses themselves. Coupled with the findings that self-rated personality does not correlate with CCICL ratings, these data show that the problems acknowledged by individuals are not figments of their imaginations, or their own self-projections. Rather, they reflect real problems that are linked to the motivational styles of their partners. Thus, the CCICL can be considered a valid index for capturing interpersonal issues that are linked to personality dispositions.

With this support in hand, we moved on to the next, and most central, question: "Are discrepancies between an observer rating of personality and the corresponding self-report indicative of the kinds of marital difficulties that the *rater* is having with his or her spouse?" Although earlier I recommended that subtracting the rating from the matching self-report score was sufficient for determining the actual difference between scales (15 T-score points was to be considered statistically significant), such a procedure does not work very well in a research context. The problem is that difference scores are not as reliable as their constituent elements (J. Cohen & Cohen, 1983). For example, say that we wish to perform a COA analysis on the Openness dimension. The reliabilities for this domain in self-report and observer versions are .87 and .89, respectively. These are quite high reliabilities for personality scales. Costa and McCrae (1992c) report spouse–self agreement on this domain as .65. Subtracting the self-report score from the rating would result in a difference

TABLE 5-2   Correlations between CCICL Ratings and NEO PI–R Self- and Observer Ratings.

NEO PI–R Domain	Emotional	Inter-personal	Flexibility	Coopera-tiveness	Personal Respon-sibility
			CCICL Category		
			Husband's CCICL Ratings		
Husband's rating of wife					
Neuroticism	.39^c	.05	.04	−.12	−.04
Extraversion	−.15	.25^b	.18	.01	−.10
Openness	−.08	.06	.41^c	.04	.11
Agreeableness	−.30^b	−.13	.16	.47^c	−.10
Conscientiousness	−.22^a	−.11	−.20^a	−.04	.37^c
Wife's self-report					
Neuroticisn	.24^b	−.07	−.11	−.12	.12
Extraversion	−.15	.24^b	.22^a	.04	−.14
Openness	−.13	.14	.39^c	−.04	.04
Agreeableness	−.10	.06	.22^a	.26^b	−.04
Conscientiousness	−.03	.08	−.13	−.15	.17
			Wife's CCICL Ratings		
Wife's rating of husband					
Neuroticism	.35^c	−.03	−.04	−.07	−.04
Extraversion	−.04	.39^c	.10	−.10	−.05
Openness	.06	.12	.22^a	.04	.06
Agreeableness	−.20^c	−.22^a	−.05	.42^c	.13
Conscientiousness	−.08	−.18	−.12	−.13	.50^c
Husband's self-report					
Neuroticism	.28^b	−.13	.02	−.03	−.15
Extraversion	−.14	.29^b	.05	−.01	−.03
Openness	.01	.05	.16	.04	−.05
Agreeableness	−.13	−.08	−.11	.22^a	.17
Conscientiousness	−.01	.05	−.08	−.06	.40^c

N = 107.
$^a p < .05$
$^b p < .01$
$^c p < .001$, two-tailed
Convergent correlations given in bold.
Note. Based on a reanalysis of data from *Criss-Cross Ratings of the Big Five Personality Dimensions as an Index of Marital Satisfaction*, by K. B. Kosek, 1996, Baltimore: Unpublished doctoral dissertation, Loyola College. Adapted with permission.

score that had a reliability of only .66. Quite a drop! Although for clinical purposes such a simple arithmetic operation will suffice, for empirical analysis a more efficient procedure is needed that still reflects the dynamic of interest.

We addressed this issue by creating a residualized rating score. This was done by use of a simple multiple regression analysis. Here, the dependent variable in the analysis was the observer rating score that was regressed on the independent variable: the self-report score on the same domain. From this analysis we saved the residual. The residual in this analysis represents that part of the observer rating that has *nothing* in common with the self-report. This score represents qualities that the rater sees in the target that are not present in the actual person (as determined by the self-report). Therefore, this residualized index represents the degree of distortion or amount of misperception the person has of the motivations of his or her partner.

This COA index should tell us two things about the person. First, these values should be related to experienced levels of marital satisfaction. Greater levels of distortion may reflect an inability of the person to either accurately anticipate or to appropriately respond to his or her partner's needs. For example, a wife may perceive her husband as being higher on Neuroticism than he admits to being. Thus, the wife may find him to be very whiny, obsessive, and moody. These behaviors upset her which may lead her to dismiss his complaints and ignore his negative feelings. This, in turn, further frustrates her husband who may feel ignored and emotionally isolated, leading him to experience and express more negative feelings. This pattern can create a negative cycle of conflict that exacerbates the situation. Further, because she feels that his negative feelings are part of an ongoing affectively distressed style, she may overlook legitimate, situationally induced stressors in his life and thus may fail to act either to mitigate their impact or to avoid their occurrence.

A second expectation is that COA scores should correlate with CCICL ratings. Thus, a man who sees his wife as more Conscientious than she admits to being, will certainly encounter issues with his wife surrounding her sense of regimentation and desire for organization. In other words, he may overinterpret the motivational significance of behaviors that surround his wife's sense of organization and persistence. Correlations between the CCICL ratings and the residualized COA index provide validating support for the utility of COA analysis by demonstrating that differences between the two sources of ratings are linked to specific points of contention in the relationship.

Tables 5-3 and 5-4 present the results of these analyses. First, as can be seen in Table 5-3, correlations between the COA indices and scores on the Locke–Wallace Marital Adjustment Scale show that the degree of distortion on *each* of the five personality domains is significantly related to levels of marital satisfaction. The pattern of these relations is similar for men and women. These results are interesting because they also show that the direction of the distortion is very important. For example, individuals are *less* satisfied with their relationship when they rate their spouse as being higher on Neuroticism than the spouse does. However, just the opposite pattern emerges on the other four domains. Individuals report *greater* marital satisfaction when they see their spouses as being higher on Extraversion, Openness, Agreeableness, and Conscientiousness.

This suggests that some types of distortion may be beneficial. Seeing one's spouse as outgoing, empathic, caring, and responsible seems to contribute to an individual's sense of satisfaction with the relationship. However, an opposite pattern—seeing the spouse as socially isolated, rigid, antagonistic, and self-centered—contributes to a greater level of dissatisfaction.

Table 5-4 presents the correlations between the COA index and scores on the CCICL. These data provide evidence for the validity of the COA index as a measure of marital conflict. As can be seen, for both men and women there is a similar pattern of association: COA index scores converge with their respective CCICL category. Thus, individuals who rate their spouse higher on Neuroticism tend to experience conflict with their spouse surrounding issues such as moodiness, jealousy, and immaturity. Conversely, when the individual rates the spouse as being lower on Neuroticism, then this person is likely to have issues with the spouse surrounding lack of emotional expression.

The bolded correlations (convergent validity coefficients) show that the discrepancies in NEO PI–R ratings on each personality domain correspond to marital issues outlined in the respective CCICL category. Notice that these correlations are the largest values in each row and column (with only one exception, found with the husband's COA rating for Extraver-

TABLE 5-3. Correlations between the Residualized COA Index and Spouses' Self-Ratings on the Locke–Wallace Marital Satisfaction Scale

Locke–Wallace Satisfaction Rating	NEO PI–R based COA Index				
	Neuroticism	Extraversion	Openness	Agreeableness	Conscientiousness
Husbands	−.29[b]	.20[a]	.25[b]	.34[c]	.39[c]
Wives	−.23[a]	.30[b]	.37[c]	.44[c]	.33[c]

$N = 107$
[a] $p < .05$
[b] $p < .01$
[c] $p < .001$, two-tailed.
Note. Based on a reanalysis of data from *Criss-Cross Ratings of the Big Five Personality Dimensions as an Index of Marital Satisfaction*, by K. B. Kosek, 1996, Baltimore: Unpublished doctoral dissertation, Loyola College. Adapted with permission.

TABLE 5-4. Correlations between CCICL Ratings and NEO PI–R Residualized
COA Index.

	CCICL Category				
NEO PI–R domain	Emotional	Inter-personal	Flexibility	Coopera-tiveness	Personal Responsibility
Husband's CCICL rating					
COA index of wife					
Neuroticism	**.31**[c]	.13	.14	−.06	−.14
Extraversion	−.07	.13	.06	−.03	−.13
Openness	−.02	−.02	**.24**[b]	.08	.11
Agreeableness	−.29[b]	−.18	.07	**.40**[c]	−.08
Conscientiousness	−.23[a]	−.17	−.15	.03	**.33**[c]
Wife's CCICL rating					
COA index of husband					
Neuroticism	**.25**[b]	.02	−.07	−.07	.12
Extraversion	.05	**.27**[b]	.09	.13	.04
Openness	.06	.11	**.16**	.01	.10
Agreeableness	−.17	−.20[a]	−.01	**.37**[c]	.07
Conscientiousness	−.08	−.23[a]	−.10	−.11	**.36**[c]

$N = 107$
[a] $p < .05$
[b] $p < .01$
[c] $p < .001$, two-tailed.
Convergent correlations given in bold.
Note. Based on a reanalysis of data from *Criss-Cross Ratings of the Big Five Personality Dimensions as an Index of Marital Satisfaction,* by K. B. Kosek, 1996, Baltimore: Unpublished doctoral dissertation, Loyola College. Adapted with permission.

sion). Further, few of the off-diagonal correlations are significant (only 4 out of 40). This provides a measure of discriminant validity to the COA ratings. These findings tell us that a rating diverging from the respective self-report indicates not only that a person is having some degree of conflict with the spouse, but that he or she is having a *specific* kind of issue with the spouse. High COA scores on Conscientiousness indicate that the person is having problems with the spouse's sense of personal responsibility, and *only* those types of issues. High COA indices on Agreeableness indicate difficulties surrounding the spouse's level of caring and nurturance. The COA score's being higher or lower than the self-report determines whether the conflict is over the spouse being too regimented and accommodating or too disorganized and antagonistic.

These data provide an empirical foundation for the convergent and discriminant validity of COA indices as a means of identifying specific aspects of marital distress and conflict. COA indices can be useful for determining the motivational bases of the conflict. These results show that certain kinds of distortions are particularly associated with lowered levels of marital satisfaction (e.g., when the person rates the spouse as being higher in Neuroticism). But all COA scores, whether they are higher or lower than the self-report rating, are associated with particular kinds of issues the person is having with the spouse. These issues become more disruptive as the overall level of marital satisfaction decreases.

Thus, COA analysis is a dynamic approach to understanding couples because it relies less on actual behaviors of the spouse and more on the subjective impact these behaviors have on the individual. It is these interpretations of the spouse's behavior that play a major role in how people respond in their relationships (Gottman, 1979; D. K. Snyder, 1982). As D. K. Snyder (1982) pointed out, "a calm discussion to one may represent veiled hostility to the other" (p. 193). By capturing these subjective interpretations, COA can allow the therapist to plan interventions that are meaningful to the couple. These interventions can take several forms. For example, in the preceding quotation it is clear that an individual perceives the low Neuroticism of his or her spouse as low Agreeableness. A therapist may wish to engage in some cognitive restructuring to help the person gain a different interpretation of the spouse's behavior, one more consistent with its underlying motivations. Or, in the case of an individual who perceives her spouse higher on a dimension that he himself already scores high on, a therapist may want to help this husband find better ways of expressing his motivations in this area, ones that are less upsetting to his mate. In either situation, the information from the COA analysis is useful for giving couples a language for talking about issues that they are eager to discuss. This language can help them to understand better their spouses' needs and can promote rapport. A successful outcome in marital therapy would be reflected by greater cross-observer agreement at the end of treatment than at the beginning.

The next section presents some case examples of using COA analyses to help better understand the dynamics of the relationship. Although there are three different comparisons that can be made from performing a COA analysis (e.g., self versus self, rating versus rating, and self versus rating), only the self-reports versus the observer rating information are presented. This provides an opportunity to become familiar with doing COA analyses. This is also an opportunity to apply the interpretive skills learned in the previous chapters for evaluating the self-report results. The reader is also encouraged to explore the interpretive and clinical value of the other two types of analyses.

CROSS-OBSERVER AGREEMENT ANALYSIS: SELECTED CASES

In performing COA analyses, there are two important steps. The first is to understand the person being *rated*. Who do they present themselves as being? What are their distinguishing personality characteristics and how would these qualities manifest themselves in an intimate relationship? The second step is to examine the points of disagreement between the self-report and the spouse's rating. On those dimensions where there is disagreement, it is important to keep in mind that the person providing the rating has an exaggerated view of those personality qualities. He or she sees the spouse as particularly evidencing the *negative* aspects of these qualities. The caveat here is that the rater is experiencing some level of dissatisfaction with the spouse and the greater the dissatisfaction, the more dysfunctionality can be inferred from the lack of convergence in the rating. However, as an aside, given the pattern of correlations presented in Table 5-3, it would be interesting to explore what divergence would represent in a rater who is experiencing satisfaction in the relationship. Perhaps divergence there may reflect sources of *satisfaction* being experienced.

It should also be kept in mind that distortions in perception are not always bidirectional. It is possible that only one partner in a relationship is experiencing distress, and that person's COA should be low. Yet, the partner may have a higher level of marital satisfaction and evidence better cross-observer congruence. Thus, COA can be useful in identifying which individual is having a problem with what type of issues. The first case history provides such an example.

Case History: Marge and Henry Dunbar

Marge and Henry are a Caucasian couple; he is 43 and she is 35. They have been married for 10 years and have two children. This is the first marriage for both. They began counseling to work on "communication problems." Henry had recently experienced the death of both his parents and he had been very unwilling to discuss this with her, although it was clear he was struggling with many issues of loss. Henry's reluctance to talk about his loss was also part of a larger pattern of unwillingness to talk about emotional issues, leaving Marge feeling isolated and alone. In response, Marge turned to someone else. Her "emotional affair" drove them to counseling. They completed the NEO PI–Rs and the CCICL 8 months into counseling, after they had made significant progress. At this time, however, Marge indicated a moderate amount of dissatisfaction in the relationship (marking a 4 on a 1 ["no dissatisfaction"] to 7 ["extreme dissatisfaction"] Likert scale). Given that Marge seems to be experiencing more difficulty with the relationship than Henry, the results of her COA are presented in Figure 5-2.

This figure presents Henry's self-report along with Marge's rating of him. As can be seen, there are several areas of disagreement. The overall profile agreement coefficient for these two sets of ratings is .34, indicating a low amount of convergence. Marge rates Henry significantly lower on Neuroticism than he rates himself, suggesting that she sees him as being very emotionally stable which is consistent with her belief that he exhibits too much emotional control. The NEO PI–R computer report indicates significant differences on the Neuroticism facets of N1 (Anxiety) and N6 (Vulnerability). Again, Marge believes that Henry's ability to deal with distress in his life is functioning too well; it prevents him from experiencing feelings that he should be sharing with her. This interpretation is consistent with her ratings on the CCICL's Emotional section: She indicates that Henry is *emotionally bland, too calm,* and exhibits *too much emotional control.*

On Extraversion, Marge sees Henry as being significantly more Gregarious than he does himself. The low Extraversion self-rating is consistent with someone who is not emotionally demonstrative and may appear to experience little joy. The E1 rating reveals what may be fueling the conflict; Marge's

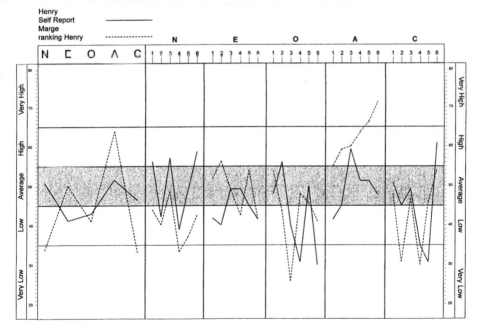

FIGURE 5-2. NEO PI–R self-rating and observer rating for Henry Dunbar.

belief that Henry spends time with friends he is close to and may be sharing his feelings with them rather than her; this belief may fuel the conflict. One may wish to explore whether Marge harbors some jealousy toward Henry's friends, who are few in number but may be very close. Although there is no significant difference between these two ratings, the E1 (Warmth) difference is interesting in this context. Henry sees himself as a mostly formal and staid individual, although Marge believes him to be quite approachable. Given this perception of him as warm and inviting to others, she may be puzzled as to why she is being excluded from his inner emotional world.

Marge's feelings of emotional abandonment are also supported by the divergence on the Openness to Feelings facet (O3; his self-rated T-score is 56 while her rated T-score is 43). A low score may indicate Marge's belief that Henry has a limited affective range as well as a belief that he does not consider emotions important. Again, this corresponds with her CCICL Flexibility rating of Henry as *lacking emotional depth*. There is also a significant difference on the O2 facet (Aesthetics). This divergence, which may at first appear odd, makes good sense here. The O2 scale evaluates the degree to which someone is not only interested in art and beauty but is emotionally moved by it as well. Henry's perceived artistic insensitivity may reflect another aspect of his personality that Marge sees as being unresponsive to external events.

The differences on Agreeableness are noteworthy, because Marge sees Henry as being much more compassionate, caring, and considerate than he sees himself. Significant differences emerge on the A1 (Trust), A2 (Straightforwardness), and A6 (Tender-Mindedness) scales. These ratings may be double-edged in reference to Marge's issues. On the one hand, the higher ratings may suggest why Marge wanted them to go to counseling. After all, she sees him as a very decent person and, perhaps, in many ways a very good spouse. Thus, she is interested in maintaining the relationship and giving it a chance to succeed despite the problems. As we noted in Table 5-3, distortions in this direction are associated with higher levels of marital satisfaction for the rater. These may be the qualities of Henry that contribute to Marge's experienced happiness with the relationship. However, these ratings may be another part of Marge's frustrations as well. She may question why a person who is trusting, straightforward, and caring would refuse to discuss his feelings with her, especially when he knows how important such revelations are to her. Why, then, does he refuse her? These kinds of perceived inconsistencies may be underlying Marge's conflicts with Henry and motivating her to seek therapy: to find the answers that seem to be eluding her.

Finally, on Conscientiousness, Marge rates Henry as being lower overall on this domain than he himself does, indicating that she may perceive Henry as being self-centered and selfish, unresponsive to the needs of others, perhaps using them for his own ends. Yet the one significant difference on this domain is found for C5 (Self-Discipline), where Marge rates him *higher* on the scale than he rates himself. Consistent with the preceding, this discrepancy may reflect Marge's perceptions of Henry as being very stoic and in control of his feelings and behaviors. He may have a sense of duty that he is trying to fulfill that keeps him from being sufficiently emotionally vulnerable to Marge. Her rating on the CCICL in the Personal Reliability section, *lets work interfere with family time,* suggests that she may think that Henry tries to escape from his feelings by immersing himself in his work.

Overall what emerges in this profile is Marge's belief that Henry is, essentially, emotionally unavailable to her. She believes that he has many important feelings hidden inside him that he seems unwilling to discuss. She may also believe that Henry has been "emotionally unfaithful" to her. She sees him as very gregarious and perhaps sharing his feelings with others rather than her. This may have provoked Marge's jealousy, leading her to, in turn, seek out others with whom to confer and find succorance.

But what appears from Henry's self-rating is an individual who is not a very emotional person. His low Extraversion score indicates that he does not experience many positive emotions and his average score on Neuroticism suggests no experiences of strong negative feelings (although any negative affect centers on Anxiety and Depression). As a result, Henry may appear quite unemotional. Feelings are something that he does not experience much, and his corresponding low scores on Openness (especially O3) indicate that feelings are also not important to him. Thus, he may appear very stoic and staid. It would certainly be difficult to get great emotional reactions from him (Marge's "emotional affair" may have been such an attempt). When he is overwhelmed with the stressors of life (high N6—Vulnerability), he may not resort to emotional outbursts to help relieve stress; rather, he is more likely to use the defense mechanisms of reaction formation and rationalization. He may even underplay his physical and emotional discomforts.

Marge certainly overemphasized the lack of emotional diversity that Henry experiences. However, his self-rated scores on N1 and N3 indicate that Henry experiences some negative affect, centering on Anxiety and Depression. It is interesting that Marge does not seem to pick this up, and this may underscore Henry's success at hiding his feelings. Perhaps there is a need for some exploration as to how Henry expresses his feelings of anxiety and depression, or for some examination as to why he may not be forthcoming in relating these feelings to his wife. This is perhaps the most germane question to our analysis. Why is Henry reluctant to share his feelings with his wife? To answer these questions, we need to turn to an examination of Marge's COA profile, which is presented in Figure 5-3.

Figure 5-3 presents Marge's self-report along with Henry's rating of her on the NEO PI-R. These two profiles converge quite well, having a profile agreement coefficient of .75, indicating a high level of agreement. This is also consistent with Henry's marital dissatisfaction rating of "2" on the CCICL. Both raters acknowledge that Marge experiences a high level of negative affect, although she thinks she copes with these feelings better than Henry thinks she does. Both agree on her overall Openness and the pattern of the facets is similar, although Marge sees herself as being more dogmatic and concrete.

Despite this overall level of agreement, there are several areas of difference that need to be considered. Overall, Henry sees Marge as much more extraverted than she sees herself, especially when it comes to her own sense of joyousness (E6). Significant differences are also noted on E2 (Gregariousness) and E5 (Excitement-Seeking). Henry does not see Marge as interpersonally isolated as she sees herself to be. This may explain Marge's need for more emotional intimacy from Henry; he does not really appreciate how few social contacts she has. He may be her sole source of emotional contact, although he may see more activity than there is, or Marge may not realize the extent of her own social world.

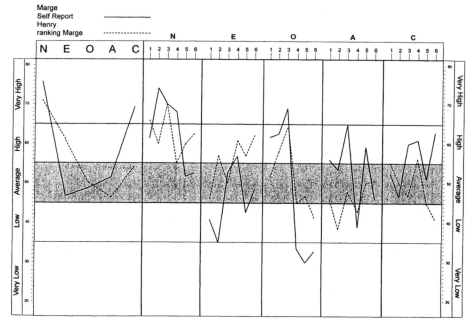

FIGURE 5-3. NEO PI-R self-rating and observer rating for Marge Dunbar.

Other differences appear on the Conscientiousness domain, on C3 (Dutifulness) and C6 (Deliberation), where Henry rates Marge lower. Henry's high ratings on N5 (Impulsiveness) and E5 (Excitement-Seeking), as well as the low rating on C6, may suggest a perception of Marge as very impulsive and perhaps reckless.

But what is important in this profile is perhaps the reason for Henry's emotional distance from Marge: Marge's high level of emotional dysphoria. Both parties agree that Marge experiences much anxiety, frustration, depression, and self-consciousness. There may be some question in Henry's mind about her ability to manage all of this dysphoria. He may be unwilling to share his strong feelings of loss and grief with his wife because he does not wish to burden her with additional, painful feelings. Despite Marge's own emphasis on emotions and feelings (see her very high O1—Fantasy, and O3—Feelings scores), he may look elsewhere for emotional expression.

This attempt at "protecting" Marge from his feelings will certainly be experienced as a serious rebuff. Marge's high score on N4 (Self-Consciousness) indicates a sensitivity to rejection. She may look to Henry for affirmation and validation, especially as a wife. The degree to which he is able to show his feelings to her may be one of her criteria for determining her success and adequacy as a partner. His turning away from her may challenge these kinds of feelings. This may lead her to be quite jealous of his other social contacts; they are perceived as taking over her own role as emotional helpmate. She may even feel threatened by his few associates. As you may recall from Figure 5-2, Marge rated Henry as being very gregarious, while she rates herself as being very low in this quality. She may see him as being quite skilled interpersonally, an area where she may feel inadequate. Marge may feel that these perceived social skills also give Henry opportunities to find better emotional contacts, opportunities that she may be unable to pursue, or create, for herself.

Thus, we can begin to see how and why Henry and Marge's issues have arisen. In therapy, one may wish to explore Henry's emotional world and help him identify and discuss various emotions more effectively. On the other hand, the therapist may wish to explore Marge's ability to cope with negative emotions. Marge's efforts to manage her own affective dysphoria may leave her little room to work with others' problems. She may have too high expectations for what she can handle herself. Thus, helping her to cope better with her own emotions may make her more available to provide assistance to Henry. One must also explore whether she really is interested in Henry's talking to her about his feelings, or whether she really wants an opportunity to talk more about her own feelings.

Given that Henry is not a very emotional man himself, it is possible that Marge overwhelms him with her own strong emotions. He may need to distance himself in order to maintain his own sense of balance and perspective. Although Henry is clearly aware of the great amount of ongoing emotional distress Marge experiences, some exploration of his responses to these feelings would be welcome. Perhaps helping Henry affirm and support Marge's personhood more clearly may assuage and comfort her feelings of inadequacy.

Another area of exploration is the value systems of these two individuals. Both present low self-report scores on O6 (Values) and acknowledge such in each other. Low values on this facet indicate that the individual has a very strong network of values, a clear sense of right and wrong. This value system is also not open to negotiation or modification; it is a rigid set of beliefs. To what degree do these two sets of values correspond with one another? What are the expectations that such values create? Is Marge trying to live up to an unrealistic image of a good wife? Has she set standards too high for their own relationship? In completing the CCICL, Henry checked only two items, *can't say "no" to others* and *sets unrealistically high standards for self*. These two items may reflect Marge's strong need to be accepted by others; she looks for validation through serving others and living up to high standards of success. Then again, what values does Henry hold about marriage? Does he believe that a man should not appear emotionally vulnerable? Does he consider discussions about his feelings inappropriate to share with his wife? These issues would need to be explored with this couple.

Overall, this case history provides us with some important concepts. First, dissatisfaction in a relationship can come from many sources. In evaluating the COA profiles for Marge, we learn that there are three areas potentially contributing to her dissatisfaction. First, her own high levels of Neuroticism speak to a general, distressed lifestyle. Insecure and anxious on the inside, she may find all of her relationships tenuous and difficult to manage. As the data presented earlier showed, individuals high on Neuroticism experience less satisfaction with life in general and their marriages in particular. Second, her perceptions of Henry are indeed skewed in certain areas, leading to interpretations of his behavior that reinforce her feelings of isolation and emotional abandonment. Finally, Henry's self-report indicates the presence of various characteristics (e.g., his own lack of emotionality, his interpersonal aloofness) that also contribute to Marge's lack of satisfaction. Obviously, all three of these areas need clinical attention.

A second insight from this case is that marital dissatisfaction does not have to be a mutual experience. Clearly Henry does not have any major issues with Marge, and finds the relationship to be meeting his needs. Given Henry's profile and his tendency to dampen emotional issues, one must raise the question as to whether Henry is merely denying some important issues in the relationship. It may also speak to his own need to avoid conflict or there may be some degree of secondary gain for him by keeping Marge feeling insecure in the relationship. These issues need to be explored as well. One benefit of Henry's high level of marital satisfaction may be his willingness to accept changes in the relationship in order to improve its quality for Marge.

Even though only one person in this relationship was experiencing marital distress, an exploration of *both* COA profiles can provide useful information about the relationship. I hope this case study begins to illustrate the usefulness of COA analyses for understanding the dynamics of any given relationship. This approach should be useful for working with premarital couples as well; they can explore the motivational expectations of their partners and begin to see the life directions each of their personalities would wish to move toward. The COA process can help support the relationship by fostering greater self-insight, greater emotional insight into the partner, and enhanced communication skills in dealing with intimate topics.

The following cases are presented to help extend your ability to evaluate COA profiles and infer useful clinical insights.

Case History: Sarah and Bob H.

This Caucasian couple has been married for 12 years, having no children. Bob is a chief counsel (lawyer) who has been unemployed for the past $2\frac{1}{2}$ years. Sarah is a human resources manager. Originally, Bob came to therapy to deal with his ongoing frustrations about being unemployed. Eventually, though, he realized that he was experiencing a great deal of friction in his relationship with his wife. He decided to bring Sarah into treatment to help manage his problems associated with being unemployed. The couple had been in treatment for 5 months when the COA profiles were obtained. Because Bob is the identified patient, his COA profiles are presented first in Figure 5-4.

On his CCICL, Bob rated a moderate amount of dissatisfaction and conflict in his relationship. Figure 5-4 presents Sarah's NEO PI–R self-report and Bob's observer rating. The profile congruence index is only .48, suggesting a low level of agreement. An evaluation of the two sets of ratings indicates differences on 12 scales. In terms of the domains, Bob rates Sarah higher on Neuroticism and Conscientiousness. As was pointed out in Chapter 4, this type of profile indicates that Bob sees Sarah as a very competitive person, one who uses her ambitiousness to compensate for internal feelings of inadequacy. Meeting her high standards of success provides some brief solace to her intrinsic feelings of unwantedness and inadequacy, while failure provides a painful deluge of feelings that confirm her worst

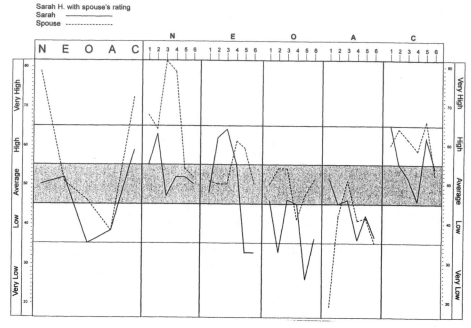

FIGURE 5-4. NEO PI–R self-rating and observer rating for Sarah H.

fears: that she is useless and of no value. Thus, there is a strong emotional edge to Sarah's ambitions. Sarah is seen as competitively climbing the professional and social ladder in order to find self-acceptance.

This interpretation is further confirmed when the facet scales are examined. Bob rated Sarah significantly higher on Depression, Self-Consciousness, and Achievement. These ratings suggest that Bob sees Sarah as a very focused and intense person who may have a very low tolerance for failure.

Another area of disagreement is on E5 (Excitement-Seeking). Sarah is seen as a risk taker and thrill seeker. Coupled with the preceding perceptions, this rating may indicate that Sarah enjoys being "where the action is." Her drive to succeed is attracted by opportunities for high profile involvement in challenging tasks. Again, this perception contrasts starkly with Bob's professionally lackluster situation.

A final difference of note is Bob's rating of Sarah on A1 (Trust). Such a score indicates a perception of Sarah as being cynical and skeptical, always assuming that others are dishonest or dangerous. This perceived inability to recognize the good in others may underscore Bob's belief that Sarah has no belief in him or his ability to find gainful employment.

Overall, Bob perceives his wife as a very ambitious woman who values success in herself and others. Distrustful of others, self-assertive, energetic, and hardheaded (low A6), Sarah is not seen as taking Bob's unemployment well. Such "failure" may be completely unacceptable to Sarah, who may see this situation as reflecting negatively on her as well. Given Sarah's perceived need to present a highly successful face to the world, Bob's unemployment may be an embarrassment to her that she is trying to distance herself from. This picture is complemented by Bob's CCICL ratings of Sarah as *feeling inadequate, can't receive criticism, hostile attitude toward others, overcontrolling, always wants to be boss, cynical, always does things her way,* and, *too neat.*

However, Sarah's self-report does not reflect many of these perceptions. She does not indicate the levels of Self-Consciousness and Achievement Striving seen in the rating. She does not see herself as "driven" to succeed in order to compensate for feelings of inadequacy. Rather, if she experiences any negative affect, it is anger and frustration. Although she feels herself quite competent (C1) and self-disciplined (C5), she does not see herself as having a very high aspirational level (C4). Although Sarah sees herself as being low on Agreeableness, her level of Trust (A1) is not as low as Bob indicates; she may be skeptical of people's motives at times but maintains a general positive attitude toward others.

These varying perceptions of Sarah are significant given Bob's current employment status. He may be very sensitive to his own failures and inability to find employment and may be projecting his own ambitiousness and self-accusatory ideations onto Sarah. She may be quite frustrated at the current situation, especially with the financial hardships Bob's unemployment has caused. As a result, she may respond with anger and hostility, but this negative affect may not stem from her own sense of personal inadequacy. Bob may interpret this anger not as frustration, but as a punitive attack on him personally. He may even believe that she is gloating over his loss of employment.

In order to better understand the areas of conflict in this relationship we need to consider the other half of this profile: Bob's self-report compared with Sarah's rating, which is presented in Figure 5-5. On the CCICL Sarah also rated a moderate amount of conflict and dissatisfaction in the relationship. The profile agreement coefficient for these two profiles is –.52, indicating a very low level of agreement. In fact, this value shows that the rating is quite the opposite of the self-report. Given the level of conflict in this relationship, this amount of discrepancy is not surprising.

Bob saw Sarah as being very ambitious and not tolerating his apparent failures very well. Looking at Bob's self-report we can see that he scores very high on Self-Consciousness (N4) and Achievement Striving (C4). Therefore, it is *he* who is ambitious and tries to succeed in order to stave off his own personal feelings of inadequacy. Failure represents an outcome that awakens very painful feelings that he may find difficult to

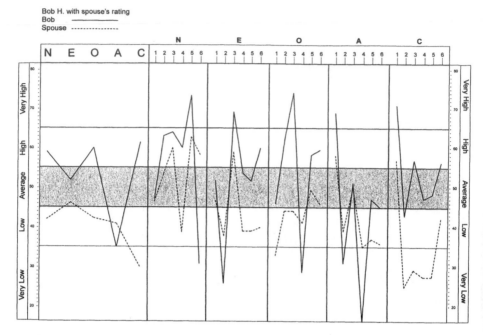

FIGURE 5-5. NEO PI–R self-report and observer rating for Bob H.

manage or even accept. Thus, our earlier hypothesis that Bob is projecting his own competitiveness and punitive feelings onto Sarah seems supported here. His externalization of his pain is placing a high degree of stress on the relationship. His repeated failures to find employment may create a number of frustrations (both interpersonal and financial) on Sarah, who may respond with anger which is interpreted by Bob as an attack on his adequacy as a person.

In Sarah's perceptions of Bob, there are a number of inconsistencies. Sarah sees Bob significantly lower on overall Neuroticism, indicating a belief that in general Bob is a rather emotionally stable individual who may not show his emotions very clearly. This is consistent with her CCICL ratings of *unconcerned about impressions made on others* and *too much emotional control*. On the facets, her rating of him on N4 is significantly lower than the self-report, suggesting that she may not see how inadequate he feels about himself. She may not recognize the effect on his self-esteem his unemployment has had. More than a professional setback, this situation affects his sense of personal adequacy.

One potential area of conflict for Sarah may center on how well Bob is able to manage the many negative feelings this situation is creating. Bob feels that he is coping well (N6) while Sarah certainly does not agree. There may be some issues surrounding the best way for the couple to manage Bob's unemployment. Looking to Openness, Sarah believes Bob to be much more closed and rigid than he sees himself, especially on facets O2 (Aesthetics), O3 (Feelings), and O6 (Values). Bob has a set way of wanting to do things (low O4) and enjoys structure and direction. However, there may be a strong reluctance on Bob's part to try things (e.g., employment opportunities) that may not conform to his expectations or that may not provide as well-defined a job description as he would like.

This may lead Bob to forgo certain opportunities that present themselves. Given the length of his unemployment, Sarah may be urging him to try new types of jobs that may be available, but Bob resists. He may be holding out for a certain type of position that Sarah may see as unrealistic or not possible at this time. As such, Sarah may be finding Bob's intransigence and unwillingness to explore new types of positions frustrating. Given his low Agreeableness scores (which she agrees with), he can be quite bullheaded and stubborn. This is consistent with her CCICL ratings of *sees the world in black or white terms, too set in his/her ways, unimaginative,* and *stubborn.*

Another interesting area of divergence concerns Conscientiousness. Overall, Sarah rates Bob significantly lower on this domain as well as lower on the facets of C3 (Dutifulness), C5 (Self-Discipline), and C6 (Deliberation). Bob sees himself as being organized, focused, and motivated. Sarah believes just the opposite: He is unorganized and unambitious. CCICL ratings on the Personal Responsibility domain were *unorganized* and *sloppy/messy.* For Sarah, Bob's behavior is more self-centered and passive. He does not seem to be energetically pursuing new career opportunities. Sarah's combined ratings of low Neuroticism and low Conscientiousness suggest that she sees Bob as being informal, noncompetitive, and easygoing. He may not share the same notions of success and material advancement that she has.

Sarah's image of Bob is one of a man who is not very ambitious or success oriented. Rather, he has some very explicit ideas about how he needs to pursue his goals which he is very committed to, but which may not be the most efficient or productive from Sarah's perspective. She does not think that his way of doing things is working well at all, yet he remains doggedly attached to that process and will not consider any alternatives. Rather than focus on the task at hand, Bob is perceived by Sarah as lashing out at her and perhaps making her responsible for his inability to find work. Although Bob sees himself as being assertive and proactive in this situation, Sarah instead sees him as becoming involved with his own feelings and circumstances and not really dealing with the issues at hand.

There is indeed much turmoil in this relationship for both individuals, and the sources of distress are different. Bob seems to be projecting his own feelings of inadequacy onto Sarah, who is perceived as being castrating and demeaning. Sarah, on the other hand, is quite frustrated at Bob's inability to organize himself to pursue employment. He seems to have locked himself into a very small subset of opportunities that may not be realistic for him at this time. Rather than acknowledging the faults with his approach, he instead attacks her emotionally.

An interesting dynamic to consider with this couple is their individual low scores on Agreeableness. Both of them are low on Compliance (A4); they both like to have things their own way. They are both low on Straight-forwardness (A2), indicating a desire to manipulate people to get what they want from them. In some sense, these two people represent an irresistible force meeting an immovable object. They are both out to have their own way and will use whatever strategies it takes to accomplish their goals. Both individuals want Bob to find a job that he is happy with, but they probably have very different ideas about how this should happen. Also, both individuals see themselves (and each other) as being quite competent, so naturally each thinks that he or she is capable of finding the solution.

Having two antagonistic individuals in a relationship will certainly lead to much conflict. After all, they are naturally confrontative individuals. They will invariably look for each other's weak spot. In this conflict, Bob seems to focus on Sarah as being inadequate and perhaps overemotional. Sarah responds by underestimating Bob's ability to really work through his problem and succeed. Bob's perceptions of affective dysphoria challenge Sarah's sense of Self-Discipline and Competence while her perceptions of low Conscientiousness may challenge Bob's sense of personal adequacy. Thus, the therapist may want to examine how these two individuals may be trying to hurt each other in an effort to manipulate the circumstances.

Case History: Alan and Karen G.

Karen G. is a 32-year-old Caucasian female who presented herself to treatment because of conflict in her marriage. She believes that her husband blames her for everything that seems to go wrong in their lives. She believes that he expects her to "bow down to his needs" in all ways. Three months into therapy her husband, Alan, joined in. He is a 33-year-old African American who complains that he does not feel he gets respect from his wife. Both parties feel that there is very little communication currently going on in the relationship and that there is a great deal of interpersonal conflict. They have been married for 11 years. They had been in treatment for 5½ months at the time they completed the COA profiles. Because Karen was the presenting client, her COA profile of Alan is presented first in Figure 5-6.

On the CCICL Karen indicates a moderate amount of dissatisfaction and conflict in the relationship. The overall profile agreement between Alan's self-report and Karen's ratings is .86, indicating a high level of agreement. Nonetheless, there were 12 scales on which there is significant difference.

On Neuroticism, Karen and Alan agree on Alan's overall low level. On the CCICL Emotional domain Karen indicated issues about Alan having *too much emotional control, never shows concern for the future,* and *seems to want to control my emotions/desires.* On the CCICL she notes that Alan "doesn't plan for much—will call at 4:00 P.M. to ask me to get a sitter for 7 P.M. so we can do whatever just came to him. But he won't PLAN a date." Thus, Karen believes Alan has a wide range of interests that he wishes to be involved in, and he wants to do it *now.* Notice Karen's high rating of Alan on N5 (Impulsiveness) along with the low ratings on C5 (Self-Discipline) and C6 (Deliberation), which are significantly lower than the self-report scores. This pattern suggests a very impulsive approach to life, one

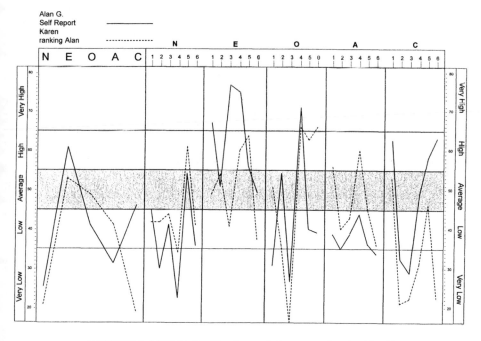

FIGURE 5-6. NEO PI–R self-rating and observer rating for Alan G.

characterized by a need for immediate gratification. He may wish to act on whatever catches his eye for the moment, making it difficult for Karen to anticipate his desires and to implement the logistical control of the household necessary to accommodate Alan's wishes.

In contrast to these very open aspects of Alan, Karen's very low rating on O3 (Feelings), shows that there are also areas of rigidity that are causing conflict. Alan does not seem to be very emotional nor to care for the feelings of others. On the CCICL Flexibility domain Karen indicates that Alan is *insensitive to the feelings of others*. The anger and frustration generated by Karen is in response to Alan's not taking her feelings seriously. Because emotions are not seen as valuable by individuals low on O3, Alan may be ignoring not only Karen's affect but its underlying message.

On Agreeableness, Karen sees Alan as being higher on A1 (Trust) and A4 (Compliance). This combination suggests a portrait of Alan as naive, gullible, and easily led. Rather than the wary, assertive individual he presents himself as, Karen sees Alan as being overly influenced by others. On the CCICL she notes Alan as being *gullible* and *overly trusting*. Karen may see Alan as giving too much consideration to the desires and wishes of his friends and ignoring her own situation and needs. Rather than respond to her needs, Alan instead expects Karen to make whatever arrangements are necessary to allow him to do what he wants.

What emerges from this profile is a picture of a man who sees himself as an assertive, dominant individual who is certainly in control of his environment. He has a very clear set of values that he relies on to provide him with a considered, well-intentioned view of the world. Although he is warm and friendly toward others (high E1), his lower Agreeableness scores indicate that he prefers to have others accommodate his needs, and he may perceive himself as the real "mover" behind any group. His low O6 (Values) score suggests a strongly held belief system, and the therapist may wish to consider what types of expectations these values may generate concerning marriage and the roles of husband and wife.

This is in contrast to what Karen sees. She does not see this masterful, ascendant individual who is in control of his environment. She perceives Alan as a passive, follower type, tending to go along with the majority, rather than as a leader. This passivity, though, does not seem to extend to his marital relationship, where he does not seem to really care about his wife's desires. Despite repeated attempts at making her wishes known, Karen feels that Alan just does not listen. This is, perhaps, what is most frustrating to Karen. Alan seems influenced by a wide range of people, *excluding* her. These contradictions in Alan also extend to his own personal motivations. On the CCICL Karen notes "lazy about 'housework' and normal maintenance and a workaholic about hobbies." Alan seems to have the time to devote to his own passions but does not seem to be interested in investing in activities that do not center around his own needs. As Karen also commented on the CCICL "doesn't seem to desire intimacy with children—or me, unless he's in need sexually."

Thus Karen's issues may center around her feeling relegated to second or third place in Alan's life. He seems to have emotionally disengaged from their relationship, except for when his needs have to be met. But Karen may not recognize the value system that Alan is working with. His very low O6 score indicates someone very much committed to a particular tradition and he may see marriage in a very different way from Karen. These value differences would certainly need to be explored. One particular area of concern would be Alan's low Dutifulness (C3) score, indicating someone who may be unreliable and undependable. Certainly this lack of follow-through on Alan's part contributes to a perception in Karen that he just does not care about, nor give much importance to, those things having to do with their home life.

In contrast, the COA profile for Karen is presented in Figure 5-7. On the CCICL Alan indicates a very high level of dissatisfaction and conflict in his marriage (a rating of 6 out of a possible 7). The profile agreement coefficient comparing the self-report and observer ratings was only .12, indicating a very low degree of agreement. As readily can be seen in Figure 5-7, Alan perceives his wife as being significantly higher on all aspects of Neuroticism. Alan's perception of Karen is as a very emotionally distressed person who is unable to manage her emotional world. Although Karen believes herself to be stable and capable of coping with a wide range of stressors, Alan believes her to be overly sensitive to life's issues. As Karen's NEO PI–R interpretive report, based on these ratings, describes her, "In coping with the stresses of everyday life, this individual is described as being likely to react with ineffective responses, such as hostile reactions towards others . . . her general defensive style can be characterized as maladaptive and self-defeating."

Much more convergence is seen on Extraversion, although there is a significant difference on E2 (Gregariousness). Karen is perceived as being much less sociable than she sees herself. On the CCICL Alan noted that Karen has *poor social skills*. These scores portray a woman who is relatively reserved and quiet, who takes a very passive role in groups. Not particularly cheerful or optimistic, Karen prefers to pursue a more mundane, low-key lifestyle. It may be that Alan's preferences for spontaneous adventures prove to be overstimulating for Karen or, given her very low scores on O4 (Actions), may threaten to disrupt her own schedule and routine. Her low scores on O5 (Ideas) and O6 (Values) suggest an individual who also has a very clear set of values that guide her perceptions of the world. She is,

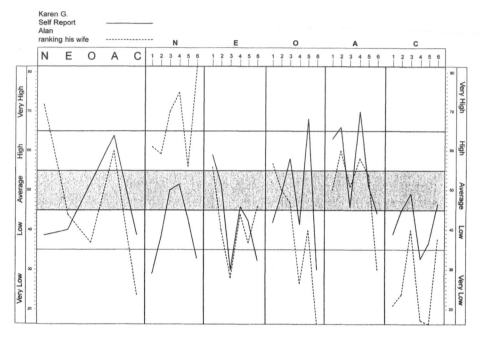

FIGURE 5-7. NEO PI–R self-report and observer rating for Karen G.

herself, quite dogmatic and has established for herself a very clear and well-delineated world. Alan's behaviors may too frequently disrupt these cherished patterns.

The Agreeableness domain portrays Karen as being quite considerate and caring. Of particular interest is her very high score on A4 (Compliance). In conjunction with the low Assertiveness (E4) rating, this indicates someone who is very passive and accommodating, who wishes to follow along with the group and do what is expected. This is curious given Karen's complaints that Alan always wants to do things his own way without much concern for her feelings. Why would such an accommodating, passive person have so much difficulty with following along with someone's requests? The answer to this question may be found in Karen's very low O4 (Actions) and O6 (Values) scores. She has certain expectations about how her clearly structured world should operate. Being asked to do things that fall outside these boundaries may be perceived as threatening or inappropriate. In response Karen may refuse to acquiesce.

Finally, on Conscientiousness, Karen is perceived as being quite low on all facets, suggesting a perception of Karen as being self-centered, careless, and disorganized. She is not seen as being very ambitious and does not always think through her situation before acting. She does not feel very competent, nor does she feel that she is in control of events in her life. She is not seen by Alan as someone who can be counted on to follow through on her commitments. Alan notes on his CCICL that Karen is *unorganized*.

Overall, Alan perceives his wife as someone who "bitches, moans, and complains about everything." She is a mostly passive individual with little drive or gumption, yet does not seem to be very receptive to his suggestions for activity in the relationship. Alan's overtures are perceived by Karen as being whimsical and unrealistic because he does not appreciate all the work that needs to be done to do what he wants, especially when it is demanded on the spur of the moment.

These COA profiles outline some important, self-maintaining areas of conflict. Alan sees himself as an active, assertive person who likes to try new and different things. Routines bore and frustrate him, so he likes to give variety a try. His requests to have Karen join him in these new undertakings may initiate a negative sequence of events. First, Karen is not a well-organized woman and is not very task oriented. Thus when Alan suggests that they go someplace different for dinner, he does not recognize that Karen does not like to have to "pick up the details" to make the suggestion work. She may doubt her ability to do it correctly or may fear making a mistake (e.g., forgetting to make the reservations at the restaurant, not calling the babysitter). Karen appears very sensitive to task requirements and feels that she may not have the energy or desire to make the necessary efforts.

A second issue is Karen's desire for structure and routine. If they are to go out to a restaurant, Karen will want to patronize her "tried and true" locations. Alan, on the other hand, will want to explore new cuisines and restaurants. This will be an ongoing source of frustration for both. Once Karen gets into her routine, she will not like to have to shift things around; this is uncomfortable for her. Karen's resistance is perceived by Alan as being an overreaction to his requests. Given Alan's very low score on O3 (Feelings), he is not very sensitive to feelings and emotions; they are mostly irrelevant to him. Thus, Karen's affective responses may overwhelm him and he may "tune out" Karen's complaints, demeaning them as just so much nonsensical ranting. Thus he rates Karen high on Neuroticism.

Not wanting to be locked into a particular pattern, Alan may retreat into his relationships with others or his personal hobbies to find the stimulation he needs. Although Karen believes that she is able to cope reasonably well with Alan's detachment, her normally compliant, externally oriented nature feels the lack of a directing force. Her attempts to obtain Alan's attention may only exacerbate the situation.

A third issue to consider is the value systems each of these individuals hold. Both have very low self-report scores on O6, indicating very rigid belief systems. Some of the conflict experienced here may be due to the varying expectations these people have of their partners. Alan expects to receive unquestioning loyalty from his wife, who should comply with all of his requests. Although Karen's low E3 and high A4 scores may not temperamentally oppose her to this expectation, demands to change the ways things have been done may create more emotional resistance.

Karen's expectations may focus on more down-to-earth tasks. Given her generally low Conscientiousness scores, she feels a need for more support from Alan around the house and in getting daily chores completed. Alan also needs to show increasing sensitivity to Karen's more gentle nature and the ways she may make requests of him; he may tend to easily dismiss her more reserved and submissive style. He needs to learn how to balance his more bottom-line–oriented information style with her more intuitive approach. Given Alan's dominant, surgent style, his lack of empathy (low O3) may lead him to unintentionally bruise Karen's feelings as well as making him insensitive to any emotional appeals she makes to him. On the other hand, Karen's more agreeable, passive nature makes her unable to break through into Alan's world. She may need to find more forceful ways of confronting Alan and communicating her needs to him.

CLINICAL YIELD FROM CROSS-OBSERVER AGREEMENT ANALYSIS

Cross-Observer Agreement analysis provides a tremendous amount of information about a couple. The contrast between the image an individual presents and the impression generated in the spouse opens a window into the personal characteristics of both individuals that may be underlying their dissatisfaction and conflict. There are three benefits of using this approach.

First, the assessment process itself provides an opportunity for individuals to clarify the images they hold of their spouses and themselves. During times of acute marital distress many dynamics may be operating and many emotions may be in play, all of which create a sometimes chaotic presenting picture. Conducting the COA analysis enables clients to sift more carefully through their feelings and then to present them in a medium very amenable to discussion.

Second, COA analysis allows a therapist to contrast various aspects of each person to their partner (e.g., self-report versus self-report; observer rating versus self-report). Each of the contrasts provides new insights into the dynamic nature of the relationship. Presenting these profiles to couples can help them engage in a systematic, focused discussion of any areas of discrepancy. Such a dialogue can help each member better understand the issues his or her partner experiences in the relationship. The five-factor model provides a clear and common language to use in this discussion. Each person should come away with a new understanding of their partner and themselves.

Finally, COA analysis provides the therapist with important information about where and how to intervene with the couple. As we saw in the previous case histories, the discrepancies between self- and observer ratings indicate specific, salient issues emerging in the relationship. These are the points at which intervention is necessary. With Alan G., the "where" of an intervention is with his low Conscientiousness ratings. A therapist may want to work toward making him appear less self-centered and fickle, and more sensitive to Karen's emotional needs and the various strategies she uses in expressing them. The "how" to intervene would want to consider this couple's low Openness scores. Such individuals may appreciate a behavioral approach rather than a cognitive or dynamic one.

COA analysis is a relatively new area. There are few data available that contrast various personality ratings. More work needs to be done to establish a better empirical foundation for using test scores in this manner. The CCICL was useful in this process: It highlighted the specific issues these couples were experiencing. Such an instrument can pinpoint areas of conflict. Although such an instrument is useful, it is by no means required for doing a COA analysis. The data presented here are encouraging and certainly showcase the heuristic value of this approach.

OBSERVER RATINGS AS PREDICTORS OF OUTCOME

As noted in the beginning of this chapter, most assessment protocols rely on self-report inventories. When we want to know something about a person or to make predictions about his or her life, we turn, naturally, to the individual for information. Other sources of information, such as observer ratings, are seen as adjuncts to assessment rather than as sources of information useful in their own right. In the first part of this chapter, observer ratings were used to show the validity of a self-report that may have been unnecessarily rejected. Then, with couples, ratings were shown to serve as a counterpoint to the self-report, outlining areas of perceived distortion between two people. In this section I take a different tack and look at an observer rating as a stand-alone source of information that can be useful in making predictions about a person.

Hogan (1991) outlined the fundamental differences between a self-report and observer rating of personality. For an observer, personality represents the target's public self or social reputation. For a self-rating, personality represents the structures, dynamics, and processes inside the person that explain why he or she acts in a certain way. Thus, information obtained from these two sources convey, to some degree, very different aspects of the individual. As Hogan noted, in some circumstances where the assessment goal is prediction of behavior (e.g., personnel selection), reputation may be a most important quality to measure. After all, the best predictor of future behavior is past behavior (Wernimont & Campbell, 1968); one's reputation, which emerges over one's history of behavior with others, should be a singularly useful predictive index.

A number of studies have evaluated the predictive utility of observer ratings. Digman (1972) reported correlations in the .50s between elementary school teachers' ratings of Conscientiousness and high school grade point average. Scheier, Buss, and Buss (1976) showed that observer ratings of personality had greater predictive validity than did self-ratings concerning the level of awareness of one's own aggressive behavior and related affective reactions. John and Robbins (1993) suggested that under highly evaluative circumstances an individual may bias his or her self-report and thus attenuate the validity of the measure. Yet an observer rating is not susceptible to the ego-involving motivations of the target, and therefore would not suffer a decline in accuracy. These authors showed that self–peer congruence declined when the rating was on an evaluative dimension while peer–peer congruence remained at comparable levels of convergence regardless of the evaluative nature of the term being rated.

Mount, Barrick, and Strauss (1994) provided the most empirically compelling support for observer ratings. They gathered a sample of 105 sales representatives who completed a self-rating on the Big Five personality domains. These individuals also had their supervisor and up to five coworkers and five customers rate them on the same personality domains as well as on several work performance indices. The results indicated two important findings. First, the observer ratings of personality were significant predictors of performance outcome (only rated Neuroticism did not correlate with any of the performance criteria). Interestingly, the only self-report score that correlated with performance was Conscientiousness. Thus, ratings may provide more criterion-relevant information in this context than self-reports.

The next finding concerned the incremental validity of the observer ratings. Incremental validity (discussed in more detail in the next chapter) determines whether a score provides any additional information over and above that already obtained by existing measures. Hierarchical multiple regression analyses were conducted in which the performance ratings were the dependent variable. On the first step of the analysis, self-reported personality scores were entered. On the second step the observer ratings were entered. A partial F-test determined whether the variables entered on Step 2 added any explanatory variance over that already accounted for on Step 1. The results showed that for the four personality domains of Extraversion, Openness, Agreeableness, and Conscientiousness, the observer ratings provided additional, explained variance in the performance criteria over and above whatever contribution was made by the self-reports.

These findings highlight the value of observer ratings as predictors in their own right. They provide useful information about an individual that is not entirely redundant with a corresponding self-report. This is because observers have a different perspective on the target than the target has of him- or herself, and these insights have their own predictive validity. Further, an observer rating is not influenced or distorted by the same kinds of motivations as a self-report. Thus, under certain circumstances one may prefer to use a rating in place of the self-report.

Concerning validity research, these data emphasize the need to distinguish between the validity of a construct and the manner in which the construct is measured. As Mount and colleagues (1994) showed, at times an observer rating was a stronger predictor of performance than a self-report. Therefore, determining the actual validity of a particular construct in predicting some outcome on the basis of only one information source (e.g., self-report) may underestimate the true strength of the relationship. As Mount and colleagues showed, the relationship between personality and performance was significantly stronger when *both* the self-report and observer ratings were included in the prediction equation.

Although these data were obtained in a work setting, the lesson should not be lost for the clinical environment. The best evaluations are those that rely on *multiple* sources of information and look for points of convergence. Obtaining similar diagnostic indicators from diverse measures and informants increases confidence in the accuracy of the inferences drawn. Observer ratings are a useful piece of any assessment process and complement information obtained from self-reports. Under circumstances where the validity of self-reported data may be questioned, obtaining information from knowledgeable informants provides a useful substitute.

Certainly more research is needed for examining the utility of observer ratings. Although ratings do not suffer from the same sources of bias and distortion as self-reports, they do have their limitations and some evaluation of their sources of bias would be helpful. Observer ratings are an assessment technology that has been underutilized. The availability of an established, normed, rating instrument in Form R of the NEO PI–R should help make this type of data more accessible, and useful, to researchers and practitioners alike.

RESEARCH APPLICATIONS WITH THE NEO PI–R

Clinical work is a very time-consuming endeavor filled with many pressures and concerns. With all the time constraints it seems reasonable to ask whether the introduction of a new assessment instrument is worth the time it consumes. Although I have already outlined how the NEO PI–R can be useful in providing clinically relevant information, there are three other benefits that also need to be considered. First, clinicians must and do have an investment in assessing the quality of their own work. How effective are one's interventions? In what ways does a therapist impact their clients? Answers to these questions help therapists fine-tune their therapeutic skills, pointing out particular strengths and weaknesses. Second, in working with clients on growth issues, it becomes important to have measures that will provide information on the adaptive capacities of the individual. Unlike many clinical instruments, the NEO PI–R can speak meaningfully about coping strategies and interpersonal styles, among other qualities. These insights focus on who a person is and the directions they are likely to move toward rather than emphasizing deficiencies and weaknesses. Finally, there are the pressures of managed care, which continually call for greater *documented* efficiency in treatment.

Although a great deal of energy is devoted to this last area, and more is said about managed care later, the first issues are quite important. Many times clinicians rely on clinical interviews to gather client information, but much of this dialogue usually surrounds finding out the problems or issues that have led the person to treatment. It is not until after therapy is well under way that attention focuses on more latent personal dimensions and their role in causing and maintaining the presenting problem. It is here that the NEO PI–R can be quite useful. It can generate tremendous amounts of information about the client's characteristic ways of living that can help both inform and direct clinical querying and intervening. Thus, the energy expended in obtaining personality assessment data is rewarded when treatment moves into its middle and end phases. This chapter provides some strategies and materials to use in meeting these challenges.

This chapter also outlines some of the ways that the NEO PI–R can be used as a research tool in areas such as cross-cultural psychology, scale validation, and program evaluation. Given the strong psychometric foundations of the instrument, it has a significant contribution to make in expanding our knowledge base in any area that concerns personality structure and development. Perhaps the two greatest potential contributions of this relatively comprehensive taxonomy is its ability to clarify the personological content of existing constructs and to point out ways of identifying new domains of individual-difference variables. This chapter outlines some of the techniques and strategies for using the NEO PI–R to realize these goals.

THE NEED AND ROLE OF RESEARCH

Overview

Today clinicians are facing great pressures from third-party payers to provide more effective services, in less time, and with lower cost. Many practitioners greet this new mental health–care landscape with frustration and nervousness. The seemingly rigid treatment standards call for interventions that do not always seem appropriate to the needs of the client. These pressures are augmented by both the growing consumer movement interested in having practitioners demonstrate some value for their services (Lyons, Howard, O'Mahoney, & Lish, 1997), and the maturing ethical dimensions of practice that call for therapists to explore and document the effectiveness of their treatments (Ogles, Lambert, & Masters, 1996).

But behind this seemingly black cloud lies an important silver lining: the need for empirical documentation of clinical outcomes. Underlying all these pressures on practice is the need for clinicians to provide greater accountability for the effectiveness of their interventions, both in terms of client satisfaction and more objective indices of relief from symptomatology. Responding to this need requires clinicians to collect data to support the value of their services. Although this may appear to be cumbersome and inconvenient in a milieu that is already overburdened with paperwork and time commitments, the fact is this need for accountability will not just go away. It provides a real impetus for the social sciences to begin to put in place a paradigm for the collection of information that can speak meaningfully to the quality of our interventions and the conditions under which they can be expected to work. All of this interest in creating greater therapist accountability has a singular focus on obtaining outcome assessment data.

Outcome assessment data speak to the very heart of practice, in that they provide information about how effective our treatments are, and with what type of clients. Collecting relevant clinical outcome data will (a) help improve the quality and efficacy of treatment, (b) enhance the empirical foundation of the clinical sciences, and (c) provide greater accountability (Barlow, Hayes, & Nelson, 1984). With so many types of professionals vying for a slice of the mental health pie the emphasis on empirical data will only grow, enabling those with the data to claim the largest share.

Thus the pressure will increase for clinicians to create a clinical environment that includes a significant assessment component. There are numerous works currently available that outline how relatively easy outcome assessments can be performed (e.g., Lyons *et al.*, 1997; Ogles *et al.*, 1996; Stout, 1997). All of these works stress the need for more information on treatment efficacy. Research has to be seen as our friend. It alone will be able to stave off the onslaught of managed care and its ubiquitous call for more efficiency. Only data will be able to speak persuasively about how much treatment various "problems" will need to receive, and how much improvement can be expected with different kinds of clients.

This need for more outcome data must be seen as an irresistible force in our field. This information must be collected and someone will have to do it; either managed care will collect its own data or we will need to do it ourselves. If it is us, social scientists, both clinicians and researchers, who undertake this research challenge, then we will receive an added bonus for our efforts: We will have the ultimate control of how we define ourselves professionally. It is the selection of variables and outcomes that will have the largest influence on marking out the territory we as social scientists call our own, the constructs we find of interest, and the goals we pursue with our interventions. It would be to our advantage if we make these selections rather than having some outside agency impose them on us.

The basic paradigm for conducting outcome research is really quite straightforward. It may consume some additional time of the client and therapist, but its payoff is certainly worth the investment. The NEO PI–R can play a pivotal role in this process. The dimensions assessed speak meaningfully about the motivations and capacities of individuals. As was highlighted in Chapter 2, the NEO PI–R facets and domains are very closely linked to a wide array of clinical dimensions and outcomes. Scores on the NEO PI–R can be used to match treatments to clients, to make differential diagnoses, and to formulate expectations of treatment outcome, to name a few of its potential benefits. But this is only the beginning.

How Clinicians Can Provide Important Insights

Clinicians are in an ideal position to collect important clinical information. Dealing directly with the consumers of their services, clinicians can collect assessments at ideal and timely moments. Although the choice of instruments to use is quite large, many of the basic tools for assessing outcome are largely context-specific questionnaires that are tailored to reflect the particular services that were rendered. The last section in this chapter provides some examples of forms that I have used in my own outcome evaluation studies. They are included to provide a template for those interested in performing their own work. Readers should feel free to modify and adapt these questionnaires to meet the needs of their own situation.

Several developments have made the current field ready for these types of investigations: first, the presence of a wide range of psychometrically useful clinical instruments that are relatively simple to administer and score; second, the availability of high-speed computers that can easily analyze data sets and support scoring programs to interpret clinical data; and, finally, the increasing sophistication of the social sciences themselves. We are building better theoretical models and employing more mature empirical designs to test them. As a consequence, the field is moving toward a new level of development, one that is far more data driven than at any time in its past. Thus the question is no longer *whether* we need to obtain clinical outcome data, but rather *when* and *how* this information will be obtained.

In order to fully enjoy the fruits that outcome research can provide for us, we need to become familiar with the many issues that emerge in doing research with the NEO PI–R. The sections that follow outline several of these, including identifying the number of factors in a data set, evaluating the generalizability of the five-factor structure in new samples, and establishing the validity of new and existing constructs. In writing this chapter I tried to balance the need to provide more technical information with the reality that many readers may be relatively unfamiliar with the quantitative bases of these techniques. The information presented here provides a blueprint to follow in using the NEO PI–R in its most empirically advantageous way.

Ultimately, though, clinicians and researchers will need to forge a new alliance that will allow for the collection of data that will help (re)establish the value of the social sciences and to document empirically the efficacy of our interventions. We need to do this in a way that maintains the integrity of our discipline and brings forth our own sense of identity, rather than having it imposed on us from outside sources. Finally, our ability to influence managed care and its reimbursement strategies will be entirely dependent on the type and quality of empirically based information that we can bring to bear on the issues of treatment and outcome. Because we are at the applied frontier of our field, we need to take a more active and involved role in this process.

ISSUES RELATING TO THE FACTOR ANALYSIS OF NEO PI–R INFORMATION

The factor structure of the NEO PI–R is well established empirically in the research literature, both for the English version (Costa & McCrae, 1992c; Costa, McCrae, & Dye, 1991; McCrae & Costa, 1987; Piedmont, 1994) and for foreign language versions (Capara, Barbaranelli, & Comrey, 1995; Katigbak, Church, & Akamine, 1996; Piedmont & Chae, 1997; Silva *et al.*, 1994; Vassend & Skrondal, 1995). Nonetheless, there remain some technical debates reverberating in the literature relating to factor analytically derived information from the NEO PI–R. This section provides an overview of the technical issues underlying these controversies and the responses that have been made to address them. The ultimate aim of this section, however, is to provide the reader with guidelines for both selecting and using factor analytic techniques with NEO PI–R data. It should be remembered that the best analytic endeavors are those that have a clear theoretical framework for guiding the investigations. This section addresses two of the more basic questions surrounding the NEO PI–R: how many factors really exist in this instrument and what is their nature?

Factor Orthogonality

Controversy continues to center on whether or not the five factors are independent of one another as claimed. On the one hand, orthogonality is a preferred quality of the data because it assures very little redundancy in content. Information obtained from one factor has nothing in common with the remaining dimensions. This assures efficacy in assessment and enables one to build useful prediction models. In response to this, some argue that such technical neatness is rarely observed in nature (e.g., J. Block, 1995). As Loevinger (1994) has stated, "There is no reason to believe that the bedrock of personality is a set of orthogonal (independent) factors, unless you think that nature is constrained to present us a world in rows and columns. That would be convenient for many purposes, particularly given the statistical programs already installed on our computers. But is it realistic?" (p. 6).

Spirrison (1994) responded that the question of orthogonality is irrelevant. The five-factor model represents an abstraction of what we refer to as personality. Whether this abstraction provides a faithful reproduction of a real entity is another question. What is important is whether this abstraction has any empirical utility, "The question is whether the rows and columns of orthogonal solutions provide an effective framework for organizing our perceptions of personality" (p. 582). From this perspective, given that personality is in and of itself an abstraction developed by psychologists to understand human behavior rather than a reflection of some real, underlying psychic reality, then the "neatness" of the model should not be grounds for dismissing it. Rather, its value should be determined by its heuristic and predictive utility.

However, given the empirical basis of both the FFM and the NEO PI–R, it seems necessary that any approach to determining factor orthogonality take an empirical route. Fortunately, whether the factors are correlated can be empirically determined. If the five factors are really correlated, then creating scales that contain that overlap should be better predictors of external criteria than scales constrained to be independent. This is because the independent factors are losing information and their construct validity will suffer. McCrae and Costa (1989b) demonstrated that when the five factors are treated as independent entities, the factors' convergent correlations with external criteria were higher than when the factors were allowed to correlate. Further, patterns of discriminant validity were also lower for the orthogonal factors.

But the persistent question is "Why do we continue to find significant correlations between the various five factors?" If the underlying structure is in fact orthogonal, why is that not witnessed in real data? There are a number of studies, usually confirmatory in nature, that show substantial overlap among factors (e.g., Mooradian & Nezlek, 1996; Vassend & Skrondal, 1995). I believe one possible reason for this observed overlap is researchers' reliance on only a single source of information for obtaining the personality ratings: self-reports. Consequently, the observed interfactor correlations may be the result of correlated method error. If this potential source of error can be controlled for, then one would expect to find that the correlations among the five domains would become zero.

This hypothesis can be tested by obtaining personality ratings from multiple information sources. I evaluated this hypothesis using a sample of 178 undergraduate and graduate students who completed the Multidimensional Personality Questionnaire (MPQ; Tellegen, 1982) and a NEO PI–R for themselves as well as having two people rate them on the observer form of the NEO PI–R (see Piedmont, 1994, for a description of the sample and methods). The purpose of these analyses was to evaluate the overlap between the Neuroticism and Extraversion domains. As was out-lined earlier, these two factors are strongly related to experienced Well-Being and there continues to be some controversy over the relationship between these two domains. Some argue that Positive and Negative Affect (Extraversion and Neuroticism, respectively) are correlated (e.g., Chen, Dai, Spector, & Jex, 1997; Green, Goldman, & Salovey, 1993), while others believe the two to be truly orthogonal (e.g., Goldstein & Strube, 1994).

The MPQ contains two global domains of interest here, Positive Affect and Negative Affect. I tested two models using LISREL 8 (Jöreskog & Sör-bom, 1993). The first model is presented in Figure 6-1, and outlines two latent dimensions, Negative Affect (NEG-AFF) and Positive Affect (POS-AFF). The former was defined by self-rated measures of Neuroticism (SELFN) and Negative Affect (NEGAFF) as well as by observer-rated Neu-roticism (RATEN). The latter latent dimension was defined by self-rated Ex-traversion (SELFE) and Positive Affect (POSAFF) and observer-rated Extraversion (RATEE). As can be seen, the estimated correlation between the two latent dimensions was –.31, suggesting that Positive and Negative Affect may reflect a singular bipolar dimension rather than two distinct do-mains. The overall model chi square with 11 degrees of freedom was 25.47 (p = .0078), suggesting a relatively poor model fit, although the Normed Fit Index (NFI), Goodness of Fit Index (GFI) and Adjusted Goodness of Fit Index (AGFI) were all over .90, indicating that the model does match the data well. This apparent inconsistency is a regular problem noted in confir-matory analyses using personality-based data and is considered later.

A second model was also tested and it is presented in Figure 6-2. Here two additional latent dimensions were included, one that represented self-report variance and the other representing observer-rating variance. These dimensions were added to represent the impact of information source on scores. The overall model chi square with 4 degrees of freedom was 2.27 (p = .69) indicating a very good fit of the model to the data. Secondary fit indices were all uniformly close to unity (NFI = .99; GFI = 1.0; AGFI = .98) This model also fits the data significantly better than the previous one ($\Delta = \chi^2 = 23.2, p < .01$).

Two conclusions can be drawn from these data. First, by including the dimensions representing the information source for the ratings (e.g., self versus observer), we obtain a model that fits the data much better than when these dimensions are not included (model chi squares of 2.27 versus 25.47, respectively). Second, the estimated correlation between the latent personality domains drops to a nonsignificant –.18, supporting the con-tention that these domains are independent. Thus, the observed covari-

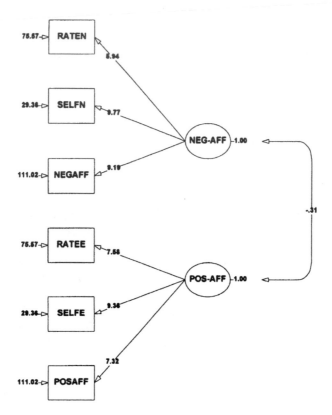

FIGURE 6-1. Estimated Confirmatory Factor Analysis Parameters for the Personality Only Model.

ance among the personality scales noted in these data can be attributed to correlated method error arising from a single information source (note that the correlation between rating sources is $r = .75$ which attests to the cross-observer validity of these personality dimensions). Thus, two personality scales will correlate both because they share substantive content and because it is the same person generating the information. Any distortions introduced in one scale by a person will also be included in all other measures he or she completes. Hence, all these measures will correlate to some degree.

These data support my contention that observed correlations among the five personality domains noted in several studies is the result of correlated error introduced by relying on a single information source. By using multiple raters and including latent dimensions that represent these

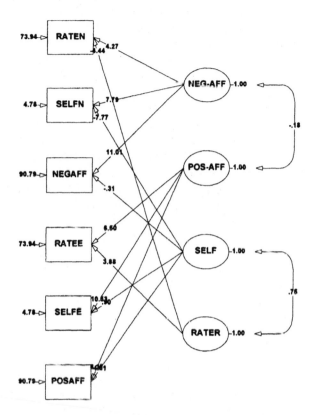

FIGURE 6-2. Estimated confirmatory factor analysis parameters for the Personality and Information Source Model.

sources of method variance in CFA models, it may be possible to remove this overlap from the estimated correlations among the substantive personality dimensions.

Thus, it appears that the five factors do represent independent aspects of personality. In order to capitalize on this reality, Costa and McCrae (1992c) provide weights for creating factor scores for each of the five factors. These factor scores are based on varimax rotations of NEO PI–R data from the standardization sample and result in factors that are indeed more orthogonal than the domain raw scores. The computer scoring program provides these values in lieu of the raw domain scores. These factors have also been shown to be better predictors of external criteria because they rely on information from all 30 facet scales. When conducting research with the NEO PI–R, it is preferable that these values be calculated and included rather than simply relying on values obtained by summing the facets for each domain.

NUMBER OF FACTORS

The issue of how many factors are needed to explain the full spectrum of personality continues to be debatable in the field. As noted in Chapter 1, there are numerous personality models advocating any number of personality domains. Discussions of the merits of these models is beyond the scope of this book, but the issue of how many factors there are does raise two concerns for us. The first issue relates to evaluating various factor structures and the second centers on one's ability to obtain the appropriate factor structure from NEO PI–R data.

Evaluating Factor Structures

In prefacing this section, a few comments on factor analysis are necessary. Factor analysis is a data reduction process. Its aim is to reduce a large set of items into homogeneous clusters of items known as factors. As is the case with all statistical analyses, such procedures are tools designed to help investigators obtain insights from a data set. As a tool, factor analysis can never provide "the answer" to a question one may hold of a data set. Rather, it can only suggest possible interpretations. A statistical test or analysis should never be seen as providing the final word; it can never do that. Even with an instrument as empirically sound as the NEO PI–R, factor analysis can never provide complete certainty for conclusions drawn from a set of data (see Vassend & Skrondal, 1995).

Also, as a tool, statistical results are only as good as the data they analyze. The term *GIGO* is appropriate here. It stands for "Garbage In, Garbage Out." Poor data, no matter how well analyzed or evaluated will always lead to poor statistical conclusions. Statistical analyses do *not* change the fundamental value of data. Instead, they merely try to make as much sense out of data as possible. In the social sciences, much of the data collected is weak. Samples are rarely randomly selected, the subjects to variables ratios are frequently low, distributions are not truly normal, and the ordinal nature of the data analyzed (to name a few problems) will always play havoc with the data analyses to an unknown degree. In terms of factor analysis, these problems manifest themselves through the non-replicability of factor structure across different samples, the emergence of method or error factors, and the encountering of anomalous statistical difficulties (e.g., negative variances, singular matrices). Therefore, great care needs to be taken in the interpretation of the results from factor analyses. Perhaps the most important criteria for evaluating the worth of any factor analysis is the degree to which the obtained structure can be replicated across different samples. Other than that, *caveat emptor*.

With that said, it should be realized that there are researchers who believe that the five factor model specifies either too many factors or too few. For example, Eysenck believed that there are only three factors: Neuroticism, Extraversion, and Psychoticism (Eysenck, 1991; Eysenck & Eysenck, 1985). Neuroticism and Extraversion correspond well to their five-factor model equivalents; however, Psychoticism is seen as a "superfactor"; it combines Agreeableness and Conscientiousness into one domain. Openness to Experience is not represented in this model. Still others believe that there should be more than five factors. For example, Jackson, Ashton, and Tomes (1996) have suggested that there are six factors. They found evidence for N, E, O, and A. Conscientiousness, however, was found to be broken into two specialized dimensions, Industriousness and Methodicalness. Tellegen and Waller (in press) believe that there are seven dimensions: the already acknowledged five plus Positive and Negative Valence (see also Almagor, Tellegen, & Waller, 1995; Benet & Waller, 1995). These additional two factors represent more of the evaluative nature of personality assessment. Unlike the adjectives that were used to generate the five-factor model, the terms subsumed by these new factors represent qualities that were originally considered unsuitable for analysis (e.g., excellent, impressive, wicked, cruel).

All of these different personality models claim support for themselves, and do so in relation to the five-factor model. Frequently supporting data is provided that includes either the NEO PI–R or markers for the five factors. How can such models exist given the very strong empirical basis of the five-factor model? Is the five-factor model incorrect in its specification of personality dimensions? These are important questions that need to be answered. But it is reassuring that these questions are empirical questions. In other words, data can be used to settle the issues that these studies raise. The way to analyze data to answer these kinds of questions is at the heart of this section.

When Five Factors Are Not Enough

In evaluating whether there are more than five factors, the first test of the larger factor set's viability should be replication: Can the factor structure be obtained in multiple samples? If the kinds of statistical artifacts mentioned earlier (e.g., low subjects to variables ratio, non-normal distributions) are operating in a data set to create additional factors, these forces will be much less influential or entirely absent in another data set containing the same variables. Thus, obtaining a similar factor structure in a different sample will be very difficult.

Factor comparability is usually obtained through the use of a congruence coefficient (see Gorsuch, 1983, for how to calculate this value and for other comparability indices). A congruence coefficient is a value between 0 and 1 that indexes the degree to which the pattern and magnitude of the factor loadings from two analyses that include the same variables measured over different samples are equivalent. Usually a value of .90 or greater is considered high enough to warrant the conclusion that two solutions are identical (i.e., the obtained factors represent equivalent entities). However, there are other methods for determining how high a congruence coefficient needs to be (see McCrae, Zonderman, *et al.*, 1996).

If a replicated factor structure can be obtained, such an event, in and of itself, does not call into question the comprehensiveness of the five-factor model. McCrae and Costa (1995) outlined three criteria that need to be met before these additional factors can be accepted as new dimensions. First, the new factor or factors must be shown to be independent of the original five. Second, the new factor or factors should be of the same general breadth as the other five; the new factor should encompass several other, more specific qualities in its range of convenience in a way similar to the way each domain of the NEO PI–R contains six facet scales. Third, the new factor should be recoverable from multiple sources of information. The qualities of personality represented in this new factor should also be recoverable from other established personality instruments. Further, these new qualities should be able to be consensually validated, being found in *both* self-reports and observer ratings. When these criteria are applied, many studies claiming more than five personality domains fail (see McCrae & Costa, 1995; Piedmont, McCrae, & Costa, 1991).

These criteria distinguish between a true, broad-based dimension of personality and more specific, unique personality descriptions. As noted in Chapter 1, there are qualities of personality that are reliably obtained, but reflect highly circumscribed aspects of personality (e.g., Goldberg, 1990). One needs to be careful not to overvalue additional, circumscribed factors that may be encountered in a data set.

When Five Factors Are Too Many

The problem of fewer than five factors provides another set of issues to be considered when working factor analytically with the NEO PI–R. As noted earlier, Eysenck has argued that there are only three factors that describe personality; Neuroticism (N), Extraversion (E), and Psychoticism (P). Clearly, in a system such as this the smaller model is either leaving out dimensions of personality or is combining some of the NEO PI–R domains into a single, more global dimension. If the smaller model is leaving out information that is contained in the NEO PI–R, then usually one can be confident that the smaller model is overlooking important aspects of personality. If it is combining domains, then some empirical considerations need to be evaluated to determine whether the smaller model is to be preferred due to its greater parsimony or whether the smaller model is inappropriately combining independent dimensions.

For the three-factor model advocated by Eysenck, both issues emerge. First, Eysenck's model leaves out the dimension of Openness to Experience. However, Eysenck (1991) has suggested that Openness is really an aspect of cognitive ability rather than personality. Although there is data showing that Openness is *not* an aspect of cognitive functioning (McCrae, 1993–1994, 1994b), let us finesse this point for now by granting the issue to Eysenck (see Costa & McCrae, 1995b, for a response). This still leaves us with the need to evaluate the worth of a system with fewer than five factors.

Several studies have shown that Eysenck's dimension of Psychoticism is inversely related to the domains of Agreeableness and Conscientiousness (e.g., Costa *et al.*, 1991; Goldberg & Rosolack, 1994) and Eysenck (1992) has interpreted this to mean that these domains are merely facets of the larger Psychoticism dimension. However, Costa and McCrae (1992b, 1995b) have argued that Psychoticism represents "a relatively arbitrary conflation of two independent dimensions" (1995b, p. 310). As noted earlier in this chapter, the question as to whether the five factors should be considered orthogonal or correlated has important conceptual implications. If the five factors are correlated, then this leaves open the possibility of obtaining "high-order factors," super dimensions that are comprised of two or more of the five. This is what Eysenck claimed. However, if the five domains are orthogonal, then no such super factors can exist (an identity matrix cannot be factored) and Costa and McCrae would be correct. Although the data suggest that orthogonal factors have better predictive validities than oblique (correlated) factors, there are other empirical criteria that can be applied for evaluating the internal quality of a factor structure.

One important way of clarifying this issue is to evaluate the pattern of external correlations these elements have. One of the important aspects of factor analysis is that it identifies homogeneous groupings of items. As in the NEO PI–R, the six facet scales are more specific articulations of the larger domain to which they belong. Thus, these scales all correlate in a similar way with relevant criteria. For example, all six Neuroticism facets are related to low psychological well-being (e.g., Costa & McCrae, 1984). Therefore, aggregating across the facets produces domain scores that are more reliable and stable than their constituent elements. If Agreeableness and Conscientiousness are merely subfacets to Psychoticism, then they should reveal a similar pattern of correlates to a given criterion and summing these two dimensions together should produce an index that is more strongly associated with this criterion than either of the domains separately.

Costa and McCrae (1995b) used this strategy in evaluating the relations between the NEO PI–R and the Eysenck Personality Profiler (EPP). Correlations between Agreeableness and Conscientious and the EPP scales showed very different patterns of correlates for the two NEO PI–R domains. Further, when Agreeableness and Conscientiousness were aggregated and then correlated to the EPP scales, the resulting correlations were *lower* than their individual associations. Thus, the Psychoticism dimension appears to inappropriately combine independent personality qualities. This forced aggregation ultimately impairs external validity, which should be regarded as an important criterion for evaluating the utility of any personality model.

What should be taken from this discussion is that empirical methods can and do generate a wide variety of statistical models for describing personality systems. Any review of the current literature will reveal numerous taxonomic models ranging from 3 to as many as 16 factors. Often, the quantitative basis of these models is quite compelling. This can leave one quite confused about the state of affairs in personality measurement. How many factors are there? But with a little care and patience, the discerning reader can begin to ask the appropriate, sophisticated questions that can provide an answer to that question. Given that the five-factor model has been shown to be a reliable description of personality variables, it can and should be the reference point for any critical evaluation of other models.

In the case of a model advocating more than five personality dimensions, the questions that need to be asked include whether the factor structure can be replicated in a new sample, the independence of the new factors from the established five, and the personological breadth of the new domains. When a model advocates fewer than five factors, it needs to be determined whether the model omits something already contained in the five-factor model. Such an omission would be sufficient evidence to reject the new model. However, if the model seems to combine two or more of the Big Five's domains, then some evaluation of the predictive utility of this global factor needs to be conducted. Does the "super factor" actually evidence higher external validity than its components? If not, then the new model does not provide an optimal specification of personality structure.

RECOVERING THE NEO PI–R STRUCTURE IN NEW SAMPLES

The NEO PI–R is extensively used in a wide array of applications, including industrial and organizational, psychotherapeutic, medical, and cross-cultural contexts. In each of these environments issues emerge concerning the psychometric properties of the instrument with these new populations. This is especially true when the scale is used internationally. An important question that emerges concerns the cross-cultural generalizability of the five-factor model: Is it as useful a description of personality when employed with individuals who do not have the same lexical and historical heritage as the West? Do the basic concepts of the five-factor model remain relevant in new cultures? Answers to these questions have important implications for those who wish to construct a unified theory of personality structure and development.

Empirically, answers to these questions involve a confirmatory data analytic approach. In these studies, data are collected on the NEO PI–R in a new sample and the questions are whether the five-factor structure can be recovered and if the obtained structure is similar to normative values. Thus, a set of observed values are compared to an *a priori* defined numerical model. The closer the obtained values come to the ideal values, the more likely that the data will be regarded as "fitting" the model. Programs such as LISREL (Jöreskog & Sörbom, 1993) are designed to mathematically evaluate this kind of model fit. The value of this approach is that one must specify some theoretical model and the relations among the respective elements prior to conducting the research. This is a much more sophisticated and powerful approach to data analysis than the usual *post hoc*, exploratory methods commonly employed. Exploratory methods capitalize heavily on chance and sample specific factors that result in poor replicability of findings.

Confirmatory Factor Analysis (CFA) has been used quite frequently in NEO PI–R research, and has generated much controversy. Of particular interest has been the apparent failure to find the anticipated five-factor structure. Borkenau and Ostendorf (1990) conducted the first CFA of NEO PI–R data and found that the observed data did not fit the expected model very well. Parker, Bagby, and Summerfeldt (1993) performed a CFA of the original NEO PI–R normative data. They tested several models, including complex ones that specified secondary loadings among the facets, and found that none of their models provided satisfactory fit. In a later study by Panter, Tanaka, and Hoyle (1994) it was found that the five factors were by no means mutually independent. That these findings are at variance with other empirical evidence that shows a clear, replicable factor structure raises two possibilities. The first is that the five-factor model does not have a robust structure. Studies finding this structure may have capitalized on sample specific variance, or the five-factor model may be a limited phenomenon, emerging only in certain segments of our society (e.g., college students). The second possibility is that CFA procedures may not be appropriate for use with personality data. Specifically, CFA may require a model to explain more variance in the data than is possible given the reliabilities of the measures used.

In order to evaluate these two possibilities, Burke and his colleagues (Church & Burke, 1994; Katigbak *et al.*, 1996) systematically evaluated both the five-factor structure in a cross-cultural sample (Filipinos) and CFA procedures relative to exploratory analyses. The first result of note in these studies was that a five-factor model did emerge from NEO PI–R data when exploratory factor analysis (EFA) was applied. This model was also found to cross-validate strongly in another sample. Thus the data clearly showed not only that the five factors are present but that their relevance emerged in a sample very different from the original derivation sample. Once this replicable structure was obtained, the data (and model) were subjected to CFA to determine fit. Given the robustness of the model in these different samples, it would not have been surprising to find convergence with the CFA results. However, the CFA results were repeatedly disappointing. As Katigbak and colleagues (1996) noted,

> In theory, confirmatory factor analysis would seem to be the ideal method for testing the cross-cultural generalizability of a personality model. However, an increasing number of studies . . . indicate that both its significance tests and conventional goodness-of-fit criteria may be too stringent. . . . Indeed, we found here that exploratory factor solutions that are highly congruent across samples . . . were judged to have at best only a fair fit when applied in these different (cross-validation) samples. (p. 111)

McCrae, Zonderman, *et al.* (1996) believed that the assumptions underlying CFA may not be appropriate to real personality-type data.

At the heart of CFA analyses is the chi square test for model fit. This is a major advantage to the approach because it allows one to evaluate how well observed data fit some *a priori* model. However, problems with the chi square test have been known for years (e.g., Bentler & Bonnett, 1980; Marsh, Balla, & McDonald, 1988). The most problematic issue concerns the sensitivity of the statistic to sample size. Given a large enough sample, any model will be rejected. As a result numerous other fit indexes have been developed to address this issue, but their interpretation and statistical properties are not fully understood. Consequently they do not have accompanying significance tests and this leaves their practical value in question. As noted earlier, a common finding in CFA analysis using personality data is that an overall chi-square fit statistic is significant (indicating that the model does not fit the data) yet secondary fit indexes show that there is a high level of congruence. This type of outcome is awkward to manage both statistically and interpretively.

Although CFA may not be the most appropriate method for evaluating how well a factor structure resembles the underlying five-factor model, users of the NEO PI–R still need to have some confirmatory-based approach for evaluating structure in new samples. EFA methods spring to mind, but they have their own limitations. First, they provide solutions that are sample specific. Given the reality that research samples rarely are representative of a population, it is possible that limited, nonreplicable factors could emerge in a specific data set. Therefore, without a clear statistical model driving the analysis itself, it becomes difficult for researchers to discern the merits among a variety of potentially acceptable solutions.

One analytic strategy, using EFA techniques, could be to extract five factors from a NEO PI–R data set in a new sample and to compare them statistically with normative values presented in the manual. Such a comparison would use congruence coefficients (Gorsuch, 1983) to assess the actual degree of comparability between the two sets of structures. Although Katigbak and colleagues (1996) saw this approach as the preferred strategy for those using personality data, they point out a disadvantage: Sample specific variation in the covariance among NEO PI–R facets may overstate differences between the observed sample and normative values. This is because the NEO PI–R does not evidence true simple structure. Many of the facet scales have significant secondary loadings on other factors. These cross-factor loadings make sense theoretically and have been replicated numerous times (e.g., Church & Burke, 1994). For example, Angry Hostility, a facet of Neuroticism, reflects one's tendency to experience anger. However, individuals low on Agreeableness also tend to experience and express anger directly; thus this facet loads negatively on Agreeableness as well. Perhaps the most problematic area concerns the facets for Extraversion and Agreeableness. These two domains comprise the interpersonal circumplex, so the facets scales form a more complex, circular pattern around these two domains. Small, sample specific changes in these scales' patterns of covariation could lead to very different factor structures for these two domains.

In order to address this problem, McCrae, Zonderman, *et al.* (1996) proposed a methodology for conducting confirmatory analyses using NEO PI–R data that allows one to determine whether an obtained data set matches a normative structure. The value of this approach is threefold. First, it relies on EFA techniques which have shown themselves to be most straightforward and useful for analyzing personality-type data. Second, it provides an a priori empirical framework for factor analyzing the data matrix. Finally, it provides useful measures of fit. The proposed methodology uses regular EFA methods for extraction of five factors, and then orthogonal Procrustes rotations to obtain final structural fit of the data.

Orthogonal Procrustean rotation is a type of targeted rotation (Schönemann, 1966). The goal is to rotate an observed set of data into a format that is determined *a priori*. The predetermined structure serves as the "target matrix" that the rotation attempts to approximate. The eigenvectors (factor loadings) of the rotated solution are then compared to the normative (targeted) values through use of congruence coefficients. These values determine how well the real data represents the model. Usually, congruence coefficients greater than .90 are considered high enough to convey adequate "fit." McCrae, Zonderman, *et al.* (1996) have developed actual significance values for these statistics.

In order to evaluate the degree of fit, congruence coefficients are calculated for not only the overall five factors, but also for the pattern of loadings for each facet scale across the five factors. It is possible for an overall factor (which is based on the loadings for 30 facet scales) to have acceptable fit, but individual facets may not show correspondence with their respective normative values. Thus, these congruence coefficients can be used as "modification" indexes for evaluating where and to what degree a particular element does not conform to its expected values. Table 6-1 presents an SPSS Matrix program for performing a Procrustean rotation of NEO PI–R data.

As can be seen, there are two principal data matrices. The *norms* matrix is already provided. These values are the factor loadings for the NEO PI–R in the normative sample. This matrix will serve as the target matrix for rotating obtained data. The other matrix, *loadings,* is for the actual data. It should be entered as a 30 (rows) by 5 (columns) matrix. The first column should be the factor loadings for each of the facet scales on Neuroticism, the next column is for Extraversion, then Openness, Agreeableness, and Conscientiousness, in that order. The entered loadings can be either rotated or unrotated loadings from the original EFA. The program will automatically print out a table of its results. It will calculate congruence coefficients for each factor and facet scale, and an overall fit congruence coefficient. McCrae, Zonderman, *et al.* (1996) provided .05 and .01 critical values for these congruence coefficients for each of these statistics. The 95th and 99th percentile cutoff values for the domain factor coefficients are .55 and .65, respectively. Similar cutoff values for the facet congruence coefficients are .86 and .94, respectively. Finally, the critical values for the overall congruence coefficient are .42 and .46, respectively.

Orthogonal Procrustes Rotations serve as a useful compromise strategy for doing confirmatory analyses using NEO PI–R data. It capitalizes on the straightforward, familiar techniques of EFA and avoids the many restrictive assumptions of CFA. Most notably, it provides a method of evaluating structural fit in a way that is not overly dependent on sample specific variance. In other words, whatever distortions may be in the data at hand, the influence on the final factor structure is minimized because the data are being rotated to a form determined *a priori.*

TABLE 6-1. SPSS Program for Conducting an Orthogonal Procrustean Rotation of NEO PI–R Factor Data

matrix.
compute   loadings={

Insert your own principal components derived, orthogonally rotated five factors
Must be a 30 (rows) by 5 (columns) matrix. Follow format of next section.
                             }.

compute   norms ={

.81,	.02,	−.01,	−.01,	−.10 ;
.63,	−.03,	.01,	−.48,	−.08 ;
.80,	−.10,	.02,	−.03,	−.26 ;
.73,	−.18,	−.09,	.04,	−.16 ;
.49,	.35,	.02,	−.21,	−.32 ;
.70,	−.15,	−.09,	.04,	−.38 ;
−.12,	.66,	.18,	.38,	.13 ;
−.18,	.66,	.04,	.07,	−.03 ;
−.32,	.44,	.23,	−.32,	.32 ;
.04,	.54,	.16,	−.27,	.42 ;
.00,	.58,	.11,	−.38,	−.06 ;
−.04,	.74,	.19,	.10,	.10 ;
.18,	.18,	.58,	−.14,	−.31 ;
.14,	.04,	.73,	.17,	.14 ;
.37,	.41,	.50,	−.01,	.12 ;
−.19,	.22,	.57,	.04,	−.04 ;
−.15,	−.01,	.75,	−.09,	.16 ;
−.13,	.08,	.49,	−.07,	−.15 ;
−.35,	.22,	.15,	.56,	.03 ;
−.03,	−.15,	−.11,	.68,	.24 ;
−.06,	.52,	−.05,	.55,	.27 ;
−.16,	−.08,	−.00,	.77,	.01 ;
.19,	−.12,	−.18,	.59,	−.08 ;
.04,	.27,	.13,	.62,	.00 ;
−.41,	.17,	.13,	.03,	.64 ;
−.04,	.06,	−.19,	.01,	.70 ;
−.20,	−.04,	.01,	.29,	.68 ;
−.09,	.23,	.15,	−.13,	.74 ;
−.33,	.17,	−.08,	.06,	.75 ;
−.23,	−.28,	−.04,	.22,	.57}.

```
compute    s=t(loadings)*norms.
compute    w1=s*t(s).
compute    v1=t(s)*s.
call    eigen(w1,w,evalw1).
call    eigen(v1,v,evalv1).
compute    o=t(w)*s*v.
compute    q1=o &/abs(o).
compute    k1=diag(q1).
compute    k=mdiag(k1).
```

(continued)

TABLE 6-1. (*Continued*)

```
compute    ww=w*k.
compute    t1=ww*t(v).
compute    procrust=loadings*t1.
compute    cm1m2=t(procrust)*norms.
compute    ca=diag(cm1m2).
compute    csum2m1=cssq(procrust).
compute    csum2m2=cssq(norms).
compute    csqrtl1=sqrt(csum2m1).
compute    csqrtl2=sqrt(csum2m2).
compute    cb=t(csqrtl1)*csqrtl2.
compute    cc=diag(cb).
compute    cd=ca&/cc.
compute    faccongc=t(cd).
compute    rm1m2=procrust*t(norms).
compute    ra=diag(rm1m2).
compute    rsum2m1=rssq(procrust).
compute    rsum2m2=rssq(norms).
compute    rsqrtl1=sqrt(rsum2m1).
compute    rsqrtl2=sqrt(rsum2m2).
compute    rb=rsqrtl1*t(rsqrtl2).
compute    rc=diag(rb).
compute    faccongr=ra&/rc.
compute    top={ca;ra}.
compute    bot={cc;rc}.
compute    ctop=csum(top).
compute    cbot=csum(bot).
compute    total=ctop/cbot.
compute    procrust={procrust,faccongr;faccongc,total}.
print      procrust /title = "FACTOR CONGRUENCE COEFFICIENTS"
     /format f5.2
     /clabels= "NEURO"  "EXTRA"  "OPEN"  "AGREE"  "CONSC"  "ITEMCONG"
     /RLABELS=  "N1"  "N2"  "N3"  "N4"  "N5"  "N6"  "E1"  "E2"  "E3"  "E4"
                "E5"  "E6"  "O1"  "O2"  "O3"  "O4"  "O5"  "O6"  "A1"  "A2"
                "A3"  "A4"  "A5"  "A6"  "C1"  "C2"  "C3"  "C4"  "C5"  "C6"
                "FACTCONG"
     /space=newpage.
END MATRIX.
```

An example of this process may help highlight the methodology. The following data are taken from Piedmont and Chae (1997), who were interested in developing a Korean version of the NEO PI–R. The emphasis was on determining whether the measure in its new form could be considered structurally equivalent to its English relative. A translated version was given to 653 native Koreans and the resulting information was factor analyzed

using EFA techniques. Five factors were extracted and rotated and the results of this analysis are presented in Table 6-2. Congruence coefficients were
calculated between this solution and factor loadings presented in the NEO
PI–R manual (Costa & McCrae, 1992c). Several findings of interest emerge.

First, the overall congruence coefficient of .82 is significant, suggesting that the general structure is comparable with normative values. In fact,
an examination of each of the five factor congruence coefficients (located at
the bottom of the columns) suggests that all five factors are recovered in a
form comparable to the normative structure. The domains of Neuroticism,
Openness, and Conscientiousness more strongly resemble their English
counterparts than do Extraversion and Agreeableness. However, an examination of the facet congruence coefficients indicates that none of the
facet scales for the latter two domains is well replicated. The insignificant
coefficients tell us that the pattern of loadings for these scales across the
five domains is different from that found in the normative structure.
Clearly, in using EFA there is a failure to replicate two of the five domains.

But there are several reasons for this apparent failure. One reason is
that the five factors do not operate in a way that was observed in America.
Given the cross-cultural nature of this sample, this different factor structure
may have something important to say about Korean culture and how personality is expressed through it. A second explanation deals with the fact
that the NEO PI–R does not have perfect simple structure and that subtle
shifts in the facet scales' interrelatedness could impact overall structure.
Given, as noted earlier, that the Extraversion and Agreeableness domains
constitute the interpersonal circumplex, a complex ordering of traits that is
designed to combine various quantities of these two dimensions, this second explanation may be likely. The only way to determine which of these
two hypotheses is correct is to conduct an Orthogonal Procrustes rotation
of the results. If such an analysis still could not recover the five domains in
a way consistent with normative data, then this would be strong evidence
that personality may indeed be organized differently in Korean culture.
However, if the normative structure could be better approximated, then the
observed distortions most likely are due to sample specific factors.

These data were then analyzed using the statistical program presented in Table 6-1. The result of this targeted rotation procedure was the
factor structure presented in Table 6-3. As can be seen, the obtained factor
structure more closely approximates normative values. The overall congruence coefficient is much higher than previously found (.96 versus .82).
The congruence coefficients for the five factors are all quite high, including
the Extraversion and Agreeableness domains, whose values have risen
to .95. Finally, the facet congruence coefficients also show significant

TABLE 6-2.. Principal Components Analysis Using a Varimax Rotation of the Korean NEO PI–R Facet Scales.

Korean NEO PI-R Facets	Varimax factor loadings					Facet congruence
	Factor 1	Factor 2	Factor 3	Factor 4	Factor 5	
N1: Anxiety	**.81**	.02	.02	−.02	−.14	.99[b]
N2: Angry Hostility	**.65**	.35	.05	−.25	−.16	.84
N3: Depression	**.82**	−.07	.09	−.11	−.19	.99[b]
N4: Self-Consciousness	**.81**	−.06	−.03	−.10	−.06	.96[b]
N5: Impulsiveness	**.52**	.36	.15	−.05	**−.49**	.95[b]
N6: Vulnerability	**.71**	−.11	−.12	−.02	**−.42**	.99[b]
E1: Warmth	−.05	.20	.19	**.79**	−.08	.68
E2: Gregariousness	−.15	**.40**	−.14	**.63**	−.12	.62
E3: Assertiveness	−.31	**.63**	.08	.09	.22	.79
E4: Activity	.13	**.63**	.08	.20	.23	.74
E5: Excitement Seeking	.09	**.61**	.18	.19	−.18	.64
E6: Positive Emotions	−.26	.35	**.41**	**.44**	−.08	.66
O1: Fantasy	.21	.10	**.53**	.01	−.32	.97[b]
O2: Aesthetics	.09	.00	**.72**	.19	.01	.98[b]
O3: Feelings	.17	.24	**.70**	.13	.11	.89[a]
O4: Actions	−.27	.31	.37	.08	−.24	.88[a]
O5: Ideas	−.10	.21	**.72**	−.05	.14	.96[b]
O6: Values	−.27	−.18	**.51**	.10	−.09	.83
A1: Trust	−.32	−.21	.09	**.60**	.24	.78
A2: Straightforwardness	−.16	**−.52**	.07	.19	.33	.57
A3: Altruism	−.08	.34	.14	**.68**	.22	.39
A4: Compliance	−.09	**−.71**	−.03	.21	−.04	.39
A5: Modesty	.23	**−.46**	−.25	.15	−.01	.60
A6: Tendermindedness	.11	−.29	.36	**.48**	.17	.56
C1: Competence	**−.48**	.18	.13	.07	**.54**	.99[b]
C2: Order	−.09	.06	−.13	−.02	**.70**	.99[b]
C3: Dutifulness	−.04	−.12	−.03	.23	**.80**	.96[b]
C4: Achievement	−.07	**.42**	.07	−.02	**.67**	.95[b]
C5: Self-Discipline	**−.43**	.04	.01	.04	**.71**	.97[b]
C6: Deliberation	−.25	−.23	.05	−.04	**.64**	.92[a]
Factor Congruence	.97[b]	.60[a]	.93[b]	.61[a]	.95[b]	.82[b]

N = 653. Loadings above |.40| are in bold.

[a]Congruence higher than that of 95% of rotations from random data.

[b]Congruence higher than that of 99% of rotations from random data McCrae, Zonderman, *et al.*

Note. From "Cross-Cultural Generalizability of the Five-Factor Model of Personality: Development and Validation of the NEO PI–R for Koreans," by R. L. Piedmont and J. H. Chae, 1997, *Journal of Cross-Cultural Psychology, 28,* p. 141. Copyright 1997 by Western Washington University. Adapted with permission.

TABLE 6.3. Principal Components Analysis Using an Orthogonal Procrustes
Rotation of the Korean NEO PI–R Facet Scales

Korean NEO PI–R Facets	Procrustean factor loadings					Facet congruence
	Factor 1	Factor 2	Factor 3	Factor 4	Factor 5	
N1: Anxiety	**.81**	.01	−.06	−.03	−.15	.99[b]
N2: Angry Hostility	**.66**	.03	.03	**−.43**	−.10	.99[b]
N3: Depression	**.82**	−.11	.02	−.02	−.21	.99[b]
N4: Self-Consciousness	**.80**	−.11	−.11	−.01	−.09	.99[b]
N5: Impulsiveness	**.54**	.23	.15	−.36	**−.42**	.95[b]
N6: Vulnerability	**.69**	−.05	−.17	.01	**−.45**	.98[b]
E1: Warmth	−.04	**.76**	.14	.33	−.04	.96[b]
E2: Gregariousness	−.17	**.75**	−.15	.03	−.06	.96[b]
E3: Assertiveness	−.28	**.43**	.12	**−.40**	.34	.98[b]
E4: Activity	.15	**.51**	.06	−.33	.34	.97[b]
E5: Excitement Seeking	.12	**.54**	.19	−.37	−.06	.98[b]
E6: Positive Emotions	−.21	**.58**	**.41**	.02	.01	.90[a]
O1: Fantasy	.26	.12	**.53**	−.06	−.27	.98[b]
O2: Aesthetics	.16	.18	**.68**	.19	.05	.97[b]
O3: Feelings	.25	.26	**.66**	−.02	.19	.94[b]
O4: Actions	−.23	.29	**.42**	−.19	−.15	.88[a]
O5: Ideas	−.02	.10	**.73**	−.10	.22	.97[b]
O6: Values	−.22	.00	**.52**	.24	−.08	.84
A1: Trust	−.32	.33	.04	**.56**	.21	.95[a]
A2: Straightforwardness	−.16	−.19	.02	**.57**	.24	.96[b]
A3: Altruism	−.08	.32	.05	**.72**	.16	.93[a]
A4: Compliance	−.11	−.25	−.07	**.67**	−.17	.94[a]
A5: Modesty	.19	−.16	−.31	**.43**	−.11	.95[b]
A6: Tendermindedness	.14	.20	.27	**.58**	.13	.94[b]
C1: Competence	**−.46**	.12	.14	−.02	**.58**	.99[b]
C2: Order	−.10	−.06	−.16	.02	**.69**	.98[b]
C3: Dutifulness	−.04	.03	−.11	.34	**.76**	.96[b]
C4: Achievement	−.05	.17	.05	−.24	**.74**	.98[b]
C5: Self-Discipline	**−.42**	−.01	.00	.09	**.71**	.96[b]
C6: Deliberation	−.24	−.23	.02	.25	**.60**	.99[b]
Factor Congruence	.98[b]	.95[b]	.94[b]	.95[b]	.97[b]	.96[b]

N = 653. Loadings above |.40| are in bold.
[a]Congruence higher than that of 95% of rotations from random data.
[b]Congruence higher than that of 99% of rotations from random data
Note. From "Cross-Cultural Generalizability of the Five-Factor Model of Personality: Development and Validation of the NEO PI–R for Koreans," by R. L. Piedmont and J. H. Chae, 1997, *Journal of Cross-Cultural Psychology, 28,* p. 142. Copyright 1997 by Western Washington University. Adapted with permission.

improvement: All of the 12 facets for Extraversion and Agreeableness now present themselves in a way that is identical to normative values. Thus, we can be confident that the NEO PI–R is quite similar structurally in both Korean and American samples. The Procrustean rotation helped disentangle sample specific error from more substantive relationships among these variables.

Those interested in evaluating the generalizability of the NEO PI–R to new samples should use this approach for several reasons. First, CFA techniques appear too stringent for use with personality data. All too often adequate fit is not found for proposed models. The resulting "modifications" that are introduced into the analyses in order to find a better solution are frequently *post hoc* in nature and, at times, theoretically uninterpretable. However, EFA techniques are not entirely appropriate either. EFA does not capitalize on the fact that an *a priori* model exists and this information does not fully inform the analytic process. Finally, this approach is the one recommended by the authors of the NEO PI–R as being the most useful (McCrae, Zonderman, *et al.*, 1996). Thus, any discussion of the factorial stability of the NEO PI–R will need to be done within this medium if it is to be seriously considered.

APPLICATION OF NEO PI–R DATA TO VALIDITY RESEARCH

Because the five-factor model represents a comprehensive framework of personality qualities, it is a useful standard for evaluating the personological content of scales. Correlating an instrument with markers of the five factors provides a personological "fingerprint," enabling users to better understand those aspects of the individual represented in the scale and the kinds of outcomes that can be anticipated. As Ozer and Riese (1994) have noted, mapping scales onto the five personality domains helps to clarify a scale's relations to other psychological constructs. As was discussed in Chapter 2, evaluating personological content solely on the basis of a scale's name can be quite misleading. The fact that two scales have the same name does not mean that they assess similar constructs. Similarly, different scale names does not mean that the scales measure different qualities. Rather, the similarity or dissimilarity between two scales can be inferred from the pattern of correlates each has to the five-factor model.

The value of the NEO PI–R in this process is that it provides measures of not only the five major personality dimensions, but also 30 facet scales that can more specifically highlight the motivational basis of scales. In this section, I expand on the value of using the NEO PI–R in validity research, especially as it pertains to the development of a scale's construct and incremental validity.

CONSTRUCT VALIDITY

The world of personality assessment is indeed very rich, if one were to use the number of existing scales as a measure of affluence. As I reviewed in Chapters 1 and 2, there are literally thousands of measures designed to capture a multitude of personality characteristics. There can be no doubt that among those instruments there is a tremendous amount of redundancy in content. Therefore, it becomes necessary for test developers to show the uniqueness of the constructs they develop. Although the NEO PI–R was not developed to replace all other assessment instruments, because it provides a relatively comprehensive sampling of personality traits it is in a unique position to enable test developers to think with more sophistication about the theoretical basis of their constructs and about the range of phenomena that the scale will predict.

Of course, forcing a greater degree of precision and accuracy into the development of scales increases the difficulty of making new instruments, but the payoff is certainly greater. It would be much to the benefit of the field to have fewer scales, with clearly understood, nonredundant personological content, than a haphazard amalgam of poorly defined measures (see Meehl, 1978, p. 823, for an excellent discussion of this and related issues). Bringing such empirical and conceptual clarity is where the NEO PI–R comes in. Its value is particularly relevant in areas where researchers are only beginning to delineate individual-difference constructs that define their field of interest. One such area is the field of religious research, which is used here to exemplify how the NEO PI–R can be fruitfully applied to the construct validation process.

Religious researchers are interested in determining how religion and spirituality influence human development and behavior. Recently this area of endeavor has literally exploded with interest, as attested by the development of literally dozens of new scales. This interest in scale development reflects a real need for researchers in this area to get a handle on the spiritual dimensions of the person. But this wholesale development of scales has proceeded without much interest in integrating all these measures into some cohesive model. Thus, researchers in this field are left with a rather chaotic mishmash of measures. The situation is so bad that Gorsuch (1988) has argued that no new religious measures be developed until the construct validity of the existing instruments can be better ascertained.

The real question in this area is whether these putatively spiritual constructs represent qualities of people that are distinct from established personality measures or are rather some new combination of them. Also, without any larger framework for classifying spiritual constructs, the possibility of redundancy in content is very high. Although the five-factor model is not religiously based, it can provide a useful starting point for evaluating the personological content of religious constructs. As I have noted elsewhere (Piedmont, 1996b), if religious variables have any overlap with personality, then correlating such scales with the five factors can help illuminate the underlying personological motivations of the scale as well as highlight the types of behavioral outcomes to be anticipated. Further, correlations with the five-factor model can also help to nomologically link religious constructs with one another.

In order to address this question, I gave the NEO PI–R along with several popularly used religious scales to a mixed-sex undergraduate sample of 493 people. The first scale was the Hood Mysticism Scale (Hood, 1975), a measure of reported mystical experiences. It contains two factors, a general mystical experience dimension and the joyful or noetic qualities associated with religious experiences. Also given was the Faith Maturity Scale (Benson, Donahue, & Erickson, 1993). It reflects "the degree to which a person embodies the priorities, commitments, and perspectives characteristic of vibrant and life-transforming faith" (p. 3). There are two subscales, the Vertical, which evaluates the degree to which one has a close relationship with God, and the Horizontal, which looks at the degree to which one's faith influences relationships with others. The third measure was the Intrinsic/Extrinsic Religiosity Scale (Gorsuch & Venable, 1983). Intrinsic Religiosity reflects a religious orientation that is internalized and done for its own sake. Extrinsic Religiosity reflects an attitude toward religious involvement for the sake of achieving some other goal. The final measure was the Spiritual Well-Being scale (Ellison, 1983). This scale attempts to measure spirituality as it speaks to overall well-being. There are two subscales, Religious Well-Being, which examines the level of satisfaction one experiences in his or her relationship with God, and Existential Well-Being, which evaluates the level of personal meaning one has derived for his or her life. The correlation of these scales to the NEO PI–R is given in Table 6-4.

Two conclusions can be drawn from these data. First, the number of significant correlations attests to the relevance of the five-factor model for understanding religious-oriented constructs. For example, the Intrinsic Religiosity scale correlated positively with Agreeableness and Conscientiousness. People who have an internalized view toward religion may be perceived by others as being moral, reverent, considerate, responsible, and dependable (Hofstee, de Raad, & Goldberg, 1992). The negative correlation

TABLE 6-4. Correlations between Select Religious Constructs and the NEO PI–R Domains

| Religious scale | NEO PI–R Domain | | | | | R^2 | α | $\alpha-R^2$ | $1-\alpha$ | ΔR^2 |
	N	E	O	A	C					
Hood Mysticism 1[a]	.02	.08	.23[e]	−.04	.02	.06[e]	.90	.84	.10	.001
Hood Mysticism 2[b]	−.04	.13[d]	.20[e]	.01	.09[c]	.06[e]	.82	.76	.18	.002
Intrinsic Religiosity	.00	−.04	−.09[c]	.09[c]	.11[c]	.03[c]	.71	.68	.29	.007
Extrinsic Religiosity	.11[c]	−.04	−.07	−.07	−.09[c]	.02	.69	.67	.31	.000
Existential Well-Being	−.51[e]	.34[e]	−.05	.20[e]	.39[e]	.35[e]	.87	.52	.13	.000
Religious Well-Being	−.04	.05	−.11[c]	.11[c]	.13[d]	.05[e]	.93	.88	.07	.001
FMS - Horizontal	−.06	.08	.17[e]	.25[c]	.16[c]	.09[e]	.74	.65	.26	.12[c]
FMS - Vertical	−.09[c]	.11[c]	.04	.13[d]	.17[e]	.05[e]	.81	.76	.19	.02[d]

[a]General Mysticism Factor
[b]Joyful Religious Expression Factor
[c]$p < .05$
[d]$p < .01$
[e]$p < .001$ (all correlations are two-tailed).
Note. "Strategies for Using the Five-Factor Model in Religious Research," by R. L. Piedmont, 1996. In R. L. Piedmont (Chair), The Five-Factor Model and Its Value for Religious Research (1996, p. 14), Toronto, Ontario, Canada, Symposium presented at the annual convention of the American Psychological Association. Copyright 1996 by Ralph L. Piedmont. Reprinted with permission.

with Openness suggest a strong commitment to the person's values. This pattern is very consistent with Gorsuch's (1994) definition of Intrinsic Religiosity, "the motivation for experiencing and living one's religious faith for the sake of the faith itself. The person's religion is an end unto itself, a goal pursued in the absence of external reinforcement" (p. 317). An Extrinsic Religious orientation reflects mostly an anxious and insecure temperament. Such individuals may engage in religious practices in an attempt to minimize or reduce ongoing feelings of guilt and inadequacy.

Correlating these measures with the NEO PI–R provides insights into their construct validity. It also enables one to look across scales to evaluate redundancy. For example, the Existential Well-Being scale clearly captures aspects of well-being and life satisfaction as evidenced by its very strong correlations with (low) Neuroticism and (high) Extraversion. However, the Religious Well-Being scale appears not to measure a similar construct. It reflects not so much well-being as a sense of commitment to core, internalized values. Thus, the scale may be misleading in its "well-being" label because it does not seem to capture those qualities that are motivationally fundamental to the experience of well-being. In fact, the Religious Well-Being scale appears personologically quite similar to the Intrinsic Religiosity scale; both measure have correlates with the same NEO PI–R domains of similar magnitude.

A similar pattern of correlates raises the real possibility of redundancy between the Religious Well-Being and Intrinsic Religiosity scales. These scales appear to reflect similar motivational qualities of the individual. If this is true, then one needs to question whether both instruments are really necessary. However, similar domain correlates may mask still more subtle differences. Any full analysis of redundancy would need to rest on a *facet analysis,* correlating each scale with all 30 NEO PI–R facet scales to garner a more nuanced interpretation of the measures. Such an analysis indicates that in terms of Openness, both scales have a single significant correlation with O6 (Openness to Values). On Agreeableness, both scales have a significant correlation with A2 (Straightforwardness), although the Intrinsic scale also correlates with A6 (Tender-Mindedness) while the Religious Well-Being scale has additional correlates with A1 (Trust) and A3 (Altruism). Finally, on Conscientiousness both scales correlate significantly with C4 (Achievement Striving) and C6 (Deliberation). Religious Well-Being also correlates with C1 (Competence).

Thus, even on the facet level these two instrument seem to reflect the same personological content. Future research will need to focus on the discriminant validity of these two scales. It may be that each predicts different types of religious–spiritual outcomes. Without any compelling evidence of this nature, one would do well to avoid using both scales in the same study. Here is another example of how instruments with very different names and intended uses capture redundant content. In fact, one would make a serious interpretive error if he or she were to conclude that a positive correlation between these two instruments (which should occur given their overlap with the five-factor model) reflected the greater spiritual satisfaction derived from those with an Intrinsic Religiosity. The correlation would not reflect the association between two separate constructs, but rather the redundancy in psychological content.

A second conclusion that can be drawn from the data in Table 6-4 is that although the religious constructs share something in common with the five-factor model, the multiple R^2's shown in the sixth column indicate that these religious constructs are not completely redundant with the model. These values were obtained by using each of the religious scales as the dependent variable in a regression equation. The five NEO PI–R domain scores were entered as a single block. The R^2 values represent the amount of variance each religious scale has in common with the NEO PI–R domain scores. Although there is a significant amount of overlap between the two sets of constructs, it is clear that each religious variable contains a significant amount of unique, reliable variance. This indicates that scores on the religious scales contain information about people that is not shared with the five-factor model. Thus, these scales have the potential to offer new insights into psychological phenomena not already assessed by traditional personality scales. However, documenting this capability requires a more rigorous empirical paradigm, one that includes the systematic evaluation of the relatedness of these two sets of variables to various criteria. This involves an *incremental validity paradigm*.

THE INCREMENTAL VALIDITY PARADIGM

With so many scales available in the marketplace today and the very real question of redundancy in content, it is critical that one evaluate the unique value of a scale; its "bang for the buck," so to speak. What does a scale tell us about some outcome that cannot be obtained from already established measures? This question is particularly salient when one is interested in developing new personality dimensions. The incremental validity paradigm is useful in determining the common and unique predictiveness of various classes of variables. Its ultimate value is that it provides a direct index of what a scale adds to our predictive ability.

For religious research, incremental validity paradigms would be helpful in outlining those individual-difference qualities distinctive to religious constructs that are predictive of important outcomes (e.g., prosocial behavior, altruism, racism, sexual behavior) over and above the more traditional personality variables as represented by the five-factor model and the NEO PI–R. In this manner, researchers can begin to articulate more clearly those aspects of human functioning that are singularly captured by religious constructs.

At the heart of this approach is stepwise regression analysis. Once a suitable criterion is selected, measures of the five-factor model (i.e., the domain scores from the NEO PI–R) can serve as markers of traditional personality qualities. They would be entered on step 1 of the analysis. Then, the religious construct or constructs of interest can be entered on step 2. This variable would then identify that variance in the criterion *not* associated with the personality traits. A partial F-test (J. Cohen & Cohen, 1983) would then determine whether the variance accounted for by the religious variable (or the construct entered on step 2) added significantly to that already accounted for by the personality dimensions entered on the first step.

The data in Table 6-4 provide a systematic evaluation of the unique variance of each of the religious constructs. The Cronbach alpha (α) for each scale is given for this sample. This value outlines the amount of reliable variance in the observed scores. The column labeled "$\alpha - R^2$" indicates the amount of unique, reliable variance in the observed scores. This value subtracts the amount of shared variance between the religious and personality constructs from the total amount of reliable variance. The larger this value, the more scores on this scale capture qualities of the individual not shared by the five-factor model. A. S. Kaufman (1975) and Silverstein

(1982) suggest that to conclude a scale has enough reliable variance to warrant a separate interpretation, its unique variance component should be larger than its error $(1 - \alpha)$ and at least 25% of the total variance. All of these scales have a pattern consistent with these guidelines. Thus, they have something to say independent of the five personality dimensions.

However, the most important question is whether this unique, reliable variance has something meaningful to contribute to the prediction of important outcomes. This is where the incremental validity paradigm comes into play. For the data presented in Table 6-4, those subjects also completed a behavior-based index of prosocial behavior. This variable served as the outcome for the stepwise regression analysis. The NEO PI–R domain scores were entered on the first step, and then each of the religious constructs was systematically entered on step 2. The last column of Table 6-4 (ΔR^2) indicates the increase in explained variance the religious constructs added to predicting prosocial behavior over personality's contribution. As can be seen, only the FMS scales added significantly to the explained variance. The other measures, despite large amounts of reliable, unique variance, had nothing to contribute uniquely to this outcome. Thus, any association between these religious constructs and prosocial behavior would be due *entirely* to variance that overlaps with the more traditional personality scales.

These findings are surprising given the importance of the religious constructs. They are measurement staples of religious research, yet any predictive value they may have in regard to nonreligious outcomes may be due to their overlap with standard personality variables. It should also be mentioned that other studies have evaluated the predictiveness of these constructs against a wide range of outcomes (e.g., burnout among clergy, racism, sexual attitudes, quality of life) and the results have been equally lackluster (Csarny, 1997; Rodgerson, 1994). The one, and to date in my research, only exception has been the Faith Maturity Scale, which has consistently shown itself to possess significant incremental validity (e.g., Chen, 1996).

The incremental validity paradigm provides an empirically sophisticated methodology for evaluating the utility of individual-difference constructs in providing additional, nonredundant information about people. It very directly assesses what a new scale tells us about others over and above what can be determined with existing scales. The NEO PI–R serves as the anchoring point in these ventures. Although in this example I used only the domain scores as the reference point, it is equally appropriate to enter the facets instead. This will generate a larger portion of variance attributable to personality. Scales that fail to improve predictiveness need to be reconsidered. As seen in the example data here, many of the religious constructs failed the incremental validity test. Thus, researchers in the area of spirituality need to demonstrate the value of many of their constructs;

their relatedness to important psychological outcomes seems to be based solely on their overlap with personality constructs. Merely repackaging established constructs under new labels does not, ultimately, serve the cause of science, the purpose of which is to expand our understanding of human nature not merely rehash it.

In all fairness, though, the Faith Maturity Scale offers promise and hope to religious researchers who are interested in identifying constructs unique to their area of inquiry. This measure, although having something in common with the NEO PI–R, does have sufficient unique variance to provide additional explanatory power for a number of psychologically relevant outcomes. Greater attention should be given to examining exactly what this uniqueness is and to plumb its personological depths empirically. It may, in time, provide a new source of individual-difference constructs with the potential to expand both our current models of personality and our ability to predict important psychological outcomes.

OUTCOME RESEARCH

An important contribution of psychological tests is their ability to help us anticipate important life outcomes. Ultimately test data need to tell us about the direction a person's life will move in and the kinds of events that he or she is likely to experience. Ideally, it would be useful if assessors could evaluate individuals on dimensions that would indicate not only the client's current strengths and weaknesses, but also the risk potential to experience certain negative life outcomes, such as health problems, poor life satisfaction, interpersonal difficulties, and so on. From my introductory remarks in this chapter, social scientists would also want to know how personality may dispose someone to experience a mental disorder, or what their suitability for therapy may be, or their potential to benefit from an intervention. These are all important questions, and the NEO PI–R has something to contribute to all of these outcomes. For the purposes of this section, I focus on using the NEO PI–R in an applied clinical context for assessing change and predicting outcome.

Conducting outcome studies is a rather straightforward process. What is needed is the ability to collect data at two points in time: at the beginning of treatment and then again at the end. Certainly, the NEO PI–R should be given at both assessment intervals. However, the NEO should not be considered all that is necessary. One would want to complement the NEO with more specific clinical measures, perhaps the Brief Symptom Inventory (BSI; Derogatis, 1993) to assess symptomalogical distress, and a measure of psychosocial issues. At the end of treatment one would repeat these measures as well as additional ratings that focus on the important therapeutic elements of the treatment. This rating form should be completed by the therapist. The form would include subjective ratings of how well the client has progressed along a number of relevant dimensions. An example of such a form I have used is presented in Figure 6-3.

This form was used in a study evaluating the efficacy of an outpatient substance abuse program that was spiritually based and vocationally focused. It dealt with chronic substance abusers who were primarily from a transient population. The program ran for 6 hours a day, 5 days a week for 6 weeks. The goal at the end of the program was to have participants secure some type of full-time employment. The program itself involved numerous types of interventions, including individual and group counseling, spiritual discussions, cultural trips, and vocational training. The form presented in Figure 6-3 was specifically designed, with consultation with the staff, to assess issues that were relevant to their own goals.

In developing any type of outcome study, one should consider the specific goals pursued, the types of clients treated, and the interventions used. This information must be included in the outcome rating survey if it is to have any relevance. Thus, the rating form in Figure 6-3 may not generalize to other clinical contexts, but readers should feel free to modify this form to address the unique features of their contexts. Nonetheless, there are some general features in the form that should be considered.

First, there are a number of simple Likert rating scales evaluating the effectiveness of various aspects of the program for the client. These include the perceived attitude of the clients toward the treatment and their success in reaching various spiritual criteria. Each of these items is valuable in its own right, because the items address very specific aspects of the intervention program. Such single-item scales carry a respectable level of reliability and validity (see Wanous, Reichers, & Hudy, 1997). However, one can build in more reliability to these assessments by aggregating multiple items to form scales and obtaining multiple ratings for each client. In collecting multiple ratings, three raters are usually optimal, but two will work very well.

A second value of this form is the presentation of a check list of various therapeutic techniques. Therapists indicate those that seemed to work well with the client by putting a "+" before it and indicate those interventions that did not seem to be as effective by placing a "−" in front of it. These types of ratings can be very useful for identifying which type of client appears to respond to which type of treatment. This person-by-treatment assessment is at the very heart of current clinical research. It represents the next step that the field will be taking as it hones its techniques and defines their range of application.

COUNSELOR'S FINAL EVALUATION

NAME: _____   DATE: _____

1. Client's attitude towards program: From "1" Very little
Acceptance to "7" Very much Accepting 1   2   3   4   5   6   7

2. Client's efforts in treatment: "1" very little effort to "7"
very diligent effort 1   2   3   4   5   6   7

3. Treatments which seemed most helpful (Place a plus sign (" + ") before all treatments that were used
SUCCESSFULLY; a minus sign ("-") before any treatments that were used UNSUCCESSFULLY.

☐ Gestalt   ☐ Vocational   ☐ Spiritual Direction   ☐ Cultural Trips
☐ Client Centered   ☐ Group Sessions   ☐ Problem Solving   ☐ Journaling
☐ Cognitive Treatment   ☐ Relaxation Sessions   ☐ Art Therapy
☐ Insight   ☐ Systematic Desens.   ☐ AA/NA Program

4. THERAPEUTIC SUBPROCESSES USED (Place a plus sign (" + ") before all subprocesses that
were used SUCCESSFULLY; a minu sign ("-") before any subprocesses that were used
UNSUCCESSFULLY.

☐ Support and reassurance   ☐ Interpretation: Current life   ☐ Cognitive restructuring
☐ Advice, problem solving   ☐ Problem solving advice   ☐ Free association
☐ Experiencing techniques   ☐ Stress management   ☐ Prayer/meditation
☐ Interpretation: early life   techniques   ☐ Spiritual readings
☐ Other: _____

5. Length of program for client (in weeks):

6. Reason for termination (check only one):

☐ relapse   ☐ other priorities   ☐ violation of program rules
☐ loss of interest   ☐ legal difficulties   ☐ completed program
☐ Other: _____

7. How successfully were treatment goals reached? "1" not
successful "4" partially successful "7" fully successful 1   2   3   4   5   6   7

8. What degree of recovery was noted? "1" likely to
relapse "4" no change "7" likely to stay clean 1   2   3   4   5   6   7

9. Spiritual development: "1" rigid (willfulness), "4" no
change "7" flexibility (willingness) 1   2   3   4   5   6   7

10. What was the client's attitude towards vocational
training? "1" resistive "4" complacent "7" proactive 1   2   3   4   5   6   7

11. How well did the client learn the job searching/
vocational techniques provided? "1" not well, "7" very
well 1   2   3   4   5   6   7

12. Overall, how much personal growth (i.e., emotional,
vocational, spiritual) did this person experience? "1" not
much growth "7" a lot of growth 1   2   3   4   5   6   7

(Continued)

13. Please rate the client's motivation to want to make a
change in their lifestyle. "1" very little motivation to
change "7" very high motivation to change 1   2   3   4   5   6   7

14. Please rate the degree to which you believe the client
CAN make a change in their lifestyle. "1" unable to make a
personal change "7" very capable of making a personal
change 1   2   3   4   5   6   7

15. Please rate the degree to which you believe the client
can maintain any change in their lifestyle. "1" unable to
maintain any changes, will revert to earlier lifestyle "7" no
difficulty in maintaining any changes 1   2   3   4   5   6   7

FIGURE 6-3. An example of a therapist's rating scale for treatment efficacy.

The size of this type of list is limited only by the kinds of interventions that are being used. This type of approach appreciates the reality that most clinicians are eclectic in their dealings with clients. Thus, rather than trying to classify therapeutic interventions by the theoretical orientation of the therapist, this type of list can provide a more detailed insight into exactly what interventions were applied.

Another useful question asked is why clients dropped out of the program. Oftentimes in clinical research one goal is to identify those who complete from those who fail to complete the course of treatment. This type of question seeks to identify the reason or reasons for early termination. Are certain types of individuals more prone to "quit" than others? But, as this item illustrates, there are numerous possible reasons for someone's dropping out. In this example, one reason could be a relapse to using drugs. Identifying those who are at risk for repeat drug use and those more likely to stick with the program is of fundamental interest to substance abuse counselors. However, people left this program for other reasons, including a loss of interest, legal problems (such as being arrested for an earlier crime) or life circumstances that took them out of the area. These types of cases should not be included in any analyses of recidivism.

A similar kind of form can also be given to clients to complete on their own. Such a questionnaire can access their perceptions of the therapeutic program and how well each element was received. Clients can also rate how successful they found the treatment to be. Other questions can be included about the client's view of a number of useful dimensions, all of which speak to his or her satisfaction with the services that were rendered. Figure 6-4 provides an example of such a questionnaire that I have used, although there are a number of standardized client satisfaction questionnaires already available (e.g., Larsen, Attkisson, Hargreaves, & Nguyen, 1979).

As can be seen in Figure 6-4, clients are directly asked to indicate how successful they found various aspects of the treatment and how much im-

PARTICIPANT'S EVALUATION

NAME: _____   DATE: _____

As part of our evaluation of the effectiveness of the CHRP program, we would like your view of the counseling you have received. Please answer the following questions.

1. How helpful did you find your participation in the CHRP program in dealing with the problem that brought you in for treatment?

☐ very helpful   ☐ somewhat helpful   ☐ not very helpful   ☐ not helpful at all

2. In general, how do you feel now compared to how you felt when you began the program?

☐ much better   ☐ better   ☐ the same   ☐ worse

3. Do you have more self-esteem and feel better about yourself?

☐ much better   ☐ better   ☐ the same   ☐ worse

4. Do you think you are able to get along better with other people?

☐ much better   ☐ better   ☐ the same   ☐ worse

5. Which aspects of the program seemed the most helpful to you? Please check one response for each aspect.

	very helpful	somewhat helpful	not helpful or don't know
Getting advice about what to do	☐	☐	☐
Feeling accepted by the group	☐	☐	☐
Learning to understand yourself in relation to the God of your understanding	☐	☐	☐
Getting reassurance and support	☐	☐	☐
Learning about other people	☐	☐	☐
Expressing your feelings	☐	☐	☐
Taking responsibility for your life	☐	☐	☐
The morning dialogue	☐	☐	☐
The employment readiness training	☐	☐	☐
The spiritual element to the program	☐	☐	☐
Learning about "Action, Attitude, Awareness"	☐	☐	☐
Learning about "Serendipity"	☐	☐	☐

If you knew someone with similar problems, would you recommend the program to them? . . . . ☐ Yes   ☐ No

FIGURE 6-4. Example of a client satisfaction questionnaire given at the end of treatment.

provement they feel they have experienced. From a consumer point of view, these types of questions provide *prima facie* evidence of treatment efficacy. If clients are not happy with what they experienced, no matter what the therapist may claim, then the value of treatment must be questioned.

This type of questionnaire can also provide very useful feedback information for therapists. A therapist may believe that a certain intervention is important or even critical to the process of therapy, but clients may indicate that it is the least useful. Finding out why such discrepancies exist can be helpful in tailoring a treatment program to better meet the needs of the clients. It may also provide insights as to why resistance may be developing in some or all clients at certain points in the program.

The utility of both these questionnaires is that they are easy to administer and interpret. They do not take much time to complete and can provide a wide range of valuable information. Given the high face validity of the items, these measures can be readily interpreted by simply reading over the responses. Further, these responses can be easily entered into data programs for later statistical analyses. These scores become very interesting when aggregated over many clients and then correlated to the psychometric information that is collected in tandem with the forms. The next sections outline some of the kinds of data I have obtained from using scales like the ones just described.

Understanding Change over Time

As we noted earlier in this book, the dimensions of the NEO PI–R remain very stable in adulthood; as Costa and McCrae (1994) noted, 25-year test–retest values hover around .80, and it is estimated that over a 50-year adult life span 60% of the variance remains stable. These stability coefficients are complemented by analyses of mean level change which also show no significant shifts over time. Based on this data Costa and McCrae noted that personality is pretty much "set like plaster" after age 30.

Such evidence for stability raises a number of theoretical, philosophical, and ideological questions. How, then, do we define the concepts of psychological growth and freedom? To what degree do individuals have the capacity to make choices? Is personality destiny? From an applied perspective, what purpose do psychological interventions serve? Should clinicians attempt to affect clients by helping them make shifts in their fundamental psychological structures or through improving their psychosocial instrumentality (e.g., coping ability)? Answers to these questions certainly address our field at its most fundamental level and force us to think most seriously about concepts of change and development (these issues were touched on in Chapter 1 in the discussion on genotypic versus phenotypic change).

But even if adulthood is not characterized by any natural psychological metamorphoses, are such transformations possible given the interdiction of certain events? There are three types of events that could arguably provide transmuting opportunities: traumatic personal experiences (e.g., war), religious conversions, and therapeutic interventions. These rather radical experiences may provide a portal into the psyche that capitalizes on our innate psychic plasticity.

In order to address the ability of individuals to experience genotypic change as a function of psychotherapy, I evaluated clients participating in a 6-week outpatient drug rehabilitation program (see Piedmont, 1996a; Piedmont & Ciarrocchi, in press). In this study I was able to measure participants on the NEO PI–R both before and after their involvement in the program. A total of 99 individuals (58 men and 41 women) successfully completed the 6-week program. All subjects had been drug-free for at least 30 days prior to entering this program. Most were alcohol and cocaine abusers with an average of 14 years of substance involvement. The treatment they received included individual sessions, CDA groups, discussions of spirituality, and vocational counseling. The program was conducted 5 days a week for 6 hours a day. The results are presented in Table 6-5.

As can be seen, over the 6-week treatment interval, significant shifts occurred in all the major domains of personality. The largest gains (about one-half standard deviation) were noticed for Neuroticism and Conscientiousness; individuals decreased their overall levels of emotional dysphoria and increased feelings of competence and self-discipline. Also, the changes in Extraversion and Agreeableness indicate a shift toward an interpersonal style characterized by greater affability and trust. The increase noted on Openness reflects greater awareness of potential opportunities and a broader awareness of values.

Overall these results are extremely encouraging. Although "normal" adulthood may not be characterized by any quantitative shifts in personal-

TABLE 6-5. t-Test Evaluating Mean Level Change in NEO PI–R Domain Scales over a 6-Week Interval.

NEO PI–R domains	Time 1	Time 2	t Difference
Neuroticism	61.34	54.22	-6.98^a
Extraversion	50.36	52.75	3.68^a
Openness to Experience	54.00	56.25	3.70^a
Agreeableness	41.69	44.44	3.77^a
Conscientiousness	41.27	46.72	5.59^a

$N = 99$
$^a p < .001$, two-tailed.
NEO PI–R scores presented as T-scores with a mean of 50 and standard deviation of 10, based on normative data from unpublished manuscript.
Note. From Psychometric Utility of the NEO PI–R in an Outpatient, Drug Rehabilitation Context (p. 32), by R. L. Piedmont and J. W. Ciarrochi (in press). Adapted with permission.

ity, those seeking changes may be able to find them. These data indicate that psychological interventions may be able to induce positive changes in one's underlying dispositions. The magnitude of these shifts is indeed quite high (see Trull, Useda, Costa, & McCrae, 1995; Bagby, Joffe, Kalemba, & Harkness, 1995 for comparisons) and suggests that the more time invested in treatment, the larger the personological gains experienced by the client.

Of course, further follow-up data is necessary to determine whether these treatment changes last. Are the noted changes temporary, with the individuals returning to premorbid levels in time? Also, we need to determine whether the NEO PI–R scores obtained at posttreatment continue to be as predictive of life outcomes as found with individuals who do not show any change. More longitudinal research with clinical samples needs to be undertaken to answer these questions. However, for our purposes, two conclusions can be gleaned from these data. First, it appears that the plaster cast can be broken. Those seeking serious changes in their lives may be able to find it through therapy. The magnitude of effect for some of the NEO PI–R domains was indeed quite large, as compared with other outcome studies using this instrument. But the intervention was quite intense; these individuals experienced 30 hours of therapy a week for 6 weeks. Individual treatment usually is not this focused and does not last so long. The 180 hours of treatment correspond to about 3 years of traditional one-on-one therapy. Thus, the more put into therapy, the more benefit that may be received.

The second value of these data is that they suggest that the NEO PI–R may be a useful measure of psychotherapy outcome. Its ability to change in response to therapy indicates that it is sensitive to treatment interventions and can be a very useful index for gauging the extent of experienced change. The fact that clients changed on Extraversion and Agreeableness makes a powerful statement about the kinds of shifts in interpersonal style. Not only do these data validate the treatment that was received, but they also establish very useful expectations for future behavior on the part of clients. With a more approachable and engaging style that will lend itself to developing more mutually satisfying emotional relationships with others, these people can anticipate a deeper and more fulfilling quality to their lives. The increased scores on Conscientiousness lead one to expect a greater capacity on the part of clients to obtain and maintain vocational opportunities.

By simply collecting NEO PI–R data pre- and posttreatment, one can obtain a useful description of where clients are at these points. Shifts on the domains and facet scales can indicate how and to what degree therapy affected clients. As I pointed out in the beginning of this chapter, this type of information can be very useful in documenting efficacy for third-party payers. It is also useful for showing the magnitude of intervention necessary to bring about useful, sustainable change in clients. The next section looks at how outcome data can be used to select treatments for clients.

SELECTING TREATMENTS FOR PERSONS

Perhaps the frontier for clinical research is found in research efforts to match treatments to persons. It is here that the greatest efficiency in providing clinical services can be found. Individuals no doubt bring their own issues to therapy, but they also bring their own characteristic ways of managing events in their environment. These styles of adaptation determine the what and how of therapy. Personality dispositions no doubt influence how clients present themselves in therapy and determine their responses to interventions. Personality styles also bring with them certain therapeutic opportunities and pitfalls. Therefore, understanding clients along the dimensions of the five-factor model can help orient treatment in ways that capitalize on clients' strengths.

Perhaps the most thorough treatment of personality by treatment interactions using the NEO PI–R is presented by Miller (1991). Drawing on information from 101 of his own clients, Miller provided useful clinical insights into how individuals high and low on each of the five domains would present themselves to therapy. He also outlines some of the key problems these clients are likely to experience along with potential treatment opportunities and pitfalls. For example, individuals high on Neuroticism present themselves with a variety of negative affects. Their presenting problems span the full spectrum of neurotic pains. Although such individuals may always experience personal pain regardless of how much therapy they receive, such emotional distress can certainly motivate patient compliance with treatment. On the other hand, those low on Neuroticism present themselves as emotionally bland. Most of their issues may arise from situational problems; these individuals can and do benefit from advice and values clarification. Therapists should be cautious not to interpret the emotional blandness as defensiveness. Table 6-6 provides the strengths and weaknesses Miller (1991) associated with each of the five factors.

Of particular interest in the Miller paper was his finding that (low) Neuroticism and (high) Conscientiousness were significantly related to positive ratings of treatment outcome. Certainly high Conscientious individuals will make efforts to improve and to comply with treatment protocols. Such efforts may not be undermined by higher levels of negative affect, which compromises self-confidence and one's ability to tolerate the personal discomfort associated with any change. The lower levels of Neuroticism may reflect clients who come to therapy to address situation-

TABLE 6-6. Clinical Issues Surrounding Each of the Five Factors.

NEO Factor	Potential Strength	Potential Weakness
Neuroticism		
High:	Psychological Pain motivates compliance	Existence likely to remain uncomfortable; high N cannot be interpreted away
Low:	Wants and can benefit from advice and values clarification	Emotional Blandness may be misunderstood as defensiveness
Extraversion		
High:	Comfortable with less structured approaches; optimistic and energetic	Talkativeness can blunt treatment focus
Low:	Comfortable with structured approaches	Lacks enthusiasm for interaction with therapist
Openness		
High:	Prefers imaginative approaches	Excessive curiosity can scatter resources
Low:	Responds well to practical approaches; Education, support, behavior therapy	Rigidity and lack of curiosity can be misunderstood as resistance
Agreeableness		
High:	Treatment alliance easily formed	Accepts interpretations uncritically. Need to please therapist interferes with disclosure of transference
Low:	Assertiveness and clear thinking about self-interest facilitate problem solving	Hostility and skepticism toward therapist; difficult to form treatment alliance
Conscientiousness		
High:	Works hard to benefit from treatment. Willing to tolerate discomfort and fustration	(possibly none)
Low:	(possibly none)	Unlikely to do homework; likely to reject interventions that require hard work or toleration of discomfort

From Miller. T. (1991). The psychotherapeutic utility of the five-factor model of personality: A clinician's experience. *Journal of Personality Assessment, 57*, 418–419. Copyright 1991 by Lawrence Erlbaum Associates, Inc., Publishers. Adapted with permission.

ally induced problems. The task with these people is to find ways of marshaling already existing personal resources to manage the new stressor, which may in time pass away. No doubt, the more personal resources a client brings to therapy, the more likely they are to experience a positive outcome. The real goal is to identify ways to engage clients with fewer psychological resources and still bring about a better clinical result.

Using the evaluation form presented in Figure 6-3, I conducted a program evaluation of an outpatient substance abuse program (Piedmont & Ciarrocchi, in press). Data from this project have been presented throughout this book. One of the interesting parts of this project was to correlate NEO PI–R scores at Time 1 (entrance into the program) with counselor ratings obtained at Time 2 (at the end of treatment). Of particular interest were the correlations with items in questions 3 and 4 in Figure 6-3. These associations speak to those initial qualities of the clients that seemed to benefit from specific treatment interventions.

Our results indicated that those high on Neuroticism benefited from client-centered therapy and systematic desensitization, while problem-solving advice was *not* seen as effective with these types of clients. Openness correlated positively with vocational techniques. Those high on Agreeableness were rated as responding well to the AA and NA programs, while those low on Agreeableness responded well to relaxation sessions, art therapy, and journaling. Those high on Conscientiousness responded well to Gestalt techniques. Openness did not correlate with any of the treatment techniques.

These results should not be interpreted as generalizing to all therapeutic contexts; more research is needed before that conclusion can be drawn. Rather, these findings represent patterns of relationships that hold for a particular program, and this is the data's greatest value. In conducting outcome evaluations, clinicians are interested in documenting the efficacy of *their* particular interventions; for determining which of *their* specific clients will respond to the presented treatments. This is why outcome research is so important for individual clinicians. It provides a framework for better understanding the nuances of their clinical practice. There are so many factors that influence how a person high on some personality dimension responds to a treatment, such as the demeanor of the therapist and the way the treatment is presented. These unique features of a therapist's treatment environment are captured in these types of ratings and provide important feedback on how well various interventions are working.

These data also provide some support for the preference of therapists for eclectic approaches to treatment. Certainly there are no generic treatment models that work for all people equally well. Therapists need to respond to a myriad of nonspecific factors that clients present in order to find an intervention that seems to be congruent with the client's needs. To date, however, there has been no systematic way of linking client characteristics to therapeutic techniques or to treatment outcomes. Using simple evaluative rating scales like the one presented in Figure 6-3, clinicians can obtain data that can be effective in identifying a wealth of curative factors previously unnoticed.

UNDERSTANDING OUR CLIENTS

Another value of the NEO PI–R is that it provides an opportunity to collect data not just on individuals, but on groups. Who, in general, are the people presenting themselves for treatment? What kinds of clients do I serve? By answering these questions, therapists can begin to understand the kinds of needs people bring for treatment. It provides a useful psychological orientation to those we treat.

For example, Table 6-7 provides an overall description of the 132 individuals who began the outpatient substance abuse program outlined earlier in this chapter. The average score for everyone on each of the 35 NEO PI–R scales was calculated and then entered into the scoring software for evaluation, using the combined norms for reference. The value of this type of analysis is that it gives an overview of the entire group's personality presentation.

The resulting profile indicates that these individuals are likely to present a defensive facade of superiority and may use defense mechanisms such as acting out and projection. These individuals may have a marginal level of life satisfaction, being more sensitive to life's problems than its rewards. Overall, these individuals may prefer an interpersonal style that can be described as cold, unfeeling, dominant, assured, and especially arrogant and calculating. As a group, this personality profile quite closely resembles that of the Borderline Personality Disorder. Thus, these individuals may be skeptical and antagonistic in treatment and reluctant to establish a treatment alliance with the therapist.

Aggregating data at the group level has three important implications. First, it allows one to appreciate who is presenting for treatment. As we see in Table 6-7, those coming for substance abuse treatment present a specific personality profile. As we saw in the previous section, these personality dimensions are differentially responsive to various treatment interventions. Therefore, certain types of interventions will be more effective than others. It was not surprising that therapists in this situation frequently used AA and NA groups, and Gestalt and client-centered techniques: These techniques seemed to have the best results with these types of clients. This information is useful for anticipating issues that will emerge over the

TABLE 6-7. Personality Characteristics of Clients
Entering an Outpatient Substance Abuse Program

NEO PI–R domain and facet	T-Score	Range
Neuroticism	60	HIGH
Anxiety	55	AVERAGE
Hostility	58	HIGH
Depression	59	HIGH
Self-Consciousness	58	HIGH
Impulsiveness	55	AVERAGE
Vulnerability to Stress	60	HIGH
Extraversion	51	AVERAGE
Warmth	45	AVERAGE
Gregariousness	49	AVERAGE
Assertiveness	48	AVERAGE
Activity	51	AVERAGE
Excitement Seeking	57	HIGH
Positive Emotions	50	AVERAGE
Openness to Experience	53	AVERAGE
Fantasy	53	AVERAGE
Aesthetics	56	HIGH
Feelings	54	AVERAGE
Actions	52	AVERAGE
Ideas	52	AVERAGE
Values	51	AVERAGE
Agreeableness	44	LOW
Trust	37	LOW
Straightforwardness	40	LOW
Altruism	45	AVERAGE
Modesty	45	AVERAGE
Compliance	50	AVERAGE
Tendermindedness	54	AVERAGE
Conscientiousness	45	AVERAGE
Competence	41	LOW
Order	50	AVERAGE
Dutifulness	37	LOW
Achievement	46	AVERAGE
Self-Discipline	43	LOW
Deliberation	44	LOW

course of therapy. Given the interpersonal style of the group, this outpatient program had to build in techniques that would address the blustery yet insecure and untrusting interpersonal nature of the group.

A second value of these types of data is that they allow clinicians to create local norms for their psychological instruments. Knowing the overall population characteristics, it becomes useful to evaluate each new client in

reference to these qualities. Yes, these clients are suspicious and nontrust-
ing, but how does this new client compare on these dimensions relative to
others who have come through the program? Is he or she more detached or
less so? These specific questions provide more texture and nuance to psychological evaluations. Developing local norms allows for a more fine-
grained analysis of personality as it applies in a *particular* treatment context.

The final value of aggregate data works out of the first two: It enables
therapists to conduct a needs assessment of their clients. Given the overall
portrait of the clients, what are the needs they bring to treatment? Certainly,
the overall profile presented here indicates individuals in need of several
things. Interpersonally, they need to learn how to better relate to others; to
be able to initiate and maintain emotionally satisfying relationships. People
cannot always be seen as threatening objects, but rather as possible sources
of support and encouragement. Intrapersonally, these individuals need to
create better self-images and to develop more efficient coping skills. They
need to become less impulsive and more self-controlled. Treatment with
these individuals needs to proceed on multiple levels simultaneously.

Group data can provide a useful summary statement of the personality qualities in one's treatment population. Such information can certainly
inform treatment selection and identify potential areas of intervention. The
use of group data can be extended to reflect different subgroups as well.
For example, it may be possible to identify normatively those who responded well to treatment and those who did not. These aggregated profiles can be used in two ways. First, the personality differences between the
two groups can be plotted and interpreted for its clinical significance. Why
do clients high on dimension X and low on dimension Y do poorly, while
those with the opposite pattern do well? Is it something about our center,
or therapist, or treatment modality?

A second way that these group profiles can be used is in the selection
of clients. Some programs, like the substance abuse treatment program discussed earlier, have limited resources and must evaluate prospective
clients prior to accepting them for treatment. The effort is to identify those
who appear most likely to benefit from the intervention. In such a situation, the profiles of new clients can then be compared to these aggregated
norms of those who successfully completed the program. The degree of fit
can be used as part of the selection process.

CONCLUSIONS

The NEO PI–R is an empirically powerful instrument that has numerous applications in both clinical and research contexts. The strength of
the instrument is its foundation in the five-factor model of personality, a

comprehensive taxonomy of personality traits. The NEO PI–R thus can be useful in evaluating the validity of new constructs and for organizing and integrating personality information in a given context. Clinically, the instrument provides a useful summary of personality dispositions that have numerous treatment implications.

The information presented in this chapter should be used as a paradigm for employing the NEO PI–R in various contexts. Strategies were given that address important questions about the underlying structure of the instrument as well as for using the measure in new areas, such as cross-cultural research. From an applied perspective, the NEO PI–R has much to contribute to the advancement of clinical practice. Clinicians should feel free to use and adapt the forms presented for assessing client satisfaction and measuring treatment outcome to suit their own particular needs.

The need for clinical data will not go away in this current managed care environment. If we are ever going to be able to stem the effects of the unmitigated pressures for cost cutting that the third-party payer system presents, then we will need to collect informative, rigorous data. Doing this requires the investment of only a minimal amount of time. The ease and simplicity of current spreadsheet programs and statistical packages makes the collection, storage, and analysis of data more user-friendly than at any other time. The benefits far outweigh these limited costs.

My purpose in writing this book was to provide a basic introduction to the NEO PI–R and its interpretive and empirical applications. The instrument can add much depth and clarity to any endeavor. Yet, the current research has only scratched the surface of what this instrument can do and new applications continue to be found. Perhaps the greatest value of the NEO PI–R is that it places the user in the very center of current personality research and theory. Although the NEO PI–R is formulated on a trait perspective, it provides a way of interfacing with any number of psychological theories or perspectives. Its robust empirical nature provides researchers with a useful reference point for evaluating constructs and their predictive utility.

Ultimately, though, as the five-factor model of personality continues to become more widely used, the social sciences may approach the goal of creating a truly cumulative knowledge base. Finally, research studies can be meaningfully related to one another by virtue of the personality domains they assess. Areas of redundancy and overlap can be quickly observed, while new dimensions of investigation can be highlighted, evaluated, and reconciled empirically to established models. The social sciences will indeed take on a greater focus and harmony.

However, one should not interpret this to mean that the five-factor model or the NEO PI–R is intended to replace all other assessment instruments. Rather, one should consider the five-factor model the first step of scientific inquiry: the accurate description of personality. By providing a common language for talking about personality-related phenomena, we lay the foundation for the development of more precise theories and more powerful empirical tests of the hypotheses these theories generate.

REFERENCES

Aldenderfer, M. S., & Blashfield, R. K. (1984). *Cluster analysis.* Beverly Hills, CA: Sage.

Allport, G. W. (1937). *Personality: A psychological interpretation.* New York: Holt.

Allport, G. W. (1961). *Pattern and growth in personality.* London: Holt, Rinehart & Winston.

Allport, G. W., & Odbert, H. S. (1936). Trait names: A psycho-lexical study. *Psychological Monographs, 47*(1, Whole No. 211).

Almagor, M., Tellegen, A., & Waller, N. G. (1995). The big seven model: A cross-cultural replication and further exploration of the basic dimensions of natural language trait descriptors. *Journal of Personality and Social Psychology, 69,* 300–307.

American Psychiatric Association. (1994). *Diagnostic and statistical manual of mental disorders* (4th ed.). Washington, DC: Author.

Andrews, F. M., & Withey, S. B. (1976). *Social indicators of well-being: Americans' perceptions of life quality.* New York: Plenum.

Arbisi, P. A., & Ben-Porath, Y. S. (1995). An MMPI-2 infrequent response scale for use with a psychopathological populations: The infrequency-psychopathology scale, F(p). *Psychological Assessment, 7,* 424–431.

Avia, M. D., Sanz, J., Sánchez-Bernardos, M. L., Martínez-Arias, M. R., Silva, F., & Graña, J. L. (1995). The five-factor model—II. Relations of the NEO-PI with other personality variables. *Personality and Individual Differences, 19,* 81–97.

Bagby, R. M., Joffe, R. T., Parker, J. D. A., Kalemba, V., & Harkness, V. (1995). Major depression and the five-factor model of personality. *Journal of Personality Disorders, 9,* 224–234.

Bailey, K. D. (1994). *Typologies and taxonomies: An introduction to classification techniques.* Thousand Oaks, CA: Sage.

Bakan, D. (1966). *The duality of human existence: Isolation and communion in Western man.* Boston: Beacon.

Bandura, A. (1989). Human agency in social cognitive theory. *American Psychologist, 44,* 1175–1184.

255

Barlow, D. H., Hayes, S. C., & Nelson, R. O. (1984). *The scientist-practitioner: Research and accountability in clinical and educational settings.* New York: Pergamon.

Barrick, M. R., & Mount, M. K. (1991). The Big Five personality dimensions and job performance: A meta-analysis. *Personnel Psychology, 44,* 1–26.

Barry, W. A. (1970). Marriage research and conflict: An integrative review. *Psychological Bulletin, 73,* 41–54.

Ben-Porath, Y. S., & Waller, N. G. (1992). Five big issues in clinical assessment: A rejoinder to Costa and McCrae. *Psychological Assessment, 4,* 23–25.

Bendig, A. W. (1958). Comparative validity of objective and projective measures of need achievement in predicting students' achievement in introductory psychology. *Journal of General Psychology, 59,* 51–57.

Benet, V., & Waller, N. G. (1995). The Big Seven factor model of personality description: Evidence for its cross-cultural generality in a Spanish sample. *Journal of Personality and Social Psychology, 69,* 701–718.

Benson, P. L., Donahue, M. J., & Erickson, J. A. (1993). The faith maturity scale: Conceptualization, measurement, and empirical validation. *Research in the Social Scientific Study of Religion, 5,* 1–26.

Bentler, P. M., & Bonett, D. G. (1980). Significance tests and goodness of fit in the analysis of covariance structures. *Psychological Bulletin, 88,* 588–606.

Bergeman, C. S., Chipuer, H. M., Plomin, R., Pedersen, N. L., McClearn, G. E., Nesselroade, J. R., Costa, P. T., Jr., & McCrae, R. R. (1993). Genetic and environmental effects on Openness to Experience, Agreeableness, and Conscientiousness: An adoption/twin study. *Journal of Personality, 61,* 159–179.

Berne, S. L. (1961). *Transactional analysis in psychotherapy.* New York: Grove.

Block, J. (1965). *The challenge of response sets: Unconfounding meaning, acquiescence, and social desirability in the MMPI.* New York: Appleton-Century-Crofts.

Block, J. (1971). *Lives through time.* Berkeley, CA: Bancroft Books.

Block, J. (1995). A contrarian view of the five-factor approach to personality description. *Psychological Bulletin, 117,* 187–215.

Block, J. H., & Block, J. (1980). The role of ego-control and ego-resiliency in the organization of behavior. In W. A. Collins (Ed.), *Minnesota symposia on child psychology* (pp. 39–101). Hillsdale, NJ: Erlbaum.

Bond, M. H. (1979). Dimensions used in perceiving peers: Cross-cultural comparisons of Hong Kong, Japanese, American, and Filipino university students. *International Journal of Psychology, 14,* 47–56.

Bond, M. H., Nakazato, H., & Shiraishi, D. (1975). Universality and distinctiveness in dimensions of Japanese person perception. *Journal of Cross-Cultural Psychology, 6,* 346–357.

Borkenau, P. (1992). Implicit personality theory and the five-factor model. *Journal of Personality, 60,* 295–327.

Borkenau, P., & Liebler, A. (1992). Trait inferences: Sources of validity at zero acquaintanceship. *Journal of Personality and Social Psychology, 62,* 645–657.

Borkenau, P., & Liebler, A. (1993). Convergence of stranger ratings of personality and intelligence with self-ratings, partner ratings, and measured intelligence. *Journal of Personality and Social Psychology, 65,* 546–553.

Borkenau, P., & Ostendorf, F. (1990). Comparing exploratory and confirmatory factor analysis: A study on the 5-factor model of personality. *Personality and Individual Differences, 11,* 515–524.

Botwin, M. (1995). Review of the NEO PI–R. In J. Conoley & J. Impara (Eds.), *Mental measurement yearbook* (12th ed., pp. 862–863). Lincoln: University of Nebraska Press.

Bouchard, T. J. (1968). Convergent and discriminant validity of the Adjective Check List and the Edwards Personal Preference Schedule. *Educational and Psychological Measurement, 28,* 1165–1171.

Bouchard, T. J., Jr., & McGue, M. (1990). Genetic and rearing environmental influence on adult personality: An analysis of adopted twins reared apart. *Journal of Personality, 58,* 263–292.

Boyle, G. J. (1989). Re-examination of the major personality-type factors in the Cattell, Comrey, and Eysenck scales: Were the factor solutions by Noller et al. optimal? *Personality and Individual Differences, 10,* 1289–1299.

Brooner, R. K., Herbst, J. H., Schmidt, C. W., Bigelow, G. E., & Costa, P. T., Jr. (1993). Antisocial personality disorder among drug abusers: Relations to other personality diagnoses and the five-factor model of personality. *Journal of Nervous and Mental Disease, 181,* 313–319.

Buros, O. K. (Ed.). (1978). *Eighth mental measurements yearbook* (Vol. 1). Highland Park, NJ: Gryphon.

Buss, D. M. (1984). Marital assortment for personality dispositions: Assessment with three different data sources. *Behavior Genetics, 14,* 111–123.

Buss, D. M. (1991a). Conflict in married couples: Personality predictors of anger and upset. *Journal of Personality, 59,* 663–688.

Buss, D. M. (1991b). Evolutionary personality psychology. In M. Rosensweig & L. Porter (Eds.), *Annual review of psychology* (pp. 459–451). Palo Alto, CA: Annual Reviews.

Buss, D. M. (1992). Manipulation in close relationships: Five personality factors in interactional context. *Journal of Personality, 60,* 477–499.

Buss, D. M., & Craik, K. H. (1980). The frequency concept of disposition: Dominance and prototypically dominant acts. *Journal of Personality, 48,* 379–392.

Buss, D. M., & Craik, K. H. (1983). The act frequency approach to personality. *Psychological Review, 90,* 105–126.

Butcher, J. N., & Rouse, S. V. (1996). Personality: Individual differences and clinical assessment. *Annual Review of Psychology, 47,* 87–111.

Butcher, J. N., Dahlstrom, W. G., Graham, J. R., Tellegen, A., & Kaemmer, B. (1989). *MMPI 2: Manual for administration and scoring.* Minneapolis: University of Minnesota Press.

Cantor, N. (1990). From thought to behavior: "Having" and "doing" in the study of personality and cognition. *American Psychologist, 45,* 735–750.

Cantor, N., Norem, J., Langston, C., Zirkel, S., Fleeson, W., & Cook-Flannagan, C. (1991). Life tasks and daily life experience. *Journal of Personality, 59,* 425–451.

Cantril, H. (1965). *The pattern of human concerns.* New Brunswick, NJ: Rutgers University Press.

Capara, G. V., Barbaranelli, C., Borgogni, L., & Perugini, M. (1993). The "Big Five Questionnaire": A new questionnaire to assess the five-factor model. *Personality and Individual Differences, 15*, 281–288.

Capara, G. V., Barbaranelli, C., & Comrey, A. L. (1995). Factor analysis of the NEO-PI inventory and the Comrey Personality Scales in an Italian sample. *Personality and Individual Differences, 18*, 193–200.

Carmichael, C. M., & McGue, M. (1994). A longitudinal family study of personality change and stability. *Journal of Personality, 62*, 1–20.

Caspi, A., & Bem, D. J. (1990). Personality continuity and change across the life course. In L. A. Pervin (Ed.), *Handbook of personality theory and research* (pp. 549–575). New York: Guilford.

Cattell, R. B. (1933). Temperament tests: II. Test. *British Journal of Psychology, 23*, 308–329.

Cattell, R. B. (1944). Interpretation of the twelve primary personality factors. *Character and Personality, 13*, 55–91.

Cattell, R. B. (1947). Confirmation and clarification of the primary personality factors. *Psychometrika, 12*, 55–91.

Cattell, R. B. (1948). The primary personality factors in women compared with those in men. *British Journal of Psychology, 38*, 114–130.

Cattell, R. B. (1994). Constancy of global, second-order personality factors over a twenty-year-plus period. *Psychological Reports, 75*, 3–9.

Chae, J-H, Piedmont, R. L., Estadt, B. K., & Wicks, R. J. (1995). Personological evaluation of Clance's Impostor Phenomenon Scale in a Korean sample. *Journal of Personality Assessment, 65*, 468–485.

Chen, M. C. (1996). *Psychosocial correlates of prosocial behavior among college students in Taiwan.* Unpublished doctoral dissertation, Loyola College, Baltimore.

Chen, P. Y., Dai, T., Spector, P. E., & Jex, S. M. (1997). Relation between negative affectivity and positive affectivity: Effects of judged desirability of scale items and respondents' social desirability. *Journal of Personality Assessment, 69*, 183–198.

Church, A. T., & Burke, P. J. (1994). Exploratory and confirmatory tests of the Big Five and Tellegen's three- and four-dimensional models. *Journal of Personality and Social Psychology, 66*, 93–114.

Clance, P. R. (1985). *The impostor phenomenon: Overcoming the fear that haunts your success.* Atlanta, GA: Peachtree.

Clance, P. R., & Imes, S. A. (1978). The impostor phenomenon in high achieving women: Dynamics and therapeutic intervention. *Psychotherapy Theory, Research and Practice, 15*, 241–247.

Clark, L. A. (1990). Toward a consensual set of symptom clusters for assessment of personality disorder. In J. Butcher & C. Spielberger (Eds.), *Advances in personality assessment* (Vol. 8, pp. 243–266). Hillsdale, NJ: Erlbaum.

Cloninger, C. R. (1987). A systematic method for clinical description and classification of personality disorders. *Archives of General Psychiatry, 44*, 573–588.

Cloninger, C. R., Svrakic, D. M., & Przybeck, T. R. (1993). A psychobiological model of temperament and character. *Archives of General Psychiatry, 50*, 975–990.

Cohen, J., & Cohen, P. (1983). *Applied multiple regression/correlation analysis for the behavioral sciences.* Hillsdale, NJ: Erlbaum.

Cohen, S., Doyle, W. J., Skoner, D. P., Fireman, P., Gwaltney, J. M., Jr., & Newsom, J. T. (1995). State and trait negative affect as predictors of objective and subjective symptoms of respiratory viral infections. *Journal of Personality and Social Psychology, 68,* 159–169.

Colvin, C. R., & Funder, D. C. (1991). Predicting personality and behavior: A boundary on the acquaintanceship effect. *Journal of Personality and Social Psychology, 60,* 884–894.

Costa, P. T., Jr. (1996). Work and Personality: Use of the NEO PI–R in Industrial/Organizational psychology. *Applied Psychology: An International Review, 45,* 225–241.

Costa, P. T., Jr., & McCrae, R. R. (1980a). Influence of extraversion and neuroticism on subjective well-being: Happy and unhappy people. *Journal of Personality and Social Psychology, 38,* 668–678.

Costa, P. T., Jr., & McCrae, R. R. (1980b). Somatic complaints in males as a function of age and neuroticism: A longitudinal analysis. *Journal of Behavioral Medicine, 3,* 245–257.

Costa, P. T., Jr., & McCrae, R. R. (1984). Personality as a lifelong determinant of well-being. In C. Z. Malatesta & C. E. Izard (Eds.), *Emotion in adult development* (pp. 141–157). Beverly Hills, CA: Sage.

Costa, P. T., Jr., & McCrae, R. R. (1985). Concurrent validation after 20 years: The implications of personality stability for assessment. In J. N. Butcher & C. D. Spielberger (Eds.), *Advances in personality assessment* (pp. 31–54). Hillsdale, NJ: Erlbaum.

Costa, P. T., Jr., & McCrae, R. R. (1986). Age, personality, and the Holtzman inkblot technique. *International Journal of Aging and Human Development, 23,* 115–125.

Costa, P. T., Jr., & McCrae, R. R. (1987). Neuroticism, somatic complaints, and disease: Is the bark worse than the bite? *Journal of Personality, 55,* 299–316.

Costa, P. T., Jr., & McCrae, R. R. (1988a). From catalogue to classification: Murray's needs and the five-factor model. *Journal of Personality and Social Psychology, 55,* 258–265.

Costa, P. T., Jr., & McCrae, R. R. (1988b). Personality in adulthood: A six-year longitudinal study of self-reports and spouse ratings on the NEO Personality Inventory. *Journal of Personality and Social Psychology, 54,* 853–863.

Costa, P. T., Jr., & McCrae, R. R. (1989a). Personality continuity and the changes of adult life. In M. Storandt & G. R. VandenBos (Eds.), *The adult years: Continuity and change* (pp. 45–77). Washington, DC: American Psychological Association.

Costa, P. T., Jr., & McCrae, R. R. (1989b). Personality, stress, and coping: Some lessons from a decade of research. In K. S. Markides & C. L. Cooper (Eds.), *Aging, stress, and health* (pp. 269–285). New York: Wiley.

Costa, P. T., Jr., & McCrae, R. R. (1990). Personality disorders and the five-factor model. *Journal of Personality Disorders, 4,* 362–371.

Costa, P. T., Jr., & McCrae, R. R. (1992a). Normal personality assessment in clinical practice: The NEO Personality Inventory. *Psychological Assessment, 4,* 5–13.

Costa, P. T., Jr., & McCrae, R. R. (1992b). Reply to Eysenck. *Personality and Individual Differences, 13,* 861–865.

Costa, P. T., Jr., & McCrae, R. R. (1992c). *Revised NEO Personality Inventory: Professional manual.* Odessa, FL: Psychological Assessment Resources.

Costa, P. T., Jr., & McCrae, R. R. (1992d). Trait psychology comes of age. In T. B. Sonderegger (Ed.), *Nebraska symposium on motivation: Psychology and aging* (pp. 169–204). Lincoln: University of Nebraska Press.

Costa, P. T., Jr., & McCrae, R. R. (1994). "Set like plaster"? Evidence for the stability of adult personality. In T. F. Heatherton & J. L. Weinberger (Eds.), *Can personality change?* Washington, DC: American Psychological Association.

Costa, P. T., Jr., & McCrae, R. R. (1995a). Domains and facets: Hierarchical personality assessment using the revised NEO Personality Inventory. *Journal of Personality Assessment, 64,* 21–50.

Costa, P. T., Jr., & McCrae, R. R. (1995b). Primary traits of Eysenck's P-E-N system: Three- and five-factor solutions. *Journal of Personality and Social Psychology, 69,* 308–317.

Costa, P. T., Jr., & McCrae, R. R. (in press). The revised NEO Personality Inventory (NEO-PI-R). In S. R. Briggs & J. Cheek (Eds.), *Personality measures* (Vol. 1). Greenwich, CT: JAI.

Costa, P. T., Jr., & Widiger T. A. (1994). *Personality disorders and the five-factor model of personality.* Washington, DC: American Psychological Association.

Costa, P. T., Jr., McCrae, R. R., & Norris, A. H. (1981). Personal adjustment to aging: Longitudinal prediction from neuroticism and extraversion. *Journal of Gerontology, 36,* 78–85.

Costa, P. T., Jr., McCrae, R. R., & Holland, J. L. (1984). Personality and vocational interests in an adult sample. *Journal of Applied Psychology, 69,* 390–400.

Costa, P. T., Jr., Zonderman, A. B., McCrae, R. R., & Williams, R. B., Jr. (1985). Content and comprehensiveness in the MMPI: An item factor analysis in a normal adult sample. *Journal of Personality and Social Psychology, 48,* 925–933.

Costa, P. T., Jr., Busch, C. M., Zonderman, A. B., & McCrae, R. R. (1986). Correlations of MMPI factor scales with measures of the five-factor model of personality. *Journal of Personality Assessment, 50,* 640–650.

Costa, P. T., Jr., McCrae, R. R., & Zonderman, A. B. (1987). Environmental and dispositional influences on well-being: Longitudinal follow-up of an American national sample. *British Journal of Psychology, 78,* 299–306.

Costa, P. T., Jr., Zonderman, A. B., McCrae, R. R., Cornoni-Huntley, J., Locke, B. Z., & Barbano, H. E. (1987). Longitudinal analyses of psychological well-being in a national sample: Stability of mean levels. *Journal of Gerontology, 42,* 50–55.

Costa, P. T., Jr., McCrae, R. R., & Dye, D. A. (1991). Facet scales for Agreeableness and Conscientiousness: A revision of the NEO Personality Inventory. *Personality and Individual Differences, 12,* 887–898.

Costa, P. T., Jr., Fagan, P. J., Piedmont, R. L., Ponticas, Y., & Wise, T. N. (1992). The five-factor model of personality and sexual functioning in outpatient men and women. *Psychiatric Medicine, 10,* 199–215.

Creamer, M., & Campbell, I. M. (1988). The role of interpersonal perception in dyadic adjustment. *Journal of Clinical Psychology, 44,* 424–430.

Crowne, D. P., & Marlowe, D. (1960). A new scale of social desirability independent of psychopathology. *Journal of Consulting Psychology, 24,* 349–354.

Csarny, R. J. (1997). *The incremental validity of religious constructs in predicting quality of life, racism, and sexual attitudes.* Unpublished doctoral dissertation, Loyola College, Baltimore.

Deniston, W. M., & Ramanaiah, N. V. (1993). California Psychological Inventory and the five-factor model. *Psychological Reports, 73,* 491–496.

Derogatis, L. R. (1993). *Brief Symptom Inventory, manual.* Minneapolis, MN: National Computer Systems.

Digman, J. M. (1972). The structure of child personality as seen in behavior ratings. In R. Dreger (Ed.), *Multivariate personality research* (pp. 587–611). Baton Rouge, LA: Claitor's.

Digman, J. M. (1989). Five robust trait dimensions: Development, stability, and utility. *Journal of Personality, 57,* 195–214.

Digman, J. M. (1990). Personality structure: Emergence of the five-factor model. *Annual Review of Psychology, 41,* 417–440.

Digman, J. M. (1996). The curious history of the five-factor model. In J. S. Wiggins (Ed.). *The five-factor model of personality.* New York: Guilford.

Digman, J. M., & Takemoto-Chock, N. K. (1981). Factors in the natural language of personality: Re-analysis, comparison, and interpretation of six major studies. *Multivariate Behavioral Research, 16,* 149–170.

Duijsens, I. J., & Diekstra, R. F. W. (1996). DSM-III-R and ICD-10 personality disorders and their relationship with the big five dimensions of personality. *Personality and Individual Differences, 21,* 119–133.

Edwards, A. L. (1957). *The social desirability variable in personality assessment and research.* New York: Dryden.

Edwards, A. L. (1959). *Edwards Personal Preference Schedule manual.* New York: Psychological Corp.

Edwards, A. L., & Heathers, L. B. (1962). The first factor of the MMPI: Social desirability or ego strength. *Journal of Consulting Psychology, 26,* 99–100.

Edwards. J. E., & Waters, L. K. (1983). Predicting university attrition: A replication and extension. *Educational and Psychological Measurement, 43,* 233–236.

Ellenberger, H. (1970). *The discovery of the unconscious.* New York: Basic Books.

Ellison, C. W. (1983). Spiritual well-being: Conceptualization and measurement. *Journal of Psychology and Theology, 11,* 330–340.

Entwisle, D. R. (1972). To dispel fantasies about fantasy-based measures of achievement motivation. *Psychological Bulletin, 77,* 377–391.

Eysenck, H. J. (1991). Dimensions of personality: 16, 5, or 3?—Criteria for a taxonomic paradigm. *Personality and Individual Differences, 12,* 773–790.

Eysenck, H. J. (1992). Four ways five factors are not basic. *Personality and Individual Differences, 13,* 667–673.

Eysenck, H. J., & Eysenck, M. W. (1985). *Personality and individual differences.* London, Plenum.

Fagan, P. J., Wise, T. N., Schmidt, C. W., Ponticas, Y., Marshall, R. D., & Costa, P. T., Jr. (1991). A comparison of five-factor personality dimensions in males with sexual dysfunction and males with paraphilia. *Journal of Personality Assessment, 57,* 434–448.

Fiske, D. W. (1949). Consistency of the factorial structure of personality ratings from different sources. *Journal of Abnormal and Social Psychology, 44*, 329–344.

Frances, A. J., First, M. B., Widiger, T. A., Miele, G. M., Tilly, S. M., Davis, W. W., & Pincus, H. A. (1991). An a to z guide to DSM-IV conundrums. *Journal of Abnormal Psychology, 100*, 407–412.

Friedman, M., & Rosenman, R. H. (1959). Association of a specific overt behavior pattern with increases in blood cholesterol, blood clotting time, incidence of arcus senilis and clinical coronary artery disease. *Journal of the American Medical Association, 2208*, 828–836.

Funder, D. C., & Colvin, C. R. (1988). Friends and strangers: Acquaintanceship, agreement, and the accuracy of personality judgment. *Journal of Personality and Social Psychology, 55*, 149–158.

Furnham, A. (1986). Response bias, social desirability, and dissimulation. *Personality and Individual Differences, 7*, 385–400.

Furnham, A. (1994). The big five versus the big four: The relationship between the Myers–Briggs Type Indicator (MBTI) and NEO-PI five factor model of personality. *Personality and Individual Differences, 21*, 303–307.

Gerbing, D. W., & Tuley, M. R. (1991). The 16PF related to the five-factor model of personality: Multiple-indicator measurement versus the a priori scales. *Multivariate Behavioral Research, 26*, 271–289.

Goldberg, L. R. (1981). Language and individual differences: The search for universals in personality lexicons. In L. Wheeler (Ed.), *Review of personality and social psychology* (pp. 141–165). Beverly Hills, CA: Sage.

Goldberg, L. R. (1982). From Ace to Zombie: Some explorations in the language of personality. In C. D. Spielberger & J. N. Butcher (Eds.), *Advances in personality assessment* (pp. 203–224). Hillsdale, NJ: Erlbaum.

Goldberg, L. R. (1990). An alternative "description of personality": The big-five structure. *Journal of Personality and Social Psychology, 59*, 1216–1229.

Goldberg, L. R. (1992). The development of markers for the big-five factor structure. *Psychological Assessment, 4*, 26–42.

Goldberg, L. R. (1993). The structure of phenotypic personality traits. *American Psychologist, 48*, 26–34.

Goldberg, L. R., & Digman, J. M. (1994). Revealing structure in the data: Principles of exploratory factor analysis. In S. Strack & M. Lorr (Eds.), *Differentiating abnormal and normal personality* (pp. 216–242). New York: Springer.

Goldberg, L. R., & Rosolack, T. K. (1994). The Big Five factor structure as an integrative framework: An empirical comparison with Eysenck's P-E-N model. In C. F. Halverson, Jr., G. A. Kohnstamm, & R. P. Martin (Eds.), *The developing structure of temperament and personality from infancy to adulthood* (pp. 7–35). Hillsdale, NJ: Erlbaum.

Goldstein, M. D., & Strube, M. J. (1994). Independence revisited: The relation between positive and negative affect in a naturalistic setting. *Personality and Social Psychology Bulletin, 20*, 57–64.

Gorsuch, R. L. (1983). *Factor analysis* (2nd ed.). Hillsdale, NJ: Erlbaum.

Gorsuch, R. L. (1988). Psychology of religion. *Annual Review of Psychology, 39*, 201–221.

Gorsuch, R. L. (1994). Toward motivational theories of intrinsic religious commitment. *Journal for the Scientific Study of Religion, 33,* 315–325.

Gorsuch, R. L. (1997). Exploratory factor analysis: Its role in item analysis. *Journal of Personality Assessment, 68,* 523–560.

Gorsuch, R. L., & Venable, G. D. (1983). Development of an "age universal" I-E scale. *Journal for the Scientific Study of Religion, 22,* 181–187.

Gottman, J. M. (1979). *Marital interaction: Experimental investigations.* New York: Academic Press.

Gough, H. B., & Hall, W. B. (1975). An attempt to predict graduation from medical school. *Journal of Medical Education, 30,* 940–950.

Gough, H. B., & Heilbrun, A. B. (1980). *The Adjective Check List manual.* Palo Alto, CA: Consulting Psychologists Press.

Gough, H. G. (1987). *California Psychological Inventory administrator's guide.* Palo Alto, CA: Consulting Psychologists Press.

Graham, J. R. (1990). *MMPI 2: Assessing personality and psychopathology.* New York: Oxford University Press.

Green, D. P., Goldman, S. L., & Salovey, P. (1993). Measurement error masks bipolarity in affect ratings. *Journal of Personality and Social Psychology, 64,* 1029–1041.

Gruber-Baldini, A. L., Schaie, K. W., & Willis, S. L. (1995). Similarity in married couples: A longitudinal study of mental abilities and rigidity–flexibility. *Journal of Personality and Social Psychology, 69,* 191–203.

Guilford, J. P., & Guilford, R. B. (1936). Personality factors S, E, and M, and their measurement. *Journal of Personality, 34,* 21–36.

Haan, N., Millsap, R., & Hartka, E. (1986). As time goes by: Change and stability in personality over fifty years. *Psychology and Aging, 1,* 220–232.

Hahn, R., & Comrey, A. L. (1994). Factor analysis of the NEO-PI and the Comrey Personality Scales. *Psychological Reports, 75,* 355–365.

Harkness, A. R. (1992). Fundamental topics in the personality disorders: Candidate trait dimensions from lower regions of the hierarchy. *Psychological Assessment, 4,* 251–259.

Harkness, A. R., & McNulty, J. L. (1994). The personality psychopathology five (PSY-5): Issue from the pages of a diagnostic manual instead of a dictionary. In S. Strack & M. Lorr (Eds.), *Differentiating normal and abnormal personality* (pp. 291–315). New York: Springer.

Hartmann, H. (1939/1958). *Ego psychology and the problem of adaptation.* New York: International Universities Press.

Heath, A. C., Neale, M. C., Kessler, R. C., Eaves, L. J., & Kendler, K. S. (1992). Evidence for genetic influences on personality from self-reports and informant ratings. *Journal of Personality and Social Psychology, 63,* 85–96.

Heaven, P. C. L., Connors, J., & Stones, C. R. (1994). Three or five personality dimensions? An analysis of natural language terms in two cultures. *Personality and Individual Differences, 17,* 181–189.

Helmes, E., & Jackson, D. N. (1994). Evaluating normal and abnormal personality using the same set of constructs. In S. Strack & M. Lorr (Eds.), *Differentiating normal and abnormal personality* (pp. 341–360). New York: Springer.

Helson, R., & Moane, G. (1987). Personality change in women from college to midlife. *Journal of Personality and Social Psychology, 53,* 176–186.

Hershberger, S. L., Plomin, R., & Pedersen, N. L. (1995). Traits and metatraits: Their reliability, stability, and shared genetic influence. *Journal of Personality and Social Psychology, 69,* 673–685.

Hirschfeld, R. M. A., Klerman, G. L., Clayton, P., Keller, M. B., McDonald-Scott, P., & Larkin, B. (1983). Assessing personality: Effects of depressive state on trait measurement. *American Journal of Psychiatry, 140,* 695–699.

Hofer, S. M., Horn, J. L., & Eber, H. W. (1997). A robust five-factor structure of the 16PF: Strong evidence from independent rotation and confirmatory factorial invariance procedures. *Personality and Individual Differences, 23,* 247–269.

Hofstee, W. K. B., de Raad, D., & Goldberg, L. R. (1992). Integration of the Big Five and circumplex approaches to trait structure. *Journal of Personality and Social Psychology, 63,* 146–163.

Hogan, R. (1991). Personality and personality measurement. In M. D. Dunnette & L. M. Hough (Eds.), *Handbook of industrial and organizational psychology* (2nd ed., pp. 873–919). Palo Alto, CA: Consulting Psychologists Press.

Hogan, R., & Hogan, J. (1989). How to measure employee reliability. *Journal of Applied Psychology, 74,* 273–279.

Hogan, R., & Hogan, J. (1992). *Hogan Personality Inventory, manual.* Tulsa, OK: Hogan Assessment Systems.

Holden, R. R. (1992). Associations between the Holden Psychological Screening Inventory and the NEO Five-Factor Inventory in a nonclinical sample. *Psychological Reports, 71,* 1039–1042.

Hood, R. W. (1975). The construction and preliminary validation of a measure of reported mystical experience. *Journal for the Scientific Study of Religion, 14,* 29–41.

Horner, M. S. (1968). *Sex differences in achievement motivation and performance in competitive and non-competitive situations.* Unpublished doctoral dissertation, University of Michigan, Ann Arbor.

Horner, M. S. (1972). Toward an understanding of achievement-related conflicts in women. *Journal of Social Issues, 28,* 157–175.

Horney, K. (1950). *Neurosis and human growth.* New York: Norton.

Horowitz, L. M. (1996). The study of interpersonal problems: A Leary legacy. *Journal of Personality Assessment, 66,* 283–300.

Hough, L. M. (1992). The "big five" personality variables—Construct confusion: Description versus prediction. *Human Performance, 5,* 139–155.

Hough, L. M., Eaton, N. K., Dunnette, M. D., Kamp, J. D., & McCloy, R. A. (1990). Criterion-related validities of personality constructs and the effect of response distortion on those validities. *Journal of Applied Psychology, 75,* 581–595.

Hsu, L. M. (1986). Implications of differences in elevations of K-corrected and non-K-corrected MMPI T scores. *Journal of Consulting and Clinical Psychology, 54,* 552–557.

Isaka, H. (1990). Factor analysis of trait terms in everyday Japanese language. *Personality and Individual Differences, 11,* 115–124.

Jackson, D. N. (1989). *Basic Personality Inventory manual*. Port Huron, MI: Sigma Assessment Systems.

Jackson, D. N., Aston, M. C., & Tomes, J. L. (1996). The six-factor model of personality: Facets from the big five. *Personality and Individual Differences, 21,* 391–402.

Jang, K. L., Livesley, W. J., & Vernon, P. A. (1996a). The genetic basis of personality at different ages: A cross-sectional twin study. *Personality and Individual Differences, 21,* 299–301.

Jang, K. L., Livesley, W. J., & Vernon, P. A. (1996b). Heritability of the Big Five personality dimensions and their facets: A twin study. *Journal of Personality, 64,* 577–591.

Jessor, R. (1983). The stability of change: Psychosocial development from adolescence to young adulthood. In D. Magnusson & V. L. Allen (Eds.), *Human development: An interactional perspective* (pp. 321–341). New York: Academic Press.

John, O. P. (1990). The "Big Five" factor taxonomy: Dimensions of personality in the natural language and in questionnaires. In L. Pervin (Ed.), *Handbook of personality theory and research* (pp. 66–100). New York: Guilford.

John, O. P., & Robbins, R. W. (1993). Determinants of inter-judge agreement on personality traits: The Big Five domains, observability, evaluativeness, and the unique perspective of the self. *Journal of Personality, 61,* 521–551.

John, O. P., Goldberg, L. R., & Angleitner, A. (1984). Better than the alphabet: Taxonomies of personality-descriptive terms in English, Dutch, and German. In J. J. C. Bonarius, G. L. M. van Heck, & N. G. Smid (Eds.), *Personality psychology in Europe: Theoretical and empirical developments* (pp. 83–100). Lisse, Switzerland: Swets & Zeitlinger.

John, O. P., Angleitner, A., & Ostendorf, F. (1988). The lexical approach to personality: A historical review of the trait taxonomic research. *European Journal of Personality, 2,* 171–203.

Jones, E. E., & Davis, K. E. (1965). From acts to dispositions: The attribution process in person perception. In L. Berkowitz (Ed.), *Advances in experimental social psychology* (Vol. 2, pp. 78–103). New York: Academic Press.

Jones, E. E., & Nisbett, R. E. (1972). The actor and the observer: Divergent perceptions of the causes of behavior. In E. E. Jones, D. E. Kanouse, H. H. Kelley, R. E. Nisbett, S. Valins, and B. Weiner (Eds.), *Attribution: Perceiving the causes of behavior* (pp. 79–94). Morristown, NJ: General Learning Press.

Jöreskog, K. G., & Sörbom, D. (1993). *LISREL 8 user's reference guide*. Chicago: Scientific Software International.

Juni, S. (1995). Review of the NEO PI–R. In J. Conoley & J. Impara (Eds.), *Mental measurement yearbook* (12th ed., pp. 863–868). Lincoln: University of Nebraska Press.

Kaiser, R. T., & Ozer, D. J. (1997). Emotional stability and goal-related stress. *Personality and Individual Differences, 22,* 371–379.

Karney, B. R., & Bradbury, T. N. (1995). The longitudinal course of marital quality and stability: A review of theory, method, and research. *Psychological Bulletin, 118,* 3–34.

Karney, B. R., & Bradbury, T. N. (1997). Neuroticism, marital interaction, and the trajectory of marital satisfaction. *Journal of Personality and Social Psychology, 72,* 1075–1092.

Katigbak, M. S., Church, A. T., & Akamine, T. X. (1996). Cross-cultural generalizability of personality dimensions: Relating indigenous and imported dimensions in two cultures. *Journal of Personality and Social Psychology, 70,* 99–114.

Kaufman, A. S. (1975). Factor analysis of the WISC-R at 11 age levels between $6\frac{1}{2}$ and $16\frac{1}{2}$ years. *Journal of Consulting and Clinical Psychology, 43,* 135–147.

Kaufman, L., & Rousseeuw, P. J. (1990). *Finding groups in data: An introduction to cluster analysis.* New York: Wiley.

Keller, M. C., Thiessen D., & Young, R. K. (1996). Mate assortment in dating and married couples. *Personality and Individual Differences, 21,* 217–221.

Kosek, R. B. (1996a). *Criss-cross ratings of the Big Five personality dimensions as an index of marital satisfaction.* Unpublished doctoral dissertation, Loyola College, Baltimore.

Kosek, R. B. (1996b). The quest for a perfect spouse: Spousal ratings and marital satisfaction. *Psychological Reports, 79,* 731–735.

Kozma, A., & Stones, M. J. (1987). Social desirability in measures of subjective well-being: A systematic evaluation. *Journal of Gerontology, 42,* 56–59.

Lanning, K. (1994). Dimensionality of observer ratings on the California adult Q-Set. *Journal of Personality and Social Psychology, 67,* 151–160.

Larsen, D. L., Attkisson, C. C., Hargreaves, W. A., & Nguyen, T. D. (1979). Assessment of client/patient satisfaction: Development of a general scale. *Evaluation and Program Planning, 2,* 197–207.

Larson, R. (1978). Thirty years of research on the subjective well-being of older Americans. *Journal of Gerontology, 33,* 109–125.

Leary, T. (1957). *Interpersonal diagnosis of personality.* New York: Ronald.

Lester, D., Haig, C., & Monello, R. (1989). Spouses' personality and marital satisfaction. *Personality and Individual Differences, 10,* 253–254.

Levin, J., & Montag, I. (1991). Relationship between the Basic Personality Inventory and the NEO-Personality Inventory in a nonpatient sample. *Psychological Reports, 69,* 1176–1178.

Levin, J., & Montag, I. (1994). The five factor model and psychopathology in non-clinical samples. *Personality and Individual Differences, 17,* 1–7.

Linehan, M. M., & Nielsen, S. L. (1983). Social desirability: Its relevance to the measurement of hopelessness and suicidal behavior. *Journal of Consulting and Clinical Psychology, 51,* 141–143.

Livesley, W. J., West, M., & Tanney, A. (1985). Historical comment on the DSM-III schizoid and avoidant personality disorders. *American Journal of Psychiatry, 142,* 1344–1347.

Livesley, W. J., Jackson, D. N., & Schroeder, M. L. (1992). Factorial structure of traits delineating personality disorders in clinical and general population samples. *Journal of Abnormal Psychology, 101,* 432–440.

Livesley, W. J., Schroeder, M. L., Jackson, D. N., & Jang, K. L. (1994). Categorical distinctions in the study of personality disorder: Implications for classification. *Journal of Abnormal Psychology, 103,* 6–17.

Locke, H. J., & Wallace, K. M. (1959). Short marital-adjustment and prediction tests: Their reliability and validity. *Marriage and Family Living, 21,* 251–255.

Loevinger, J. (1994). Has psychology lost its conscience? *Journal of Personality Assessment, 62,* 2–8.

Lorr, M. (1996). The Interpersonal Circle as a heuristic model for interpersonal research. *Journal of Personality Assessment, 66,* 234–239.

Lorr, M., & Strack, S. (1993). Some NEO PI five-factor personality profiles. *Journal of Personality Assessment, 60,* 91–99.

Lorr, M., Youniss, R. P., & Kluth, C. (1992). The Interpersonal Style Inventory and the five-factor model. *Journal of Clinical Psychology, 48,* 202–206.

Lubin, B., Larsen, R. M., & Matarazzo, J. D. (1984). Patterns of psychological test usage in the United States: 1935–1982. *American Psychologist, 39,* 451–454.

Lyons, J. S., Howard, K. I., O'Mahoney, M. T., & Lish, J. D. (1997). *The measurement and management of clinical outcomes in mental health.* New York: Wiley.

Marsh, H. W., Balla, J. R., & McDonald, R. P. (1988). Goodness-of-fit indexes in confirmatory factor analysis: The effect of sample size. *Psychological Bulletin, 103,* 391–410.

Marshall, G. N., Wortman, C. B., Vickers, R. R., Jr., Kusulas, J. W., & Hervig, L. K. (1994). The five-factor model of personality as a framework for personality-health research. *Journal of Personality and Social Psychology, 67,* 278–286.

McAdams, D. P. (1992). The five-factor model *in* personality: A critical appraisal. *Journal of Personality, 60,* 329–361.

McClelland, D. C., Atkinson, J. W., Clark, R. W., & Lowell, E. L. (1953). *The achievement motive.* New York: Appleton-Century-Crofts.

McCrae, R. R. (1982). Consensual validation of personality traits: Evidence from self-reports and ratings. *Journal of Personality and Social Psychology, 43,* 292–303.

McCrae, R. R. (1986). Well-being scales do not measure social desirability. *Journal of Gerontology, 41,* 390–393.

McCrae, R. R. (1989). Why I advocate the five-factor model: Joint factor analyses of the NEO-PI with other instruments. In D. Buss & N. Cantor (Eds.), *Personality psychology: Recent trends and emerging directions* (pp. 237–245). New York: Springer-Verlag.

McCrae, R. R. (1990). Traits and trait names: How well is Openness represented in natural languages? *European Journal of Personality, 4,* 119–129.

McCrae, R. R. (1993). Moderated analyses of longitudinal personality stability. *Journal of Personality and Social Psychology, 65,* 577–585.

McCrae, R. R. (1993–1994). Openness to experience as a basic dimension of personality. In K. S. Pope & J. L. Singer (Eds.), *Imagination, cognition, and personality: Consciousness in theory–research–clinical practice* (Vol. 13, pp. 39–55). Amityville, NY: Baywook.

McCrae, R. R. (1994a). The counterpoint of personality assessment: Self-reports and observer ratings. *Assessment, 1,* 151–164.

McCrae, R. R. (1994b). Openness to experience: Expanding the boundaries of factor V. *European Journal of Personality, 8,* 251–272.

McCrae, R. R. (1994c). Psychopathology from the perspective of the five-factor model. In S. Strack & M. Lorr (Eds.), *Differentiating normal and abnormal personality* (pp. 26–39). New York: Springer.

McCrae, R. R., & Costa, P. T., Jr. (1983a). Psychological maturity and subjective well-being: Toward a new synthesis. *Developmental Psychology, 19,* 243–248.

McCrae, R. R., & Costa, P. T., Jr. (1983b). Social desirability scales: More substance than style. *Journal of Consulting and Clinical Psychology, 51,* 882–888.

McCrae, R. R., & Costa, P. T., Jr. (1985a). Comparison of EPI and Psychoticism scales with measures of the five-factor model of personality. *Personality and Individual Differences, 6,* 587–597.

McCrae, R. R., & Costa, P. T., Jr. (1985b). Openness to experience. In R. Hogan & W. H. Jones (Eds.), *Perspectives in personality* (Vol. 1, pp. 145–172). Greenwich, CT: JAI.

McCrae, R. R., & Costa, P. T., Jr. (1987). Validation of the five-factor model of personality across instruments and observers. *Journal of Personality and Social Psychology, 52,* 81–90.

McCrae, R. R., & Costa, P. T., Jr. (1988). Psychological resilience among widowed men and women: A 10-year follow-up of a national sample. *Journal of Social Issues, 44,* 129–142.

McCrae, R. R., & Costa, P. T., Jr. (1989a). Reinterpreting the Myers–Briggs Type Indicator from the perspective of the five-factor model of personality. *Journal of Personality, 57,* 17–40.

McCrae R. R., & Costa, P. T., Jr. (1989b). Rotation to maximize the construct validity of factors in the NEO Personality Inventory. *Multivariate Behavioral Research, 57,* 17–40.

McCrae, R. R., & Costa, P. T., Jr. (1989c). The structure of interpersonal traits: Wiggins's circumplex and the five-factor model. *Journal of Personality and Social Psychology, 56,* 586–595.

McCrae, R. R., & Costa, P. T., Jr. (1992). Discriminant validity of the NEO-PIR facet scales. *Educational and Psychological Measurement, 52,* 229–237.

McCrae, R. R., & Costa, P. T., Jr. (1994). Does Lorr's Interpersonal Style Inventory measure the five-factor model? *Personality and Individual Differences, 16,* 195–197.

McCrae, R. R., & Costa, P. T., Jr. (1995). Positive and negative valence within the five-factor model. *Journal of Research in Personality, 29,* 443–460.

McCrae, R. R., & Costa, P. T., Jr. (1996). Toward a new generation of personality theories: Theoretical contexts for the five-factor model. In J. S. Wiggins (Ed.), *The five-factor model of personality: Theoretical perspectives* (pp. 51–87). New York: Guilford.

McCrae, R. R., & Costa, P. T., Jr. (1997). Personality trait structure as a human universal. *American Psychologist, 52,* 509–516.

McCrae, R. R., & John, O. P. (1992). An introduction to the five-factor model and its applications. *Journal of Personality, 60,* 175–215.

McCrae, R. R., Costa, P. T., Jr., & Busch, C. M. (1986). Evaluating comprehensiveness in personality systems: The California Q-Set and the five factor model. *Journal of Personality, 54,* 430–446.

McCrae, R. R., Costa, P. T., Jr., Dahlstrom, W. G., Barefoot, J. C., Siegler, I. C., & Williams, R. B., Jr. (1989). A caution on the use of the MMPI K-correction in research on psychosomatic medicine. *Psychosomatic Bulletin, 51,* 58–65.

McCrae, R. R., Costa, P. T., Jr., & Piedmont, R. L. (1993). Folk concepts, natural language, and psychological constructs: The California Personality Inventory and the five-factor model. *Journal of Personality, 61*, 1–26.

McCrae, R. R., Costa, P. T., Jr., Piedmont, R. L., Chae, J-H, Caprara, G. V., Barbaranelli, C., Marusic, I., & Bratko, D. (1996, November). *Personality development from college to mid-life: A cross-cultural comparison.* Paper presented at the 49th annual meeting of the Gerontological Society of America, Washington, DC.

McCrae, R. R., Costa, P. T., Jr., Stone, S. V., & Fagan, P. J. (1996, August). *Some reasons for disagreement between spouses in personality assessment.* Poster presented at the 104th annual convention of the American Psychological Association, Toronto, Ontario, Canada.

McCrae, R. R., Zonderman, A. B., Costa, P. T., Jr., Bond, M. H., & Paunonen, S. V. (1996). Evaluating replicability of factors in the Revised NEO Personality Inventory: Confirmatory factor analysis and Procrustes rotation. *Journal of Personality and Social Psychology, 70*, 552–566.

Meehl, P. E. (1978). Theoretical risks and tabular asterisks: Sir Karl, Sir Ronald, and the slow progress of soft psychology. *Journal of Consulting and Clinical Psychology, 46*, 806–834.

Megargee, E. I. (1972). *The California Psychological Inventory handbook.* San Francisco: Jossey-Bass.

Megargee, E. I., & Parker, G. V. C. (1968). An exploration of the equivalent of Murrayian needs as assessed by the Adjective Check List, the TAT, and Edwards Personal Preference Schedule. *Journal of Clinical Psychology, 24*, 47–51.

Miller, T. (1991). The psychotherapeutic utility of the five-factor model of personality: A clinician's experience. *Journal of Personality Assessment, 57*, 415–433.

Millon, T. (1990). *Towards a new personology: An evolutionary model.* New York: Wiley.

Mischel, W. (1968). *Personality assessment.* New York: Wiley.

Mooradian, T. A., & Nezlek, J. B. (1996). Comparing the NEO-FFI and Saucier's mini-markers as measures of the Big Five. *Personality and Individual Differences, 21*, 213–215.

Mount, M. K., & Barrick, M. R. (1995). The big five personality dimensions: Implications for research and practice in human resources management. *Research in Personnel and Human Resources Management, 13*, 153–200.

Mount, M. K., Barrick, M. R., & Strauss, J. P. (1994). Validity of observer ratings of the Big Five personality factors. *Journal of Applied Psychology, 79*, 272–280.

Murray, H. A. (1938). *Explorations in personality.* New York: Oxford University Press.

Muten, E. (1991). Self-reports, spouse ratings, and psychophysiological assessment in a behavioral medicine program: An application of the five-factor model. *Journal of Personality Assessment, 57*, 574–583.

Myers, I. B., & McCaulley, M. H. (1985). *A guide to the development and use of the Myers–Briggs Type Indicator.* Palo Alto, CA: Consulting Psychologists Press.

Narayanan, L., Shanker, M., & Levine, E. L. (1995). Personality structure: A culture-specific examination of the five-factor model. *Journal of Personality Assessment, 64*, 51–62.

Nicholson, R. A., & Hogan, R. (1990). The construct validity of social desirability. *American Psychologist, 45,* 290–292.

Norman, W. T. (1963). Toward an adequate taxonomy of personality attributes: Replicated factor structure in peer nomination personality ratings. *Journal of Abnormal and Social Psychology, 66,* 574–583.

Ogles, B. M., Lambert, M. J., & Masters, K. S. (1996). *Assessing outcome in clinical practice.* Boston: Allyn & Bacon.

Ones, D. S. (1993). *The construct validity of integrity tests.* Unpublished doctoral dissertation, University of Iowa, Iowa City.

Ormel, J., & Wohlfarth, T. (1991). How neuroticism, long-term difficulties, and life situation change influence psychological distress: A longitudinal model. *Journal of Personality and Social Psychology, 60,* 744–755.

Ozer, D. J., & Riese, S. P. (1994). Personality assessment. *Annual Review of Psychology, 45,* 357–388.

Panter, A. T., Tanaka, J. S., & Hoyle, R. H. (1994). Structural models for multimode designs in personality and temperament research. In C. F. Halverson, G. A. Kohnstamm, & R. P. Martin (Eds.), *The developing structure of temperament and personality from infancy to adulthood* (pp. 111–138). Hillsdale, NJ: Erlbaum.

Parker, J. D. A., Bagby, R. M., & Summerfeldt, L. J. (1993). Confirmatory factor analysis of the Revised NEO Personality Inventory. *Personality and Individual Differences, 15,* 463–466.

Paunonen, S. V., Jackson, D. N., Trzebinski, J., & Forsterling, F. (1992). Personality structure across cultures: A multi-method evaluation. *Journal of Personality and Social Psychology, 62,* 447–456.

Peabody, D., & Goldberg, L. R. (1989). Some determinants of factor structures from personality-trait descriptors. *Journal of Personality and Social Psychology, 57,* 552–567.

Piedmont, R. L. (1988a). An interactional model of achievement motivation and fear of success. *Sex Roles, 19,* 467–490.

Piedmont, R. L. (1988b). The relationship between achievement motivation, anxiety, and situational characteristics on performance on a cognitive task. *Journal of Research in Personality, 22,* 177–187.

Piedmont, R. L. (1993). A longitudinal analysis of burnout in the health care setting: The role of personal dispositions. *Journal of Personality Assessment, 61,* 457–473.

Piedmont, R. L. (1994). Validation of the rater form of the NEO PI–R for college students: Towards a paradigm for measuring personality development. *Assessment, 1,* 259–268.

Piedmont, R. L. (1995). Another look at fear of success, fear of failure, and test anxiety: A motivational analysis using the five-factor model. *Sex Roles, 32,* 139–158.

Piedmont, R. L. (1996a). *Cracking the plaster cast: Big 5 personality change due to outpatient drug rehabilitation counseling.* Paper presented at the 67th annual meeting of the Eastern Psychological Association, Philadelphia.

Piedmont, R. L. (1996b, August). Strategies for using the five-factor model in religious research. In R. L. Piedmont (Chair), *The five-factor model and its value for religious research.* Symposium presented at the annual convention of the American Psychological Association, Toronto, Ontario, Canada.

Piedmont, R. L. (1997a, August). Development and validation of the Spiritual Transcendence Scale: A measure of spiritual experience. In J. E. G. Williams (Chair), *Spiritual experience and the five-factor model of personality*. Symposium presented at the annual convention of the American Psychological Association, Chicago.

Piedmont, R. L. (1997b). Test review: The NEO PI–R. *Newsnotes, 32*(4), 3–4.

Piedmont, R. L., & Chae, J-H. (1997). Cross-cultural generalizability of the five-factor model of personality: Development and validation of the NEO PI–R for Koreans. *Journal of Cross-Cultural Psychology, 28*, 131–155.

Piedmont, R. L., & Ciarrocchi, J. W. (in press). Psychometric utility of the NEO PI–R in an outpatient, drug rehabilitation context. *Psychology of Addictive Behavior*.

Piedmont, R. L., & McCrae, R. R. (1998). *Are validity scales valid? Evidence from self-reports and observer ratings in a volunteer sample*. Manuscript under review. Unpublished manuscript, Baltimore, MD.

Piedmont, R. L., & Piedmont, R. I. (1996). *Couples critical incidents check list, manual*. Baltimore: Author.

Piedmont, R. L., & Weinstein, H. P. (1993). A psychometric evaluation of the new NEO-PI–R facet scales for Agreeableness and Conscientiousness. *Journal of Personality Assessment, 60*, 302–318.

Piedmont, R. L., & Weinstein, H. P. (1994). Predicting supervisor ratings of job performance using the NEO Personality Inventory. *Journal of Psychology, 128*, 255–265.

Piedmont, R. L., DiPlacido, J., & Keller, W. (1989). Assessing gender-related differences in achievement orientation using two different achievement scales. *Journal of Personality Assessment, 53*, 229–238.

Piedmont, R. L., McCrae, R. R., & Costa, P. T., Jr. (1991). Adjective check list scales and the five-factor model. *Journal of Personality and Social Psychology, 60*, 630–637.

Piedmont, R. L., McCrae, R. R., & Costa, P. T., Jr. (1992). An assessment of the Edwards Personal Preference Schedule from the perspective of the five-factor model. *Journal of Personality Assessment, 58*, 67–78.

Pincus, A. L. (1994). The interpersonal circumplex and the interpersonal theory: Perspectives on personality and its pathology. In S. Strack & M. Lorr (Eds.), *Differentiating normal and abnormal personality* (pp. 114–136). New York: Springer.

Pincus, A. L., & Wiggins, J. S. (1990). Interpersonal problems and conceptions of personality disorders. *Journal of Personality Disorders, 4*, 342–352.

Plomin, R., & Daniels, D. (1987). Why are children in the same family so different from one another? *Behavioral and Brain Sciences, 10*, 1–16.

Plomin, R., Chipuer, H. M., & Loehlin, J. C. (1990). Behavioral genetics and personality. In L. A. Pervin (Ed.), *Handbook of personality: Theory and research* (pp. 225–243). New York: Guilford.

Ptacek, J. T., & Dodge, K. L. (1995). Coping strategies and relationship satisfaction in couples. *Personality and Social Psychology Bulletin, 21*, 76–84.

Reynolds, W. M., & Kobak, K. A. (1995). *Hamilton Depression Inventory, manual*. Odessa, FL: Psychological Assessment Resources.

Rodgerson, T. E. (1994). *The relation between situation, personality, and religious problem-solving in the prediction of burnout among American Baptist clergy.* Unpublished doctoral dissertation, Loyola College, Baltimore.

Russell, R. J. H., & Wells, P. A. (1994). Predictors of happiness in married couples. *Personality and Individual Differences, 17,* 313–321.

Saklofske, D. H., Kelly, I. W., & Janzen, B. L. (1995). Neuroticism, depression, and depression proneness. *Personality and Individual Differences, 18,* 27–31.

Saucier, G. (1994). Mini-markers: A brief version of Goldberg's unipolar Big-Five markers. *Journal of Personality Assessment, 63,* 506–516.

Scheier, M. F., Buss, A. H., & Buss, D. M. (1976). Self-consciousness, self-report of aggressiveness, and aggression. *Journal of Research in Personality, 44,* 637–644.

Schinka, J. A. (1985). *Personal Problems Check List for Adults.* Odessa, FL: Psychological Assessment Resources.

Schmeck, R. R., & Grove, E. (1979). Academic achievement and individual differences in the learning process. *Applied Psychological Measurement, 3,* 43–49.

Schönemann, P. H. (1966). A generalized solution of the orthogonal Procrustes problem. *Psychometrika, 31,* 1–10.

Schroeder, D. H., & Costa, P. T., Jr. (1984). Influence of life event stress on physical illness: Substantive effects or methodological flaws? *Journal of Personality and Social Psychology, 46,* 853–863.

Schroeder, M. L., Wormworth, J. A., & Livesley, W. J. (1992). Dimensions of personality disorder and their relationships to the Big Five dimensions of personality. *Psychological Assessment, 4,* 47–53.

Schinka, J. A., Kinder, B. N., and Kremer, T. (1997). Research validity scales for the NEO PI–R: Developmental and initial validation. *Journal of Personality Assessment, 68,* 127–138.

Shock, N. W., Greulick, R. C., Andres, R., Arenberg, D., Costa, P. T., Jr., Lakatta, E. G., & Tobin, J. D. (1984). *Normal human aging: The Baltimore Longitudinal Study of Aging* (NIH Publication No. 84-2450). Bethesda, MD: National Institutes of Health.

Siegler, I. C., Zonderman, A. B., Barefoot, J. C., Williams, R. B., Jr., Costa, P. T., Jr., & McCrae, R. R. (1990). Predicting personality in adulthood from college MMPI scores: Implications for follow-up studies in psychosomatic medicine. *Psychosomatic Medicine, 52,* 644–652.

Silva, F., Avia, D., Sanz, J., Martínez-Arias, M. R., Graña, J. L., & Sánchez-Bernardos, L. (1994). The five-factor model—I. Contributions to the structure of the NEO-PI. *Personality and Individual Differences, 17,* 741–753.

Silver, R. J., & Sines, L. K. (1962). Diagnostic efficiency of the MMPI with and without the K correction. *Journal of Clinical Psychology, 18,* 312–314.

Silverstein, A. B. (1982). Factor structure of the Wechsler Adult Intelligence Scale–Revised. *Journal of Consulting and Clinical Psychology, 50,* 661–664.

Snyder, D. K. (1982). Advances in marital assessment: Behavioral, communications, and psychometric approaches. In C. D. Spielberger & J. N. Butcher (Eds.), *Advances in personality assessment* (Vol. 1, pp. 169–201). Hillsdale, NJ: Erlbaum.

Snyder, M. (1983). The influence of individuals on situations: Implications for understanding the links between personality and social behavior. *Journal of Personality, 51,* 497–516.

Spielberger, C. D., Gorsuch, R. L., & Lushene, R. E. (1970). *State–Trait anxiety inventory.* Palo Alto, CA: Consulting Psychologists Press.

Spirrison, C. L. (1994). Factorial hue and cry: Comments on Jane Loevinger's "Has psychology lost its conscience?" *Journal of Personality Assessment, 63,* 579–583.

Stagner, R. (1937). *Psychology of personality.* New York: McGraw-Hill.

Steers, K. M. (1975). Task-goal attributes, nAchievement, and supervisory performance. *Organizational Behavior and Human Performance, 13,* 392–403.

Stout, C. E. (1997). *Psychological assessment in managed care.* New York: Wiley.

Strack, S., & Lorr, M. (1994). *Differentiating normal and abnormal personality.* New York: Springer.

Taylor, R. M., & Morrison, L.P. (1984). *Taylor–Johnson Temperament Analysis manual.* Los Angeles, CA: Psychological Publications.

Tellegen, A. (1982). *Brief manual of the Multidimensional Personality Questionnaire.* Unpublished manuscript, University of Minnesota, Minneapolis.

Tellegen, A. (1988). The analysis of consistency in personality assessment. *Journal of Personality, 56,* 621–663.

Tellegen, A. (1993). Folk concepts and psychological concepts of personality and personality disorder. *Psychological Inquiry, 4,* 122–130.

Tellegen, A., & Waller, N. G. (in press). Exploring personality through test construction: Development of the Multidimensional Personality Questionnaire. In S. R. Briggs & J. M. Cheek (Eds.), *Personality measures: Development and evaluation* (Vol. 1). Greenwich, CT: JAI.

Tharp, R. G. (1963). Psychological patterning in marriage. *Psychological Bulletin, 60,* 97–117.

Thurstone, L. L. (1951). The dimensions of temperament. *Psychometrika, 16,* 11–20.

Tresemer, D. (1976). The cumulative record of research on fear of success. *Sex Roles, 2,* 217–235.

Trull, T. J. (1992). DSM-III-R personality disorders and the five-factor model of personality: An empirical comparison. *Journal of Abnormal Psychology, 101,* 553–560.

Trull, T. J., & Sher, K. J. (1994). Relationship between the five-factor model of personality and Axis I disorders in a nonclinical sample. *Journal of Abnormal Psychology, 103,* 350–360.

Trull, T. J., Useda, D., Costa, P. T., Jr., & McCrae, R. R. (1995). Comparison of the MMPI-2 Personality Psychopathology Five (PSY-5), the NEO-PI, and the NEO PI-R. *Psychological Assessment, 7,* 508–516.

Tupes, E. C., & Christal, R. E. (1961). *Recurrent personality factors based on trait ratings* (USAF ASD Technical Report No. 61-97). Lackland Air Force Base, TX: U.S. Air Force.

Vassend, O., & Skrondal, A. (1995). Factor analytic studies of the NEO Personality Inventory and the five-factor model: The problem of high structural complexity and conceptual indeterminacy. *Personality and Individual Differences, 19,* 135–147.

Viken, R. J., Rose, R. J., Kaprio, J., & Koskenvuo, M. (1994). A developmental genetic analysis of adult personality: Extraversion and Neuroticism from 18 to 59 years of age. *Journal of Personality and Social Psychology, 66,* 722–730.

Wanous, J. P., Reichers, A. E., & Hudy, M. J. (1997). Overall job satisfaction: How good are single-item measures? *Journal of Applied Psychology, 82,* 247–252.

Watkins, C. E., & Campbell, V. L. (1989). Personality assessment and counseling psychology. *Journal of Personality Assessment, 53,* 296–307.

Watson, D., & Clark, L. A. (1991). Self- versus peer ratings of specific emotional traits: Evidence of convergent and discriminant validity. *Journal of Personality and Social Psychology, 60,* 927–940.

Watson, D., & Clark, L. A. (1992). On traits and temperament: General and specific factors of emotional experience and their relation to the five-factor model. *Journal of Personality, 60,* 441–476.

Watson, D., Clark, L. A., & Harkness, A. R. (1994). Structures of personality and their relevance to psychopathology. *Journal of Abnormal Psychology, 103,* 18–31.

Webb, E. (1915). Character and intelligence. *British Journal of Psychology Monographs, 1*(3), 1–99.

Welsh, G. S. (1975). *Creativity and intelligence: A personality approach.* Chapel Hill: University of North Carolina, Institute for Research in Social Sciences.

Wernimont, P. F., & Campbell, J. P. (1968). Signs, samples, and criteria. *Journal of Applied Psychology, 57,* 120–128.

Widiger, T., & Corbitt, E. M. (1994). Normal versus abnormal personality from the perspective of the DSM. In S. Strack & M. Lorr (Eds.), *Differentiating normal and abnormal personality* (pp. 158–175). New York: Springer.

Widiger, T. A., & Costa, P. T., Jr. (1994). Personality and personality disorders. *Journal of Abnormal Psychology, 103,* 78–91.

Widiger, T. A., & Frances, A. (1985). The DSM-III personality disorders: Perspectives from psychology. *Archives of General Psychiatry, 42,* 615–623.

Widiger, T. A., & Frances, A. (1994). Toward a dimensional model for the personality disorders. In P. T. Costa, Jr, & T. A. Widiger (Eds.), *Personality disorders and the five-factor model of personality* (pp. 19–40). Washington, DC: American Psychological Association.

Widiger, T. A., & Shea, T. (1991). Differentiation of Axis I and Axis II disorders. *Journal of Abnormal Psychology, 100,* 399–406.

Widiger, T. A., & Trull, T. J. (1992). Personality and psychopathology: An application of the five-factor model. *Journal of Personality, 60,* 363–393.

Wiggins, J. S. (1979). *Personality and prediction: Principles of personality assessment.* Reading, MA: Addison-Wesley.

Wiggins, J. S. (1980). Circumplex models of interpersonal behavior. In L. Wheeler (Ed.), *Review of personality and social psychology* (Vol. 1, pp. 265–293). Beverly Hills, CA: Sage.

Wiggins, J. S. (1995). *Interpersonal Adjective Scales: Professional manual.* Odessa, FL: Psychological Assessment Resources.

Wiggins, J. S. (1996). An informal history of the Interpersonal Circumplex Tradition. *Journal of Personality Assessment, 66,* 217–233.

Wiggins, J. S., & Pincus, A. L. (1989). Conceptions of personality disorders and dimensions of personality. *Psychological Assessment: A Journal of Consulting and Clinical Psychology, 1,* 305–316.

Wiggins, J. S., & Trapnell, P.D. (1996). A dyadic-interactional perspective on the five-factor model. In J. S. Wiggins (Ed.), *The five-factor model of personality: Theoretical perspectives* (pp. 88–162). New York: Guilford.

Winch, R. F. (1958). *A study of complementary needs.* New York: Harper.

Worthington, D. L., & Schlottman, R. S. (1986). The predictive validity of subtle and obvious empirically derived psychological test items under faking condition. *Journal of Personality Assessment, 50,* 171–181.

Wrobel, T. A., & Lachar, D. (1982). Validity of the Wiener subtle and obvious scales for the MMPI: Another example of the importance of inventory-item content. *Journal of Consulting and Clinical Psychology, 50,* 469–470.

Zonderman, A. B., Costa, P. T., Jr., & McCrae, R. R. (1989). Depression as a risk for cancer morbidity and mortality in a nationally representative sample. *Journal of the American Medical Association, 262,* 1191–1195.

Zonderman, A. B., Herbst, J. H., Schmidt, C., Jr., Costa, P. T., Jr., & McCrae, R. R. (1993). Depressive symptoms as a non-specific, graded risk for psychiatric diagnoses. *Journal of Abnormal Psychology, 102,* 544–552.

AUTHOR INDEX

277

SUBJECT INDEX